Sleep Disorders
SOURCEBOOK

Fourth Edition

Health Reference Series

Fourth Edition

Sleep Disorders

SOURCEBOOK

Basic Consumer Health Information about Sleep Disorders, including Insomnia, Sleep Apnea and Snoring, Jet Lag and Other Circadian Rhythm Disorders, Narcolepsy, and Parasomnias, Such as Sleepwalking and Sleep Paralysis, and Featuring Facts about Other Health Problems That Affect Sleep, Why Sleep Is Necessary, How Much Sleep Is Needed, the Physical and Mental Effects of Sleep Deprivation, and Pediatric Sleep Issues

Along with Tips for Diagnosing and Treating Sleep Disorders, a Glossary of Related Terms, and a List of Resources for Additional Help and Information

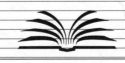

OMNIGRAPHICS

615 Griswold, Ste. 901, Detroit, MI 48226

Bibliographic Note
Because this page cannot legibly accommodate all the copyright notices, the Bibliographic
Note portion of the Preface constitutes an extension of the copyright notice.

* * *

Health Reference Series
Keith Jones, *Managing Editor*
***

OMNIGRAPHICS
A PART OF RELEVANT INFORMATION
***

Copyright © 2016 Omnigraphics
ISBN 978-0-7808-1474-5
E-ISBN 978-0-7808-1473-8

Library of Congress Cataloging-in-Publication Data

Names: Omnigraphics, Inc., issuing body.

Title: Sleep disorders sourcebook: basic consumer health information about sleep
disorders, including insomnia, sleep apnea and snoring, jet lag and other circadian
rhythm disorders, narcolepsy, and parasomnias, such as sleepwalking and sleep
paralysis, and featuring facts about other health problems that affect sleep, why
sleep is necessary, how much sleep is needed, the physical and mental effects of
sleep deprivation, and pediatric sleep issues; along with tips for diagnosing and
treating sleep disorders, a glossary of related terms, and a list of resources for
additional help and information.

Description: Fourth edition. | Detroit, MI : Omnigraphics, [2016] | Series: Health
reference series | Includes bibliographical references and index.

Identifiers: LCCN 2016027915 (print) | LCCN 2016029435 (ebook) | ISBN
9780780814745 (hardcover : alk. paper) | ISBN 9780780814738 (ebook) | ISBN
9780780814738 (eBook)

Subjects: LCSH: Sleep disorders. | Consumer education.

Classification: LCC RC547 .S536 2016 (print) | LCC RC547 (ebook) | DDC
616.8/498--dc23

LC record available at https://lccn.loc.gov/2016027915

Table of Contents

Part IV: Other Health Problems That Often Affect Sleep

Part VI: A Special Look at Pediatric Sleep Issues

Part VII: Clinical Trials on Sleep Disorders

Part VIII: Additional Help and Information

Preface

About This Book

Sleep is increasingly being recognized as important to public health. In the most recent Sleep Health Index™ published by the National Sleep Foundation, overall health was highly associated with sleep quality. According to Centers for Disease Control and Prevention (CDC), well over 50 million U.S. adults have sleep or wakefulness disorder with sleep insufficiency linked to motor vehicle crashes, industrial disasters, and medical and other occupational errors. Persons experiencing sleep insufficiency are also more likely to suffer from chronic diseases such as hypertension, diabetes, depression, and obesity, as well as from cancer, increased mortality, and reduced quality of life and productivity.

Sleep Disorders Sourcebook, Fourth Edition, offers basic consumer health information about common sleep disorders, including insomnia, sleep apnea, narcolepsy, circadian rhythm disorders, and parasomnias, and other health problems that affect sleep, such as cancer, pain, and respiratory disorders. It explains how much sleep is needed, the causes and consequences of sleep deprivation, and the methods used to prevent, diagnose, and treat sleep disorders. Pediatric sleep issues are also discussed that impact children from infancy through the teen years. A glossary of terms related to sleep disorders and a list of resources for further help and information are also included.

How to Use This Book

This book is divided into parts and chapters. Parts focus on broad areas of interest. Chapters are devoted to single topics within a part.

Part I: Sleep Basics presents facts about why and how people sleep, including an explanation of circadian rhythms, the physical characteristics of sleep, the benefits of napping, and what is known about dreaming. It describes gender differences in sleep, explains how aging affects sleep patterns, and discusses myths related to sleep.

Part II: The Causes and Consequences of Sleep Deprivation defines sleep deprivation, and talks about the people most at risk for sleep deprivation. It provides information on why your brain and body need sleep. It also describes the molecular link between lack of sleep and weight gain. The part concludes with information on the connection between sleep deprivation and learning.

Part III: Sleep Disorders describes disorders that directly affect the ability to sleep. These include disorders, such as sleep apnea, snoring, insomnia, circadian rhythm disorders, and parasomnias. Narcolepsy and other disorders associated with excessive sleeping are also discussed.

Part IV: Other Health Problems that Often Affect Sleep provides information about disorders that often impact sleep quality, including cancer, fibromyalgia, headaches, respiratory disorders, and mental health concerns. The symptoms that disrupt sleep are described, and suggestions for lessening their impact are provided.

Part V: Preventing, Diagnosing, and Treating Sleep Disorders identifies common sleep disruptors and explains the importance of a proper sleep environment. It describes how sleep studies work and details treatment options, including medications, dietary supplements, continuous positive airway pressure, and other complementary and alternative medications.

Part VI: A Special Look at Pediatric Sleep Issues describes sleep disturbances in infancy, childhood, and adolescence. It discusses safe sleeping environments for infants and explains sudden infant death syndrome. It provides information on how to get children into bed and offers facts about bedwetting, sleepwalking, and teeth grinding.

Part VII: Clinical Trials on Sleep Disorders describes what clinical trials are and provides information on some of the more recent clinical trials related to sleep disorders.

Part VIII: Additional Help and Information includes a glossary of terms related to sleep and sleep disorders and a directory of resources for additional help and support.

Bibliographic Note

This volume contains documents and excerpts from publications issued by the following U.S. government agencies: Agency for Healthcare Research and Quality (AHRQ); Centers for Disease Control and Prevention (CDC); ClinicalTrails.gov; *Eunice Kennedy Shriver* National Institute of Child Health and Human Development (NICHD); Federal Aviation Administration (FAA); Genetic and Rare Diseases Information Center (GARD); Genetic Home Reference (GHR); Genetics Home Reference (GHR); National Cancer Institute (NCI); National Cancer Institute (NCI); National Center for Complementary and Integrative Health (NCCIH); National Heart, Lung, and Blood Institute (NHLBI); National Highway Traffic Safety Administration (NHTSA); National Institute of Arthritis and Musculoskeletal and Skin Diseases (NIAMS); National Institute of Diabetes and Digestive and Kidney Diseases (NIDDK); National Institute of Mental Health (NIMH); National Institute of Neurological Disorders and Stroke (NINDS); National Institute on Aging (NIA); National Institute on DrugAbuse (NIDA); National Institutes of Health (NIH); National Science Foundation (NSF); Office of Dietary Supplements (ODS); Office of Disease Prevention and Health Promotion (ODPHP); Office on Women's Health (OWH); Substance Abuse and Mental Health Services Administration (SAMHSA); U.S. Department of Veterans Affairs (VA); and U.S. Food and Drug Administration (FDA).

In addition, this volume contains copyrighted documents from the following organization: The Nemours Foundation

It may also contain original material produced by Omnigraphics and reviewed by medical consultants.

About the Health Reference Series

The *Health Reference Series* is designed to provide basic medical information for patients, families, caregivers, and the general public. Each volume takes a particular topic and provides comprehensive coverage. This is especially important for people who may be dealing with a newly diagnosed disease or a chronic disorder in themselves or in a family member. People looking for preventive guidance, information about disease warning signs, medical statistics, and risk factors for health problems will also find answers to their questions in the *Health Reference Series*. The *Series*, however, is not intended to serve as a tool for diagnosing illness, in prescribing treatments, or as a substitute for the physician/patient relationship. All people concerned about medical symptoms or the possibility of disease are encouraged to seek professional care from an appropriate health care provider.

A Note about Spelling and Style

Health Reference Series editors use *Stedman's Medical Dictionary* as an authority for questions related to the spelling of medical terms and the *Chicago Manual of Style* for questions related to grammatical structures, punctuation, and other editorial concerns. Consistent adherence is not always possible, however, because the individual volumes within the *Series* include many documents from a wide variety of different producers, and the editor's primary goal is to present material from each source as accurately as is possible. This sometimes means that information in different chapters or sections may follow other guidelines and alternate spelling authorities.

Medical Review

Omnigraphics contracts with a team of qualified, senior medical professionals who serve as medical consultants for the *Health Reference Series*. As necessary, medical consultants review reprinted and originally written material for currency and accuracy. Citations including the phrase, "Reviewed (month, year)" indicate material reviewed by this team. Medical consultation services are provided to the *Health Reference Series* editors by:

Dr. Vijayalakshmi, MBBS, DGO, MD
Dr. Senthil Selvan, MBBS, DCH, MD
Dr. K. Sivanandham, MBBS, DCH, MS (Research), PhD

Our Advisory Board

We would like to thank the following board members for providing initial guidance on the development of this series:

- Dr. Lynda Baker, Associate Professor of Library and Information Science, Wayne State University, Detroit, MI

- Nancy Bulgarelli, William Beaumont Hospital Library, Royal Oak, MI

- Karen Imarisio, Bloomfield Township Public Library, Bloomfield Township, MI

- Karen Morgan, Mardigian Library, University of Michigan-Dearborn, Dearborn, MI

- Rosemary Orlando, St. Clair Shores Public Library, St. Clair Shores, MI

Health Reference Series *Update Policy*

The inaugural book in the *Health Reference Series* was the first edition of *Cancer Sourcebook* published in 1989. Since then, the *Series* has been enthusiastically received by librarians and in the medical community. In order to maintain the standard of providing high-quality health information for the layperson the editorial staff at Omnigraphics felt it was necessary to implement a policy of updating volumes when warranted.

Medical researchers have been making tremendous strides, and it is the purpose of the *Health Reference Series* to stay current with the most recent advances. Each decision to update a volume is made on an individual basis. Some of the considerations include how much new information is available and the feedback we receive from people who use the books. If there is a topic you would like to see added to the update list, or an area of medical concern you feel has not been adequately addressed, please write to:

Managing Editor
Health Reference Series
Omnigraphics
615 Griswold, Ste. 901
Detroit, MI 48226

Part One

Sleep Basics

Chapter 1

Understanding Sleep

Chapter Contents

Section 1.1

Why Do We Sleep?

This section includes text excerpted from "Sleep: Overview,"
Eunice Kennedy Shriver National Institute of Child
Health (NICHD), July 9, 2013.

What Is Sleep?

Sleep is a period of unconsciousness during which the brain remains highly active. It is a complex biological process that helps people process new information, stay healthy, and rejuvenate. During sleep, the brain will cycle through five distinctive phases: stage 1, 2, 3, 4, and rapid eye movement (REM) sleep.

Why Is Sleep Important?

Each phase is important to ensure that the mind and body are completely rested. Certain phases are needed to help you feel rested and energetic the next day, while other phases help you learn information and form memories.

Inadequate sleep contributes, in the short term, to problems with learning and processing information, and it can have a harmful effect on long-term health and well-being. According to the Centers for Disease Control and Prevention, more than 25% of U.S. adults believe they get insufficient sleep at least 15 of every 30 days.

Sleep affects performance on daily tasks, mood, and health in the following ways:

- **Performance.** Cutting back on sleep by as little as 1 hour can make it difficult to focus the next day and can slow your response time. Insufficient sleep can also make you more likely to take risks and make bad decisions, according to the National Heart, Lung, and Blood Institute (NHLBI).

- **Mood.** Sleep affects your mood. Insufficient sleep can cause irritability that can lead to trouble with relationships, particularly for children and teens. Also, people who don't get enough sleep are more likely to become depressed, according to the NHLBI.

- **Health.** Sleep is important for good health, according to the NHLBI. Lack of sleep or lack of quality sleep increases your risk for high blood pressure, heart disease, and other medical conditions. The quality of your sleep is affected by environmental factors, such as disturbances while you are sleeping and whether you remain asleep the entire night. Also, during sleep the body produces hormones that help children grow and, throughout life, help build muscle, fight illnesses, and repair damage to the body. Growth hormone, for example, is produced during sleep. It is essential for growth and development. Some hormones produced during sleep affect the body's use of energy. This may be how inadequate sleep leads to obesity and diabetes.

What Makes Us Sleep?

Patterns of sleep are regulated by two processes working together: sleep drive and the circadian clock.

- **Sleep drive.** The need for sleep is driven by the length of time you are awake. The longer you are awake, the greater your drive or "need" to sleep. The drive to sleep continues to build within your body until you are able to sleep.

- **Circadian clock.** Your body has a natural clock, called a "circadian clock," which helps you regulate your sleep. The word "circadian" refers to rhythmic biological cycles that repeat at approximately 24-hour intervals. These cycles are also referred to as circadian rhythms. Your circadian clock is strongly influenced by light, which is the reason that people living in different regions have different sleeping schedules. This is also the reason that your sleeping patterns tend to vary due to the amount of light and darkness present.

At bedtime, when your drive to sleep is greatest, your sleep drive and circadian clock work together to allow you to fall asleep. After you have slept for a while, when your drive to sleep is lower, your circadian clock allows you to stay asleep until the end of the night.

What Happens during Sleep?

When a person is sleeping, the brain cycles through five distinct phases: stage 1, 2, 3, 4, and rapid eye movement (REM) sleep. Each phase helps to ensure that the mind and body are rested. Certain phases are needed to help you feel rested and energetic the next day, while other phases help you learn information and form memories.

Sleep phases progress in a cycle from stage 1 to REM sleep, and then the cycle starts over again with stage 1. Some of the characteristics of each phase are shown below.

- **Non-REM sleep (75% of sleep):** As you begin to fall asleep, you enter non-REM, which consists of stages 1 through 4, as follows:

  - Stage 1

    - You are between being awake and falling asleep.

    - You may start to lightly sleep.

  - Stage 2

    - You fall into a deeper sleep.

    - You become disengaged from your surroundings.

    - Your body temperature becomes slightly lower.

  - Stages 3 and 4

    - Your deepest and most restorative sleep occurs.

    - Your blood pressure drops.

    - Your breathing rate slows.

    - Your muscles relax.

    - Your body increases the supply of blood to your muscles.

    - Your body performs tissue growth and repair.

    - Your energy is restored.

    - Your body releases hormones.

- **REM sleep (25% of sleep):** Approximately 70 to 90 minutes after you fall asleep, and then at successive intervals of about 90 to 110 minutes, you enter REM sleep. REM sleep becomes longer later into the night. REM is characterized as follows:

  - Your brain and body are energized.

  - Your daytime performance is supported.

  - Your brain is active, and dreaming occurs.

  - Your eyes dart back and forth.

- Your body becomes immobile and relaxed.
- Your body temperature is not as tightly regulated

The duration of sleep phases change during a given night's sleep. For example, near the beginning of a night of sleep, the body cycles through relatively short periods of REM sleep and long periods of deep sleep. As time proceeds throughout the night, periods of REM sleep increase and those of deep sleep decrease. Near the end of a night of sleep, a person spends nearly all of their time in stages 1 and 2 and REM.

How Much Sleep Do I Need?

According to the National Institute of Neurological Disorders and Stroke (NINDS), the amount of sleep people needs depends on several factors, including their age, individual requirements, and whether they have been getting adequate sleep.

In 2015, researchers affiliated with the National Sleep Foundation released revised recommendations for sleep duration by age. The revisions, included below, were based on a review of more than 300 research studies:

Table 1.1. Amount of Sleep required based on Age Group

Age Group	Amount of Sleep Needed
Newborns (0 to 3 months)	14 to 17 hours per day
Infants (4 to 11 months)	12 to 15 hours
Toddlers (1 to 2 years)	11 to 14 hours
Preschoolers (3 to 5 years)	10 to 13 hours
School-Age Children (6 to 13 years)	9 to 11 hours
Teenagers (14 to 17 years)	8 to 10 hours
Adults (18 to 64 years)	7 to 9 hours
Pregnant Women	During pregnancy, women may need a few more hours of sleep per night or a few short naps during the day.
Older Adults (65 years and older)	7 to 8 hours

Section 1.2

Circadian Rhythms

This section includes text excerpted from "Brain Basics:
Understanding Sleep," National Institute of Neurological
Disorders and Stroke (NINDS), July 25, 2014.

Sleep and Circadian Rhythms

Circadian rhythms are regular changes in mental and physical characteristics that occur in the course of a day (*circadian* is Latin for "around a day"). Most circadian rhythms are controlled by the body's biological "clock." This clock, called the *suprachiasmatic nucleus* or *SCN*, is actually a pair of pinhead-sized brain structures that together contain about 20,000 neurons. The SCN rests in a part of the brain called the *hypothalamus*, just above the point where the optic nerves cross. Light that reaches photoreceptors in the retina (a tissue at the back of the eye) creates signals that travel along the optic nerve to the SCN.

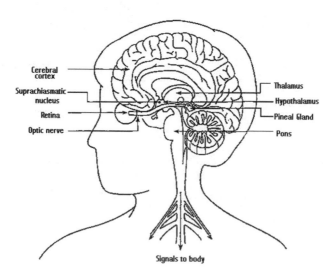

Figure 1.1. *Circadian Rhythms*

Signals from the SCN travel to several brain regions, including the *pineal gland*, which responds to light-induced signals by switching off production of the hormone melatonin. The body's level of melatonin normally increases after darkness falls, making people feel drowsy. The SCN also governs functions that are synchronized with the sleep/wake cycle, including body temperature, hormone secretion, urine production, and changes in blood pressure.

By depriving people of light and other external time cues, scientists have learned that most people's biological clocks work on a 25-hour cycle rather than a 24-hour one. But because sunlight or other bright lights can reset the SCN, our biological cycles normally follow the 24-hour cycle of the sun, rather than our innate cycle. Circadian rhythms can be affected to some degree by almost any kind of external time cue, such as the beeping of your alarm clock, the clatter of a garbage truck, or the timing of your meals. Scientists call external time cues *zeitgebers* (German for "time givers").

When travelers pass from one time zone to another, they suffer from disrupted circadian rhythms, an uncomfortable feeling known as jet lag. For instance, if you travel from California to New York, you "lose" 3 hours according to your body's clock. You will feel tired when the alarm rings at 8 a.m. the next morning because, according to your body's clock, it is still 5 a.m. It usually takes several days for your body's cycles to adjust to the new time.

To reduce the effects of *jet lag*, some doctors try to manipulate the biological clock with a technique called light therapy. They expose people to special lights, many times brighter than ordinary household light, for several hours near the time the subjects want to wake up. This helps them reset their biological clocks and adjust to a new time zone.

Symptoms much like jet lag are common in people who work nights or who perform shift work. Because these people's work schedules are at odds with powerful sleep-regulating cues like sunlight, they often become uncontrollably drowsy during work, and they may suffer insomnia or other problems when they try to sleep. Shift workers have an increased risk of heart problems, digestive disturbances, and emotional and mental problems, all of which may be related to their sleeping problems. The number and severity of workplace accidents also tend to increase during the night shift. Major industrial accidents attributed partly to errors made by fatigued night-shift workers include the Exxon Valdez oil spill and the Three Mile Island and Chernobyl nuclear power plant accidents. One study also found that medical interns working on the night shift are twice as likely as others to misinterpret hospital test records, which could endanger their patients. It may be possible to reduce shift-related fatigue by using bright lights in the workplace, minimizing shift changes, and taking scheduled naps.

Many people with total blindness experience life-long sleeping problems because their retinas are unable to detect light. These people have a kind of permanent jet lag and periodic insomnia because their circadian rhythms follow their innate cycle rather than a 24-hour one. Daily supplements of melatonin may improve night-time sleep for such patients. However, since the high doses of melatonin found in most supplements can build up in the body, long-term use of this substance may create new problems. Because the potential side effects of melatonin supplements are still largely unknown, most experts discourage melatonin use by the general public.

Section 1.3

Is Sleeping a Dynamic Activity?

This section includes text excerpted from "Brain Basics: Understanding Sleep," National Institute of Neurological Disorders and Stroke (NINDS), July 25, 2014.

Sleep: A Dynamic Activity

Until the 1950s, most people thought of sleep as a passive, dormant part of our daily lives. We now know that our brains are very active during sleep. Moreover, sleep affects our daily functioning and our physical and mental health in many ways that we are just beginning to understand.

Nerve-signaling chemicals called *neurotransmitters* control whether we are asleep or awake by acting on different groups of nerve cells, or neurons, in the brain. Neurons in the brainstem, which connects the brain with the spinal cord, produce neurotransmitters such as serotonin and norepinephrine that keep some parts of the brain active while we are awake. Other neurons at the base of the brain begin signaling when we fall asleep. These neurons appear to "switch off" the signals that keep us awake. Research also suggests that a chemical called adenosine builds up in our blood while we are awake and causes drowsiness. This chemical gradually breaks down while we sleep.

Phases of Sleep

During sleep, we usually pass through five phases of sleep: stages 1, 2, 3, 4, and *REM* (rapid eye movement) sleep. These stages progress in a cycle from stage 1 to REM sleep, then the cycle starts over again with stage 1. We spend almost 50 percent of our total sleep time in stage 2 sleep, about 20 percent in REM sleep, and the remaining 30 percent in the other stages. Infants, by contrast, spend about half of their sleep time in REM sleep.

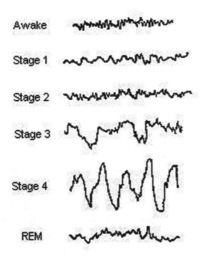

Figure 1.2. *Five Phases of Sleep*

During stage 1, which is light sleep, we drift in and out of sleep and can be awakened easily. Our eyes move very slowly and muscle activity slows. People awakened from stage 1 sleep often remember fragmented visual images. Many also experience sudden muscle contractions called *hypnic myoclonia,* often preceded by a sensation of starting to fall. These sudden movements are similar to the "jump" we make when startled. When we enter stage 2 sleep, our eye movements stop and our brain waves (fluctuations of electrical activity that can be measured by electrodes) become slower, with occasional bursts of rapid waves called *sleep spindles.* In stage 3, extremely slow brain waves called *delta waves* begin to appear, interspersed with smaller, faster waves. By stage 4, the brain produces delta waves almost exclusively. It is very difficult to wake someone during stages 3 and 4, which together are called *deep sleep.* There is no eye movement or muscle activity. People awakened during deep sleep do not adjust immediately and often feel groggy and disoriented for several minutes after they wake up. Some children experience bedwetting, night terrors, or sleepwalking during deep sleep.

When we switch into REM sleep, our breathing becomes more rapid, irregular, and shallow, our eyes jerk rapidly in various directions, and our limb muscles become temporarily paralyzed. Our heart rate increases, our blood pressure rises, and males develop penile erections. When people awaken during REM sleep, they often describe bizarre and illogical tales—dreams.

The first REM sleep period usually occurs about 70 to 90 minutes after we fall asleep. A complete sleep cycle takes 90 to 110 minutes on average. The first sleep cycles each night contain relatively short REM periods and long periods of deep sleep. As the night progresses, REM sleep periods increase in length while deep sleep decreases. By morning, people spend nearly all their sleep time in stages 1, 2, and REM.

People awakened after sleeping more than a few minutes are usually unable to recall the last few minutes before they fell asleep. This sleep-related form of amnesia is the reason people often forget telephone calls or conversations they've had in the middle of the night. It also explains why we often do not remember our alarms ringing in the morning if we go right back to sleep after turning them off.

Since sleep and wakefulness are influenced by different neurotransmitter signals in the brain, foods and medicines that change the balance of these signals affect whether we feel alert or drowsy and how well we sleep. Caffeinated drinks such as coffee and drugs such as diet pills and decongestants stimulate some parts of the brain and can cause *insomnia*, or an inability to sleep. Many antidepressants suppress REM sleep. Heavy smokers often sleep very lightly and have reduced amounts of REM sleep. They also tend to wake up after 3 or 4 hours of sleep due to nicotine withdrawal. Many people who suffer from insomnia try to solve the problem with alcohol—the so-called night cap. While alcohol does help people fall into light sleep, it also robs them of REM and the deeper, more restorative stages of sleep. Instead, it keeps them in the lighter stages of sleep, from which they can be awakened easily.

People lose some of the ability to regulate their body temperature during REM, so abnormally hot or cold temperatures in the environment can disrupt this stage of sleep. If our REM sleep is disrupted one

12

night, our bodies don't follow the normal sleep cycle progression the next time we doze off. Instead, we often slip directly into REM sleep and go through extended periods of REM until we "catch up" on this stage of sleep.

People who are under anesthesia or in a coma are often said to be asleep. However, people in these conditions cannot be awakened and do not produce the complex, active brain wave patterns seen in normal sleep. Instead, their brain waves are very slow and weak, sometimes all but undetectable.

How Much Sleep Do We Need?

The amount of sleep each person needs depends on many factors, including age. Infants generally require about 16 hours a day, while teenagers need about 9 hours on average. For most adults, 7 to 8 hours a night appears to be the best amount of sleep. Women in the first 3 months of pregnancy often need several more hours of sleep than usual. The amount of sleep a person needs also increases if he or she has been deprived of sleep in previous days. Getting too little sleep creates a "sleep debt," which is much like being overdrawn at a bank. Eventually, your body will demand that the debt be repaid. We don't seem to adapt to getting less sleep than we need; while we may get used to a sleep-depriving schedule, our judgement, reaction time, and other functions are still impaired.

People tend to sleep more lightly and for shorter time spans as they get older, although they generally need about the same amount of sleep as they needed in early adulthood. About half of all people over 65 have frequent sleeping problems, such as insomnia, and deep sleep stages in many elderly people often become very short or stop completely. This change may be a normal part of aging, or it may result from medical problems that are common in elderly people and from the medications and other treatments for those problems.

Experts say that if you feel drowsy during the day, even during boring activities, you haven't had enough sleep. If you routinely fall asleep within 5 minutes of lying down, you probably have severe sleep deprivation, possibly even a sleep disorder. *Microsleeps*, or very brief episodes of sleep in an otherwise awake person, are another mark of sleep deprivation. In many cases, people are not aware that they are experiencing microsleeps. The widespread practice of "burning the candle at both ends" in western industrialized societies has created so much sleep deprivation that what is really abnormal sleepiness is now almost the norm.

13

Many studies make it clear that sleep deprivation is dangerous. Sleep-deprived people who are tested by using a driving simulator or by performing a hand-eye coordination task perform as badly as or worse than those who are intoxicated. Sleep deprivation also magnifies alcohol's effects on the body, so a fatigued person who drinks will become much more impaired than someone who is well-rested. Driver fatigue is responsible for an estimated 100,000 motor vehicle accidents and 1500 deaths each year, according to the National Highway Traffic Safety Administration. Since drowsiness is the brain's last step before falling asleep, driving while drowsy can–and often does–lead to disaster. Caffeine and other stimulants cannot overcome the effects of severe sleep deprivation. The National Sleep Foundation says that if you have trouble keeping your eyes focused, if you can't stop yawning, or if you can't remember driving the last few miles, you are probably too drowsy to drive safely.

What Does Sleep Do for Us?

Although scientists are still trying to learn exactly why people need sleep, animal studies show that sleep is necessary for survival. For example, while rats normally live for two to three years, those deprived of REM sleep survive only about 5 weeks on average, and rats deprived of all sleep stages live only about 3 weeks. Sleep-deprived rats also develop abnormally low body temperatures and sores on their tail and paws. The sores may develop because the rats' immune systems become impaired. Some studies suggest that sleep deprivation affects the immune system in detrimental ways.

Sleep appears necessary for our nervous systems to work properly. Too little sleep leaves us drowsy and unable to concentrate the next day. It also leads to impaired memory and physical performance and reduced ability to carry out math calculations. If sleep deprivation continues, hallucinations and mood swings may develop. Some experts believe sleep gives neurons used while we are awake a chance to shut down and repair themselves. Without sleep, neurons may become so depleted in energy or so polluted with byproducts of normal cellular activities that they begin to malfunction. Sleep also may give the brain a chance to exercise important neuronal connections that might otherwise deteriorate from lack of activity.

Deep sleep coincides with the release of growth hormone in children and young adults. Many of the body's cells also show increased production and reduced breakdown of proteins during deep sleep. Since proteins are the building blocks needed for cell growth and for repair of damage from factors like stress and ultraviolet rays, deep sleep may truly be "beauty sleep." Activity in parts of the brain that control emotions, decision-making processes, and social interactions is drastically reduced during deep sleep, suggesting that this type of sleep may help people maintain optimal emotional and social functioning while they are awake. A study in rats also showed that certain nerve-signaling patterns which the rats generated during the day were repeated during deep sleep. This pattern repetition may help encode memories and improve learning.

Section 1.4

How Much Sleep Do You Need?

This section includes text excerpted from "Get Enough Sleep,"
Office of Disease Prevention and Health Promotion
(ODPHP), February 24, 2016.

The Basics

Everyone needs to get enough sleep. Sleep helps keep your mind and body healthy.

How Much Sleep Do I Need?

Most adults need 7 to 8 hours of good quality sleep on a regular schedule each night. Make changes to your routine if you can't find enough time to sleep.

Getting enough sleep isn't only about total hours of sleep. It's also important to get good quality sleep so you feel rested when you wake up.

If you often have trouble sleeping–or if you don't feel well rested after sleeping–talk with your doctor.

How Much Sleep Do Children Need?

Kids need even more sleep than adults.

• Teens need at least 9 hours of sleep each night.

• School-aged children need at least 10 hours of sleep each night.

- Preschoolers need to sleep between 11 and 12 hours a day.

- Newborns need to sleep between 16 and 18 hours a day.

Why Is Getting Enough Sleep Important?

Getting enough sleep has many benefits. It can help you:

- Get sick less often

- Stay at a healthy weight

- Lower your risk of high blood pressure and diabetes

- Reduce stress and improve your mood

- Think more clearly and do better in school and at work

- Get along better with people

- Make good decisions and avoid injuries (For example, sleepy drivers cause thousands of car crashes every year.)

Does It Matter When I Sleep?

Yes. Your body sets your "biological clock" according to the pattern of daylight where you live. This helps you naturally get sleepy at night and stay alert during the day.

When people have to work at night and sleep during the day, they can have trouble getting enough sleep. When people travel to a different time zone, they can also have trouble sleeping.

Why Can't I Fall Asleep?

Many things can make it harder for you to sleep, including:

- Stress

- Pain

- Certain health conditions

- Some medicines

- Caffeine (usually from coffee, tea, and soda)

- Alcohol and other drugs

- Untreated sleep disorders, like sleep apnea or insomnia

If you are having trouble sleeping, make changes to your routine to get the sleep you need. For example, try to:

- Follow a regular sleep schedule

- Stay away from caffeine in the afternoon
- Take a hot bath before bed to relax

How Can I Tell If I Have a Sleep Disorder?

Signs of a sleep disorder can include:

- Difficulty falling asleep
- Trouble staying asleep
- Sleepiness during the day that makes it difficult to do tasks like driving a car
- Frequent loud snoring
- Pauses in breathing or gasping while sleeping
- Pain or itchy feelings in your legs or arms at night that feel better when you move or massage the area

If you have any of these signs, talk to a doctor or nurse. You may need to be tested or treated for a sleep disorder.

Take Action!

Making small changes to your daily routine can help you get the sleep you need.

Change What You Do during the Day

- Exercise earlier in the day, not right before you go to bed.
- Stay away from caffeine (including coffee, tea, and soda) late in the day.
- If you have trouble sleeping at night, limit daytime naps to 20 minutes or less.
- If you drink alcohol, drink only in moderation. This means no more than 1 drink a day for women and no more than 2 drinks a day for men. Alcohol can keep you from sleeping soundly.
- Don't eat a big meal close to bedtime.
- Quit smoking. The nicotine in cigarettes can make it harder for you to sleep.

Create a Good Sleep Environment

Make sure your bedroom is dark. If there are street lights near your window, try putting up light-blocking curtains.

- Keep your bedroom quiet.

  - Consider keeping electronic devices–like TVs, computers, and smart phones–out of the bedroom.

Set a Bedtime Routine

- Go to bed at the same time every night.
- Get the same amount of sleep each night.
- Avoid eating, talking on the phone, reading, or watching TV in bed.
- Try not to lie in bed worrying about things.

If you are still awake after staying in bed for more than 20 minutes, get up. Do something relaxing, like reading or meditating, until you feel sleepy.

If You Are Concerned about Your Sleep, See a Doctor

Talk with a doctor or nurse if you have any of the following signs of a sleep disorder:

- Frequent, loud snoring
- Pauses in breathing during sleep
- Trouble waking up in the morning
- Pain or itchy feelings in your legs or arms at night that feel better when you move or massage the area
- Trouble staying awake during the day

Even if you aren't aware of problems like these, talk with a doctor if you feel like you often have trouble sleeping.

Keep a sleep diary for a week and share it with your doctor. A doctor can suggest different sleep routines or medicines to treat sleep disorders. Talk with a doctor before trying over-the-counter sleep medicine.

Section 1.5

Sleep: Other FAQs

This section includes text excerpted from "Sleep: Other FAQs,"
Eunice Shriver Kennedy National Institute of Child Health and
Human Development (NICHD), July 9, 2013.

Why Are Sleep Patterns Sometimes Thrown off after Traveling across Time Zones?

Circadian rhythms are disrupted when people travel from one time zone to another. The feeling that you experience when your circadian rhythms (biological cycles) are disrupted is called "jet lag." The reason for jet lag is the change in time zones. For example, in traveling from California to New York, you will "lose" 3 hours according to your body's biological clock. When you are in New York and your alarm rings at 8:00 a.m., you will feel tired and groggy because your body is still on California time, which would be 5:00 a.m. It will take your body a few days to adjust to the new time zone, but the adjustment will eventually take place. After a couple of days, you will find that 8:00 a.m. feels like the correct time to wake up if that is part of your normal schedule and you have had adequate sleep.

Some studies have shown that supplements of melatonin, a natural hormone that is produced by the body and sold as a treatment for insomnia, can help in treating jet lag. This supplement has been especially effective for people crossing five or more time zones and for those traveling east. However, additional studies are needed to test the safety and effectiveness of melatonin for insomnia and jet lag; few studies are available, and it has not been tested for long-term use. Before you take any kind of supplement, be sure to check with your healthcare provider.

What Are Some Tips for a Good Night's Sleep?

Sleep experts recommend that you try several approaches if you have trouble falling asleep:3

- **Set a schedule.** Go to bed at the same time each night and wake up at the same time each morning.

- **Exercise 20 to 30 minutes each day.** Regular daily exercise can help people sleep, as long as it is not done too close to bedtime.

- **Avoid caffeine, nicotine, and alcohol.** Caffeine acts as a stimulant and can keep you awake. Caffeine is found in coffee, chocolate, soft drinks, certain teas, diet drugs, and pain relievers. Nicotine affects the depth of sleep, and smokers tend to sleep very lightly. Alcohol prevents people from entering deep sleep (sleep stages 3 and 4) and rapid eye movement (REM) sleep.

- **Relax before bed.** Try taking a warm bath, reading, or drinking warm herbal tea before falling asleep. You can train yourself to associate these types of restful activities with sleep, particularly if you make them part of your nighttime ritual.

- **Sleep until sunlight.** Try to wake up with the sunrise, if possible. If this is not possible, use very bright lights in the morning. Sunlight (or bright light) helps the body's internal biological clock reset itself each day. Experts recommend an hour of exposure to morning sunlight for people having problems falling asleep.

- **Don't lie in bed awake.** If you are unable to fall asleep, try doing something else, like reading, watching television, or listening to music, until you feel tired. The anxiety you feel when you are unable to fall asleep further contributes to insomnia. Therefore, lying in bed waiting to fall asleep can worsen the problem of insomnia.

- **Control your room temperature.** Maintain a comfortable temperature in your bedroom. Temperature extremes can disrupt sleep or prevent you from falling asleep.

- **Know when it is time to see a healthcare provider.** You should visit your doctor or a sleep specialist if you continue to have problems sleeping. If you have trouble falling asleep night after night, or if you always feel tired during the next day, you may have a sleep disorder and should see a healthcare provider.

What Is Sudden Infant Death Syndrome (SIDS)?

SIDS is the sudden, unexplained death of an infant younger than 1 year old. It is the leading cause of death in children between 1 month and 1 year of age.

Healthcare providers don't know what exactly causes SIDS, but they do know certain things can help reduce the risk of SIDS:

- Always place infants on their backs to sleep. Infants who sleep on their backs are less likely to die of SIDS than infants who sleep on their stomachs or sides. Placing your baby on his or her back to sleep is the number one way to reduce the risk of SIDS.

- Use the back sleep position every time. Infants who usually sleep on their backs but who are then placed on their stomachs, such as for a nap, are at very high risk of SIDS. So it is important for infants to sleep on their backs every time, for naps and at night.

- Place your baby on a firm sleep surface, such as a safety-approved crib mattress covered with a fitted sheet. Never place a baby to sleep on a pillow, quilt, sheepskin, or other soft surface.

- Keep soft objects, crib bumpers, toys, and loose bedding out of your baby's sleep area; don't use pillows, blankets, quilts, sheepskins, or pillow-like bumpers in your baby's sleep area. Keep all items away from the baby's face.

- Avoid letting your baby overheat during sleep; dress your baby in no more than one layer more than an adult would wear to be comfortable and keep the room at a temperature that is comfortable for an adult.

- Give your baby a dry pacifier that is not attached to a string for naps and at night to reduce the risk of SIDS. But don't force the baby to use it. (If you're breastfeeding, wait until your child is 1 month old or is used to breastfeeding before using a pacifier.)

Chapter 2

Sleep Disorders in Women

Sleep and Women

A healthy sleeping pattern is particularly important for women, as it has a direct bearing on the quality of their lives. Unlike their predecessors, today's women are faced with the challenge of balancing home and career, and getting adequate sleep—in terms of both quantity and quality—is particularly important in order to recharge depleted energy stores in the body and brain cells and to lay the foundation for a productive day.

Studies have proved that the circadian rhythm, a 24-hour cycle that is internally generated in many organisms, including humans, has a deep impact on the sleep-wake cycle. Clinical evidence points to significant differences in the way men and women sleep, and in recent years there has been growing interest in how gender influences sleep pathologies. While much is known about the mechanisms that link sleep and circadian rhythms, research on the way gender may affect sleep is still in its nascent stage but is vital to how we understand and treat sleep-related disorders.

Clinical studies across a broad range of ages have shown that women sleep longer but report poorer sleep quality than men. Women may also complain of sleep problems when there is no measurable evidence of sleep disturbance. This reflects a *sleep state misperception* (SSM), also known as pseudo or paradoxical insomnia, a condition recognized as an intrinsic sleep disorder by the *International Classification of Sleep*

Disorders (ICSD), which is a widely accepted tool for clinical practice and research in sleep-disorder medicine. The higher incidence of SSM in women may, in part, be attributed to the statistically higher incidence of anxiety, mood, and affective disorders in women.

Despite clinical evidence pointing to a higher incidence of SSM in women compared to men, there also exist data that support the fact that women are, in fact, more prone to sleep disorders than men. The risk ratio for sleep problems increases with age and is seen to be more apparent after puberty, indicating that reproductive hormones may affect sleep patterns and circadian rhythms in women. Changes in the ovarian hormonal milieu across the lifespan would also explain how age influences sleep patterns and circadian rhythms in women.

Menstrual Cycle and Sleep

A report suggests that more than two-thirds of women experience disrupted sleep patterns during their menstrual cycles. These changes in sleep patterns manifest as part of premenstrual syndrome (PMS), a group of symptoms that occur about a week to ten days before menstruation. Although PMS may affect individuals differently, it is generally associated with mood changes, depression, irritability, fatigue, and insomnia. For some, disturbed sleep patterns may continue even during periods, with abdominal cramping and other symptoms associated with menstruation affecting sleep quality. Studies show a reduction in REM sleep in the first few days of the menstrual cycle, while progesterone, the hormone whose levels spike in the latter half of the cycle, has a soporific effect and has been shown to help women sleep better.

Pregnancy and Sleep

It has been reported that more than three-quarters of women experience sleep problems during pregnancy. While insomnia is common, other sleep-related issues may include sleep apnea, restless leg syndrome, and periodic limb movement disorder. Pregnancy places considerable demands on the body, and so pregnant women may need a few extra hours of sleep, particularly during the last trimester. But during pregnancy a number of conditions can impede a good night's sleep. These include increased heart rate, dyspnea (shortness of breath), anxiety, stress, and heartburn.

Women typically gain around 30 pounds of weight during pregnancy, and this puts extra pressure on the pelvis and spine. Consequently, pregnant women frequently experience aches in the legs and back, which often disrupt sleep. The kidneys also overwork during pregnancy, since there is a marked increase in the filtration rate, and this results in frequent urination, meaning more trips to the bathroom at night. Unsurprisingly, sleep issues tend to continue for most women even after childbirth. The stress involved in caring for the newborn and waking up frequently to nurse the baby make it difficult to get through the night without sleep interruptions.

Menopause and Sleep

Many women face increased sleep issues during and after menopause. In fact, some women begin to experience sleep problems even during perimenopause, the natural transition from a woman's reproductive phase to the cessation of menstrual periods. Sleep issues in menopause are closely linked to altered levels of hormones. A drop in estrogen level often causes hot flashes and night sweats, which can greatly disrupt sleep, depending on the severity and frequency of symptoms. Decrease in hormone levels can also lead to an increased heart rate and vaginal dryness, and these symptoms may exacerbate anxiety and stress, which may aggravate sleep problems further. There may also be other physical factors that could impact sleep in menopausal women. Arthritis and heartburn, for example, could keep women awake during the night, and the resulting sleep deprivation could lead to fatigue and further aggravate problems like anxiety and depression.

Managing Sleep Disorders in Women

The protocol for treating insomnia and other sleep-related disorders is, by and large, the same for men and women and generally includes over-the-counter and prescription medications; cognitive behavioral therapy; complementary and alternative treatments; and recommended lifestyle changes. That said, clinicians need to consider medical, social, and specific biological factors, such as pregnancy and menopause, to determine the type of treatment required for managing sleep disorders in women.

Healthy Sleep Tips for Women

Lifestyle changes may be particularly useful in dealing with insomnia and sleep issues during pregnancy and menopause. While a balanced diet, adequate physical activity, and effective coping strategies are key recommendations to deal with general sleep-related problems, specific medical conditions—such as osteoarthritis, anxiety, and depression, which may co-occur with sleep disorders, particularly in older women—need to be addressed, as well.

Following good nighttime practices can establish a regular wake-sleep pattern and help women deal with sleep issues. Avoiding heavy and spicy food just before bed can help reduce the chances of heartburn and sleep problems precipitated by it. Stimulants like caffeine, alcohol, and nicotine can make it difficult to fall asleep, so those with sleep issues should avoid these stimulants in the late-afternoon and evening. Practicing relaxation techniques during menstruation could help deal with sleep problems associated with menstrual cycles. Exposure to daylight has been shown to release melatonin, a hormone that regulates the sleep and wake cycles and also enhances appetite and mood.

Failure to get a good night's sleep is a common enough problem today, and most people experience it at some time in their lives. These problems may hardly ever require medical attention and may be easily managed by lifestyle modifications. However, serious sleep disorders can have a detrimental effect on your physical, mental, and social wellbeing and do require medical attention. A sleep specialist can help diagnose sleep problems and develop a treatment plan best suited for you.

References

1.   "Sleep and Women," UCLASleepCenter, n.d.

2.   "Women and Sleep," The National Sleep Foundation, n.d.

3.   "Sleep, Rhythms, and the Endocrine Brain: Influence of Sex and Gonadal Hormones," The Journal of Neuroscience, November 9, 2011.

4.   Hedaya, Robert J. "PMS and Insomnia: What to do?" Psychology Today, May 4, 2010.

Chapter 3

Sleep Disorders in Men

Sleep and Men

Many men consider sleep to be just one more chore on a list of things to do during the course of a 24-hour period. Some may even consider it a waste of time that could be put to better use. But this attitude might be preventing them from harnessing the power of a well-rested mind and body.

Sleep should be considered to be one of the body's most valuable daily requirements. A sound investment in sleep provides valuable benefits to many other aspects of life. During sleep the body recharges itself and prepares for another productive day. A good night's rest allows the human body to feel, think, and perform better, and a well-rested individual will find that he has more time and energy at his disposal during the day.

Causes of Sleeplessness in Men

A variety of factors may cause sleeplessness in men and prevent them from getting the amount of rest required for the body and mind to recharge. These can include:

Lack of Awareness

Many men simply aren't aware of the importance of sleep. Some may even view it as an indication of not working enough and believe

---

"Sleep Disorders in Men" @ 2016 Omnigraphics 2016. Reviewed July 2016.

they have to fight the urge to sleep. Although the amount of sleep required varies from person to person, in general adults need at least seven to eight hours of sleep per night. But many people do not get enough sleep and consequently don't have optimal levels of energy and concentration to perform their daily activities.

Some signs that you are not sleeping enough:

- Feeling of tiredness and lack of energy throughout the day

- Difficulty concentrating

- Slow to get started in the morning

- Irritability

- Dozing off during the day

Sleeping late is not an option for people who have to be at work early, and most work policies don't allow for naps on the job. The only solution is to go to sleep earlier. Plan to get eight hours of sleep per night, and prioritize this to make it a goal.

Work Demands

Extra hours at work, the need to work during weekends, long commutes to work, and paperwork at home consume much of our time in the modern world. After checking e-mails and answering mobile phones, it is often past the ideal bedtime. Stress at the workplace and anxiety about the next day can also result in disturbed sleep. The body wants to sleep, but the mind remains awake, and you may toss and turn in bed.

Try to leave your work behind when you come home. Maintain boundaries between work and personal time. And working from home—as is common these days—can make the situation even worse. Talking to friends or co-workers about your work life may help relieve stress, as can meditation or physical exercise. Make your bed a place to relax and not to worry.

Full Schedules

Men have busy schedules these days, with many more planned activities in their lives than just work. After work, they might be playing sports or watching their favorite teams in action. They could be doing pet projects or be involved in clubs, civic groups, fraternities, or church activities. Single men could be going out on dates or spending time with friends. Married men might be picking their kids up from school or helping them with their homework.

The key is to prioritize the important things and balance time effectively. Not everything needs to be done each day. Scale back on the number of things you are doing, rearrange tasks, and eliminate less important ones. These can be done when you have free time on other days. When listing and prioritizing activities, make sure sleeping is ranked high on the list.

Life Changes

Changes in life have the potential to affect your sleep dramatically. These changes may come quite by surprise, or you might have been expecting them. Negative changes tend to be most disruptive to your sleep, but positive change could have this effect, as well, because of the excitement it causes. Some changes may bring new duties and responsibilities, which could increase stress and keep you up at night.

Some negative changes that could affect your sleep include:

- The death of a loved one

- Becoming unemployed

- Getting divorced

- Being involved in an accident

- Becoming aware of a major illness

- Having a lawsuit filed against you

- An investment that has turned bad

Some such positive changes include:

- Getting married

- Having a baby

- Getting a promotion or a new job

- Moving or relocating

Some changes may cause men to experience depression, which can have a major impact on sleep patterns. You could toss and turn in bed without sleeping much or you could sleep longer with little motivation to get out of bed. Depression can also cause men to stop taking care of themselves. They may stop eating, grooming, and exercising. Abuse

29

of alcohol and drugs is common with depression, and there could be a loss of interest in day to day activities.

Men often find it difficult to talk about depression and may find it preferable not to seek help from counselors. But they need to be aware that their condition could be hazardous to their health and detrimental to their daily lives. They could begin by talking about the problem to a friend, spouse, doctor or minister. These people could help them seek help from a counselors when they've made the decision to do so. It is advisable not to face the situation on your own.

Bad Habits

Poor sleep can be the result of bad habits or routines. These include the consumption of alcohol, nicotine, and coffee in the late afternoon, in the evening, or just before bedtime. Eating big meals or exercising before bedtime can also disturb your sleep. You might tend to have a big meal at night if you were busy during the evening. Instead, try and have a good lunch so that you are satisfied with a smaller dinner. Exercise before work or during your lunch break.

Going to sleep at irregular times and waking up at different times daily could disrupt your internal body clock and prevent you sleeping soundly. To set your body's clock properly, try to wake up at a set time every day, including weekends and holidays. Avoid sleeping late on weekends to catch up on lost sleep. This doesn't work. Instead, go to bed earlier at night. Also, limit naps to an hour in order to avoid disrupting sleep at night.

Medical Conditions

Any number of medical conditions may result in poor sleep. The effects could be temporary, as with a sprained ankle, flu, or surgery, while others may be chronic and require long-term treatment. Some medical conditions become more common with increasing age, and they or their medications could begin to interfere with sleep.

The following are a few medical conditions could result in poor sleep patterns:

- Epilepsy
- Asthma
- Other respiratory diseases
- Heart disease
- Arthritis

Some medications may hinder sleep and keep you jittery through the night. Others may cause sleepiness during the day. Talk to your doctor about your medication; there may be alternatives that could eliminate these types of side-effects. The time at which you take your medicine and the dosage could also have a significant effect on the quality of your sleep.

Sleep Disorders that Affect Men

Many people spend enough time lying in bed but do not get quality sleep. Their sleep could be disturbed and broken, or they may sleep through the night but wake up tired. These are indications of an underlying sleep disorder. Sleep disorders are common, but many people who are afflicted with them remain unaware of the condition, and some may shy away from seeking help. But diagnosing and treating sleep disorders can result in a dramatic improvement in sleep, helping to establish healthy sleep patterns and allowing you to be at your best during the day.

The following are some sleep disorders commonly diagnosed among men:

Obstructive Sleep Apnea (OSA)

During sleep, muscles in the throat become relaxed. Sometimes the tissue in the mouth may collapse and prevent air from entering the lungs, or the tongue could fall back and block the airway. This is a disorder known as Obstructive Sleep Apnea (OSA), a condition that affects one in four men. This blockage could occur a few times during the night or many hundreds of times. Breathing pauses for a moment when this happens, and you tend to wake up. Someone with OSA often feels very tired during the day. Men are twice as likely as women to have OSA. Obesity and a larger neck girth increase the likelihood of having OSA, since the larger amount of fatty tissue in the neck can block the airway.

In addition to sleepiness during the day, another sign of OSA is loud snoring, which is caused by a partially blocked airway passage. The intensity of snoring could range from mild to severe. Simple snoring is generally normal and harmless, but loud and severe snoring accompanied by gasping for air is a cause for concern. Men are often not aware that they snore. It usually becomes evident when a spouse or sleep partner notices it. Left untreated, sleep apnea carries with it the risk of lung disease, diabetes, and hypertension.

Talk to you doctor if you snore loudly in the night. He or she may refer you to a sleep specialist who can test for sleep apnea. Losing weight and sleeping on the side, rather than the back, are remedies that you can try on your own. But medical treatment is essential for more serious sleep apnea.

Continuous Positive Air Pressure (CPAP) is one treatment that can be used to treat sleep apnea. A mask worn on the face during sleep delivers a steady flow of air through the nose. This keeps the airway open and prevents pauses in breathing. The use of an oral device, similar to a mouth guard, could bring relief to people with OSA. And some cases surgery may be recommended.

Narcolepsy

Narcolepsy is a chronic brain disorder that causes extreme sleepiness during day-to-day activities, like eating, walking, or driving. It causes people to fall asleep suddenly for a few seconds to several minutes. Narcolepsy commonly begins between the ages of 12 and 20, although in some cases it may begin later in life. The condition cannot be cured, but it can be controlled with treatment.

If you feel as if you could fall asleep at any time, talk to your doctor. He or she may refer you to a sleep specialist who will make a proper diagnosis. Narcolepsy can be treated using medication that will restore your sleep and wakefulness cycle to a normal pattern.

Delayed Sleep Phase Disorder

Delayed Sleep Phase Disorder (DSPD)—also called Delayed Sleep Phase Syndrome (DSPS)—is a condition characterized by the tendency to go to sleep and wake up later than what is considered normal, usually by a couple of hours. Every person has an internal clock that prompts the body to sleep and wake up at a given time. Getting into the habit of going to sleep late at night can throw the body clock out of balance, preventing you from falling asleep at the right time.

To counteract DSP, stay away from bright lights during the late afternoon and evening. Use dim lighting in your house, and switch off the lights in the bedroom at when it's time to sleep. It's also important to get enough daylight in the morning and afternoon. This sends signals to the brain to set the body clock properly.

Jet Lag Disorder and Shift Work Disorder

Jet lag disorder is caused by traveling long distances by air. This disrupts your body clock, because you might reach your destination when your body expects you to sleep, but in reality it could be daytime there, and you may need to be awake. Your body clock is not able to adjust itself because of the speed of travel involved, and this may make it hard for you to sleep.

Shift work disorder can occur in men who work late-night shifts or in rotating shifts and often need to work when the body senses that it's time to sleep. After work, these individuals feel that they want to sleep when it is actually the time for the body to remain awake. This results in tiredness and the inability to sleep properly.

Melatonin supplements have been shown to improve jet lag among travellers. Melatonin is a hormone that is released by the body at night and helps induce sleep. Light therapy has shown positive benefits on both jet lag disorder and shift work disorder. In light therapy the eyes are exposed to bright light at a regular time and for a specific duration. This mimics the effect of sunlight on the body's internal clock. Consult your doctor to see if melatonin or light therapy could be beneficial in your case.

How Can Men Sleep Better?

Developing good sleep practices is the first step in allowing men to sleep better. You can build these good habits by following some basic tips that will result in healthy sleep patterns and learning counter-productive practices to avoid.

One common misconception among men is that alcohol helps them sleep better. Alcohol might help you get to sleep, but it often causes you to wake up during the night. Many men who drink in the evening wake up very early in the morning and experience sleeplessness. To develop good sleep hygiene, refrain from drinking at least six hours before bedtime. Limit how much you drink and how frequently you drink. The heavy use of alcohol is detrimental to overall good health, as well as good sleep.

Men sometimes use prescription sleeping pills as a solution to sleep problems. These drugs help to an extent, but they shouldn't be used as a long-term solution. Because of the danger of developing a dependency, doctors generally do not prescribe sleep medication beyond a few weeks at a time.

Over-the-counter sleep medicines are readily available at drug-stores. These formulations often use antihistamines to induce drowsiness. Even though they allow you to sleep, they can make you groggy during the day and may result in slow response times. They should be used sparingly and with caution.

If you have not been sleeping well for more than a month, it is a good idea to consult a doctor. Do not ignore the problem thinking it will disappear. Your physician will likely refer you to a sleep specialist who will diagnose the cause of the problem. Before visiting a sleep specialist, it can be useful to keep a sleep diary for two weeks. This will help the specialist understand your sleep patterns, provide clues about what is hindering your sleep, and assist him or her in suggesting remedies.

Sleep is crucial to your well-being, and it touches every other aspect of your life. Do not ignore signs of trouble when there is so much to gain from consulting a doctor for diagnosis and treatment.

References

1. "Sleep and Men," UCLA Health. n.d.

2. "Sleep Apnea and Insomnia in Men," BodyLogicMD.com. n.d.

3. "Sleep Disorders," Bon Secours for Men. n.d.

Chapter 4

Napping: A Healthy Habit

Chapter Contents

Section 4.1

What Is Napping?

Most mammals are polyphasic sleepers, which mean they sleep or nap multiple times during a 24-hour period. Humans, on the other hand, are monophasic sleepers since they have distinct, alternate phases of sleeping and waking. Whether this forms the natural sleep pattern for humans has not been clearly established, however, napping is an integral part of many cultures, globally.

The United States is fast becoming a nation of deprived sleepers, due primarily to a culture that often promotes a hectic lifestyle. Napping could be a solution, since sleeping for 20-30 minutes during normal waking hours has been shown to result in remarkable improvements in mood, alertness and performance.

Types of Napping

There are three different ways that we usually nap:

- *Planned napping*: Also known as preparatory napping, this involves taking a nap before you are sleepy in anticipation of going to bed late. This helps you avoid feeling tired because of inadequate sleep later on.

- *Emergency napping*: You may take an emergency nap when you feel tired and unable to continue the task you were engaged in. This type of napping is very useful when you have been driving and are feeling drowsy or when you need to counter fatigue when operating dangerous machinery.

- *Habitual napping*: This is the practice of taking naps as a regular routine at a particular time of the day. Young children nap this way, and it is not uncommon in many cultures for adults to a nap after lunch.

Recommendations for Napping

- A nap of 20-30 minutes is optimal. It tends not to interfere with your regular sleep pattern and generally doesn't make you groggy.

- Sleep in a comfortable place with moderate room temperature and without much noise or light filtering in. It is most beneficial to sleep rather than just lie in bed resting.

- Do not take a nap too late in the day, because it will affect your regular sleep at night. Do not nap early in the day, either, since you may not be able to sleep well.

Seven Steps to Have the Perfect Nap

Just lying down, closing your eyes and hoping for the best won't necessarily help you nap. You should think it out and employ a strategy to help you nap better. The following steps will help you get the perfect nap:

Step 1

Decide how long you want to nap. Different durations confer their own benefits.

- 6 minutes: Provides improvement in memory functions.

- 10-15 minutes: Improves focus and productivity.

- 20-30 minutes: Optimum nap time, which results in alertness, concentration, and sharp motor skills.

- 40-60 minutes: Boosts brain power, consolidates memory for facts, places and faces, and improves learning ability.

- 90 to 120 minutes: Improves creativity and emotional and procedural memory.

Step 2

Nap between 1 pm and 3 pm.

The body has an inherent biological clock that controls the sleep-wake cycle, known as the circadian rhythm. Humans experience intense sleep in two periods every 24 hours. One is between 1 and 3 pm and the other is from 2 to 4 am. Alertness, reaction time, coordination, and mood are decreased during these periods. The lethargy experienced after lunch is actually biological in nature. A nap around this time will put you back on track. Napping between 1 and 3 pm will generally not disturb regular sleep. If you work a night shift, the best time to take a nap would be 6 to 8 hours after waking.

Step 3

Create a conducive atmosphere.

If you are unable to fall asleep during the day, you may not be approaching napping the right way. Lighting is an important factor, since light inhibits melatonin, the sleep regulation hormone. Darken your room with window shades or use an eye mask. Lie down, rather than sitting, when you take a nap. You will fall asleep 50 percent faster. Many people find that a hammock is the best place to nap because of the gentle swaying motion that promotes sleep.

Step 4

Use an alarm.

You will need to wake up in time to get back to work after a snooze, so set an alarm to wake you up.

Step 5

Try a coffee nap.

If you are concerned about becoming sleepy in the afternoon, try having a cup of coffee and taking a nap. Caffeine kicks into the body in 20 to 30 minutes. This should give you enough time to take a nap and get rejuvenated. Combining coffee and napping can be more beneficial than doing either of them alone.

Step 6

Avoid the blahs after napping.

Make sure you avoid sleep inertia. If you take a long nap, you may feel groggy after waking up, because a full sleep cycle was not completed. Avoid this by having coffee, washing your face, or exposing yourself to bright light. An alternative is to complete a full sleep cycle by taking a nap for at least 90 minutes.

Step 7

Get adequate sleep at night.

Nothing replaces a good night's sleep, and emergency napping cannot be a long-term substitute for regular, deep sleep. Inadequate sleep on a regular basis can result in hypertension, diabetes, weight gain, depression, and a general feeling of unease.

Pros of Napping

- Napping improves alertness and performance levels. It reduces mistakes and accidents. A NASA study conducted on military pilots showed that 40 minutes of napping increased alertness by 100 percent and performance by 34 percent.

- Naps improve alertness for some duration after the nap and often increase alertness to some extent over the entire day.

- Napping results in relaxation and rejuvenation. It is a luxurious and pleasant experience, something similar to a mini vacation.

- Taking a nap when you are feeling drowsy behind the wheel can help you regain alertness so that you can continue to drive safely.

- Night-shift workers who nap have been shown to experience improved alertness on the job.

- A 45-minute daytime nap improves memory functioning.

- Napping reduces blood pressure.

- It reduces the risk of cardiovascular diseases.

- Temporary sleep issues due to jet lag, stress, or illnesses can often be remedied by napping.

- A quick nap is very good for mental and physical stamina.

- Napping improves mental acuity and overall health.

Cons of Napping

- The stigma associated with napping is probably the biggest downside of napping.
    - It may be equated with laziness.
    - It is often associated with lack of ambition and low standards.
    - Napping may be seen as normal only for children, the sick, and the elderly.

- Napping can be counterproductive for people with sleep disorders or those with irregular sleep patterns.

- Naps are often not recommended for people with sleep apnea.

References

1. "Napping," National Sleep Foundation, n.d.

2. Belsky, Gail. "The Pros and Cons of Napping," Health, n.d.

3. Brown, Brendan. "A How-To Guide to the Perfect Nap [Infographic]," Art of Wellbeing, February 16, 2016.

Section 4.2

Benefits of Napping

This section includes text excerpted from "Sleep Researchers Home in on the Benefits of Napping," U.S. Department of Veterans Affairs (VA), February 11, 2014.

Napping for Better Health

Getting a good night's sleep is important for everyone. Good sleep refreshes people, helps them perform better, and contributes significantly to health and happiness. For many veterans, however, getting a good night's sleep is extremely difficult.

Sleep disturbances are common in patients suffering from bipolar disorder, substance abuse, major depression, panic disorder, and chronic pain disorders. Sleep disorders following recent exposure to traumatic events can predict the later development of posttraumatic stress disorder (PTSD).

Disrupted sleep, or the inability to get a full night's sleep without interruption, is a very common negative consequence of PTSD. According to VA's National Center for PTSD, nightmares are one of the 17 symptoms of the disorder, and as many 71 percent of those with the illness reported experiencing nightmares, sometimes or more frequently, compared to only 3 percent of those who did not serve.

For some who simply cannot get a good night's sleep, there is a way to avoid many of the consequences of sleeplessness. "Napping has been shown to alleviate the negative physical and psychological symptoms of disrupted sleep," says Elizabeth A. McDevitt, a graduate student in the department of psychology at the University of California, Riverside. At the time the research was conducted, McDevitt was affiliated with the San Diego VA Medical Center and the University of California, San Diego (UCSD).

According to a study recently published online in the *Journal of Physiology and Behavior* by McDevitt and two colleagues from the San Diego VA and UCSD, napping is especially helpful to manage circadian disruption (problems related either from changes in a person's sleep-wake cycle, such as jet lag, daylight saving time, or between workweeks and weekends; or through the inability to get enough sleep in the time allotted for sleep.) In healthy, well-rested subjects, napping has also been shown to improve performance across a range of performance tasks.

Despite the benefits of napping, however, some people report that they simply cannot nap, or don't want to nap. In their study, McDevitt and her colleagues set out to determine why some people nap and others do not.

She and her colleagues asked 27 healthy, non-smoking college students between the ages of 18 and 35 to participate in an experiment. All of them spent between seven and nine hours in bed every night, and none of them had a sleep disorder. They were asked to keep a diary of their sleep habits for a week, including their daily naps if they took them, and wore special actigraph wristwatches (small, wristwatch shaped devices that record motion and are used to assess sleep by determining whether a person is active or inactive) to verify what they had put down in their diaries.

After a week of measurements, each participant reported to the Laboratory for Sleep and Behavioral Neuroscience at the San Diego VA. Their level of sleepiness was measured at 9 a.m., 11 a.m., 4:30 p.m., and 6:30 p.m. At 1:30 p.m., they were all asked to take a nap, and were allowed to sleep for a maximum of 90 minutes—but they were given no more than 120 minutes in bed, whether they napped or not. While they napped, their brain waves were monitored through electrodes to see how deeply they were sleeping.

By correlating the information in the subjects' diaries, and analyzing the brain wave information they obtained, the team found that people who nap frequently sleep more lightly during their naps than those who usually never nap at all. In sleeping, the body progresses through a series of five stages, from light sleep through dreaming, called the sleep cycle. (Sleep does not progress through these stages in order, however.)

Those who had taken three to four naps in the week before the brain wave tests took place had the least amount of slow wave sleep (scientist's term for stage 3, or deep sleep) and the most amount of stage 1, or light sleep; those who took one to two naps a week had the most amount of stage 2 sleep, which is somewhat deeper, and those who never napped at all had the highest amount of stage 3 sleep while in the laboratory, meaning they slept the most deeply. The naps that people of all groups took did not measurably affect their sleep at night.

Using this data, the team developed two hypotheses. First, that some people avoid napping because of the high levels of deep sleep that they fall into when they do nap—meaning that, when they wake up, they feel groggy and tired instead of rested and refreshed. And second, people who choose to nap may just be sleepier people than those who do not.

"Individuals who frequently nap may generally be sleepier people who are self-treating their sleepiness with daytime naps," said McDevitt. "They might be predisposed to be good daytime nappers, or they have learned to become skilled nappers through practice."

The team suggested that future studies should consider the possibility of nap practice or nap training to maximize the benefits of napping, and examine how differences in sleep associated with nap behavior may influence changes in performance following a nap.

Chapter 5

Benefits of Slumber

Why You Need a Good Night's Sleep

We have so many demands on our time—jobs, family, errands—not to mention finding some time to relax. To fit everything in, we often sacrifice sleep. But sleep affects both mental and physical health. It's vital to your well-being.

Of course, sleep helps you feel rested each day. But while you're sleeping, your brain and body don't just shut down. Internal organs and processes are hard at work throughout the night.

"Sleep services all aspects of our body in one way or another: molecular, energy balance, as well as intellectual function, alertness and mood," says Dr. Merrill Mitler, a sleep expert and neuroscientist.

When you're tired, you can't function at your best. Sleep helps you think more clearly, have quicker reflexes and focus better. "The fact is, when we look at well-rested people, they're operating at a different level than people trying to get by on 1 or 2 hours less nightly sleep," says Mitler.

"Loss of sleep impairs your higher levels of reasoning, problem-solving and attention to detail," Mitler explains. Tired people tend to be less productive at work. They're at a much higher risk for traffic accidents. Lack of sleep also influences your mood, which can affect how you interact with others. A sleep deficit over time can even put you at greater risk for developing depression.

This chapter includes text excerpted from "The Benefits of Slumber," National Institutes of Health (NIH), April 2013.

But sleep isn't just essential for the brain. "Sleep affects almost every tissue in our bodies," says Dr. Michael Twery, a sleep expert at NIH. "It affects growth and stress hormones, our immune system, appetite, breathing, blood pressure and cardiovascular health."

Research shows that lack of sleep increases the risk for obesity, heart disease and infections. Throughout the night, your heart rate, breathing rate and blood pressure rise and fall, a process that may be important for cardiovascular health. Your body releases hormones during sleep that help repair cells and control the body's use of energy. These hormone changes can affect your body weight.

"Ongoing research shows a lack of sleep can produce diabetic-like conditions in otherwise healthy people," says Mitler.

Recent studies also reveal that sleep can affect the efficiency of vaccinations. Twery described research showing that well-rested people who received the flu vaccine developed stronger protection against the illness.

A good night's sleep consists of 4 to 5 sleep cycles. Each cycle includes periods of deep sleep and rapid eye movement (REM) sleep, when we dream. "As the night goes on, the portion of that cycle that is in REM sleep increases. It turns out that this pattern of cycling and progression is critical to the biology of sleep," Twery says.

Although personal needs vary, on average, adults need 7 to 8 hours of sleep per night. Babies typically sleep about 16 hours a day. Young children need at least 10 hours of sleep, while teenagers need at least 9 hours. To attain the maximum restorative benefits of sleep, getting a full night of quality sleep is important, says Twery.

Sleep can be disrupted by many things. Stimulants such as caffeine or certain medications can keep you up. Distractions such as electronics—especially the light from TVs, cell phones, tablets and e-readers—can prevent you from falling asleep.

As people get older, they may not get enough sleep because of illness, medications or sleep disorders. By some estimates, about 70 million Americans of all ages suffer from chronic sleep problems. The 2 most common sleep disorders are insomnia and sleep apnea.

People with insomnia have trouble falling or staying asleep. Anxiety about falling asleep often makes the condition worse. Most of us have occasional insomnia. But chronic insomnia—lasting at least 3 nights per week for more than a month—can trigger serious daytime problems such as exhaustion, irritability and difficulty concentrating.

Common therapies include relaxation and deep-breathing techniques. Sometimes medicine is prescribed. But consult a doctor before trying even over-the-counter sleep pills, as they may leave you feeling unrefreshed in the morning.

People with sleep apnea have a loud, uneven snore (although not everyone who snores has apnea). Breathing repeatedly stops or becomes shallow. If you have apnea, you're not getting enough oxygen, and your brain disturbs your sleep to open your windpipe.

Apnea is dangerous. "There's little air exchange for 10 seconds or more at a time," explains Dr. Phyllis Zee, a sleep apnea expert at Northwestern University. "The oxygen goes down and the body's fight or flight response is activated. Blood pressure spikes, your heart rate fluctuates and the brain wakes you up partially to start your breathing again. This creates stress."

Apnea can leave you feeling tired and moody. You may have trouble thinking clearly. "Also, apnea affects the vessels that lead to the brain so there is a higher risk of stroke associated with it," Zee adds.

If you have mild sleep apnea, you might try sleeping on your side, exercising or losing weight to reduce symptoms. A CPAP machine, which pumps air into your throat to keep your airway open, can also help. Another treatment is a bite plate that moves the lower jaw forward. In some cases, however, people with sleep apnea need surgery.

"If you snore chronically and wake up choking or gasping for air, and feel that you're sleepy during the day, tell your doctor and get evaluated," Zee advises.

Good sleep is critical to your health. To make each day a safe, productive one, take steps to make sure you regularly get a good night's sleep.

Chapter 6

Dreaming

Chapter Contents

Section 6.1

Dreaming and Rapid Eye Movement (REM) Sleep: The Science behind Dreams

This section includes text excerpted from "Brain Basics: Understanding Sleep," National Institute of Neurological Disorders and Stroke (NINDS), July 25, 2014.

Dreaming and REM Sleep

We typically spend more than 2 hours each night dreaming. Scientists do not know much about how or why we dream. Sigmund Freud, who greatly influenced the field of psychology, believed dreaming was a "safety valve" for unconscious desires. Only after 1953, when researchers first described REM in sleeping infants, did scientists begin to carefully study sleep and dreaming. They soon realized that the strange, illogical experiences we call dreams almost always occur during REM sleep. While most mammals and birds show signs of REM sleep, reptiles and other cold-blooded animals do not.

REM sleep begins with signals from an area at the base of the brain called the *pons*. These signals travel to a brain region called the *thalamus*, which relays them to the *cerebral cortex*–the outer layer of the brain that is responsible for learning, thinking, and organizing information. The pons also sends signals that shut off neurons in the spinal cord, causing temporary paralysis of the limb muscles. If something interferes with this paralysis, people will begin to physically "act out" their dreams–a rare, dangerous problem called *REM sleep behavior disorder*. A person dreaming about a ball game, for example, may run headlong into furniture or blindly strike someone sleeping nearby while trying to catch a ball in the dream.

REM sleep stimulates the brain regions used in learning. This may be important for normal brain development during infancy, which would explain why infants spend much more time in REM sleep than adults. Like deep sleep, REM sleep is associated with increased production of proteins. One study found that REM sleep affects learning of certain mental skills. People taught a skill and then deprived of

48

non-REM sleep could recall what they had learned after sleeping, while people deprived of REM sleep could not.

Some scientists believe dreams are the cortex's attempt to find meaning in the random signals that it receives during REM sleep. The cortex is the part of the brain that interprets and organizes information from the environment during consciousness. It may be that, given random signals from the pons during REM sleep, the cortex tries to interpret these signals as well, creating a "story" out of fragmented brain activity.

Section 6.2

Nightmares

This section contains text excerpted from the following sources: Text under the heading "Sleep Problems and Nightmares" is excerpted from "Sleep Problems and Nightmares," U.S. Department of Veterans Affairs (VA), August 2011. Reviewed July 2016; Text under the heading "Nightmares and PTSD" is excerpted from "Nightmares and PTSD," U.S. Department of Veterans Affairs (VA), August 13, 2015.

Sleep Problems and Nightmares

Ongoing sleep problems can harm relationships and the ability to work and concentrate It is not unusual to have nightmares during times of stress. For combat veterans, these nightmares may include combat scenes. If you have frequent and distressing nightmares, please talk to your medical or mental health provider. Frequent nightmares may be a sign of a more serious problem. Nightmares interfere with sleep and can be a sign of other problems There are treatments that can help with sleep problems and nightmares.

Nightmares

It is not unusual to have nightmares during times of stress. For combat veterans, these nightmares may include combat scenes. If you have frequent and distressing nightmares, please talk to your medical or mental health provider. Frequent nightmares may be a sign of a more serious problem.

Tips for Coping with Nightmares

- The morning after a nightmare, spend some time thinking about what might be causing increased stress in your life. Even positive stress (such as getting married, a new job, moving) can cause anxiety that may result in nightmares.

- Practice some form of relaxation every night before bed. Try imagining yourself in a calming or relaxing place, practice deep slow breathing, or listen to soothing music or sounds.

- Make your bedroom as soothing and comfortable as possible. Think about leaving a dim light or nightlight on to help you recognize your surroundings more quickly if you wake up from a nightmare.

Nightmares and PTSD

Nightmares are dreams that are threatening and scary. Nearly everyone has had a nightmare from time to time.

For trauma survivors, though, nightmares are a common problem. Along with flashbacks and unwanted memories, nightmares are one of the ways in which a trauma survivor may relive the trauma for months or years after the event.

How Common Are Nightmares after Trauma?

Among the general public, about 5% of people complain of nightmares. Those who have gone through a trauma, though, are more likely to have distressing nightmares after the event. This is true no matter what type of trauma it is.

Those trauma survivors who get PTSD are even more likely to complain of nightmares. Nightmares are one of the 17 symptoms of PTSD. For example, a study comparing Vietnam Veterans to civilians showed that 52% of combat Veterans with PTSD had nightmares fairly often. Only 3% of the civilians in the study reported that same level of nightmares.

Other research has found even higher rates of nightmares. Of those with PTSD, 71% to 96% may have nightmares. People who have other mental health problems, such as panic disorder, as well as PTSD are more likely to have nightmares than those with PTSD alone.

Not only are trauma survivors more likely to have nightmares, those who do may have them quite often. Some survivors may have nightmares several times a week.

What Do Nightmares That Follow Trauma Look Like?

Nightmares that follow trauma often involve the same scary elements that were in the trauma. For example, someone who went through Hurricane Katrina may have dreams about high winds or floods. They may dream about trying to escape the waters or being in a shelter that does not feel safe. A survivor of a hold-up might have nightmares about the robber or about being held at gunpoint.

Not all nightmares that occur after trauma are a direct replay of the event. About half of those who have nightmares after trauma have dreams that replay the trauma. People with PTSD are more likely to have dreams that are exact replays of the event than are survivors without PTSD.

Lab research has shown that nightmares after trauma are different in some ways from nightmares in general. Nightmares after trauma may occur earlier in the night and during different stages of sleep. They are more likely to have body movements along with them.

Nightmares and Cultural Differences

Nightmares may be viewed differently in different cultures. For example, in some cultures, nightmares are thought to mean that the dreamer is open to physical or spiritual harm. In other cultures, it is believed that the dreams may contain messages from spirits or may forecast the future. These beliefs may lead those with nightmares to use certain practices in an effort to protect themselves.

Are There Any Effective Treatments for Posttraumatic Nightmares?

Nightmare symptoms often get better with standard PTSD treatment. If nightmares persist, there are treatments that can reduce how often they occur.

One treatment is Imagery Rehearsal Therapy (IRT). In IRT, the person who is having nightmares, while awake, changes how the nightmare ends so that it no longer upsets them. Then the person replays over and over in their minds the new dream with the non-scary ending. Research shows that this type of treatment can reduce how often nightmares occur.

Also, treatment for breathing problems that occur during sleep may reduce the nightmares that follow trauma. High levels of sleep-disordered breathing have been seen in trauma survivors. In one study, patients given a treatment to improve their breathing during sleep no longer had violent, scary dreams.

Little research exists on the use of medicines to treat nightmares from trauma. The medicine with the most promise is prazosin. Two studies have found that prazosin reduces nightmare symptoms. More research on prazosin is under way.

Section 6.3

Night Terrors

This section includes text excerpted from "Night Terrors,"
© 1995–2016. The Nemours Foundation/KidsHealth®.
Reprinted with permission.

What Are Night Terrors?

Most parents have comforted their child after the occasional nightmare. But if your child has ever experienced what's known as a night terror (or sleep terror), his or her fear was likely inconsolable, no matter what you tried.

A night terror is a sleep disruption that seems similar to a nightmare, but with a far more dramatic presentation. Though night terrors can be alarming for parents who witness them, they're not usually cause for concern or a sign of a deeper medical issue.

During a typical night, sleep occurs in several stages. Each is associated with particular brain activity, and it's during the rapid eye movement (REM) stage that most dreaming occurs.

Night terrors happen during deep non-REM sleep. Unlike nightmares (which occur during REM sleep), a night terror is not technically a dream, but more like a sudden reaction of fear that happens during the transition from one sleep phase to another.

Night terrors usually occur about 2 or 3 hours after a child falls asleep, when sleep transitions from the deepest stage of non-REM sleep to lighter REM sleep, a stage where dreams occur. Usually this transition is a smooth one. But rarely, a child becomes agitated and frightened—and that fear reaction is a night terror.

During a night terror, a child might suddenly sit upright in bed and shout out or scream in distress. The child's breathing and heartbeat might be faster, he or she might sweat, thrash around, and act upset and scared. After a few minutes, or sometimes longer, a child simply calms down and returns to sleep.

Unlike nightmares, which kids often remember, kids don't have any memory of a night terror the next day because they were in deep sleep when it happened—and there are no mental images to recall.

What Causes Night Terrors?

Night terrors are caused by over-arousal of the central nervous system (CNS) during sleep. This may happen because the CNS (which regulates sleep and waking brain activity) is still maturing. Some kids may inherit a tendency for this over-arousal—about 80% who have night terrors have a family member who also experienced them or sleepwalking (a similar type of sleep disturbance).

Night terrors have been noted in kids who are:

- overtired or ill, stressed, or fatigued
- taking a new medication
- sleeping in a new environment or away from home

Night terrors are relatively rare—they happen in only 3–6% of kids, while almost every child will have a nightmare occasionally. Night terrors usually occur between the ages of 4 and 12, but have been reported in kids as young as 18 months. They seem to be a little more common among boys.

A child might have a single night terror or several before they cease altogether. Most of the time, night terrors simply disappear on their own as the nervous system matures.

Coping with Night Terrors

Night terrors are caused by over-arousal of the central nervous system (CNS) during sleep. This may happen because the CNS (which regulates sleep and waking brain activity) is still maturing. Some kids may inherit a tendency for this over-arousal—about 80% who have night terrors have a family member who also experienced them or sleepwalking (a similar type of sleep disturbance).

Night terrors have been noted in kids who are:

- overtired or ill, stressed, or fatigued

- taking a new medication

- sleeping in a new environment or away from home

Night terrors are relatively rare—they happen in only 3–6% of kids, while almost every child will have a nightmare occasionally. Night terrors usually occur between the ages of 4 and 12, but have been reported in kids as young as 18 months. They seem to be a little more common among boys.

A child might have a single night terror or several before they cease altogether. Most of the time, night terrors simply disappear on their own as the nervous system matures.

Chapter 7

Sleep and Aging

Does Your Need for Sleep Change as You Get Older?

Sleep needs change over a person's lifetime. Children and adolescents need more sleep than adults. Interestingly, older adults need about the same amount of sleep as younger adults–seven to nine hours of sleep per night.

Unfortunately, many older adults often get less sleep than they need. One reason is that they often have more trouble falling asleep. A study of adults over 65 found that 13 percent of men and 36 percent of women take more than 30 minutes to fall asleep.

Also, older people often sleep less deeply and wake up more often throughout the night, which may be why they may nap more often during the daytime. Nighttime sleep schedules may change with age too. Many older adults tend to get sleepier earlier in the evening and awaken earlier in the morning.

What Are the Consequences of Poor Sleep for Older Adults?

Older adults who have poor nighttime sleep are more likely to have attention and memory problems, a depressed mood, excessive daytime sleepiness, more nighttime falls, and use more over-the-counter or

This chapter includes text excerpted from "Sleep and Aging," National Institute of Aging (NIA), National Institutes of Health (NIH), December 2012. Reviewed July 2016.

prescription sleep aids. Poor sleep is also associated with a poorer quality of life.

I Have Trouble Falling Asleep at Night. Is That Just a Normal Part of Aging?

Many people believe that poor sleep is a normal part of aging, but it is not. In fact, many healthy older adults report few or no sleep problems. Sleep patterns change as we age, but disturbed sleep and waking up tired every day are not part of normal aging.

What Is the Most Common Reason Older Adults Wake up at Night?

The most common reason older adults wake up at night is to go to the bathroom. Prostate enlargement in men and continence problems in women are often the cause. Unfortunately, waking up to go to the bathroom at night also places older adults at greater risk for falling.

What Are the Most Common Sleep Disorders among Older Adults?

The most common sleep disorders among older adults are insomnia, sleep-disordered breathing, such as sleep apnea, as well as movement disorders like restless legs syndrome.

At What Point Should I See a Doctor About a Sleeping Problem?

If you are often tired during the day and don't feel that you sleep well, you should discuss this with your doctor or healthcare provider. Many primary care providers can diagnose sleep disorders and offer suggestions and treatments that can improve your sleep.

As I Get Older, Why Do I Tend to Become Tired Earlier in the Evening?

As people age, their sleeping and waking patterns tend to change. Older adults usually become sleepier earlier in the evening and wake up earlier in the morning. If they don't adjust their bedtimes to these changes, they may have difficulty falling and staying asleep.

Chapter 8

Sleep Myths

What Are Some Myths about Sleep?

There are several common myths about sleep, including the following:

Myth 1: Snoring is a common problem, especially among men, but it isn't harmful.

Although snoring might be harmless for most people, for some it is a symptom of a life-threatening disorder called sleep apnea. People who snore and experience daytime sleepiness, one of the symptoms of sleep apnea, should be concerned about this disorder and speak with a health professional.

Those with sleep apnea have brief pauses in breathing that prevent air from moving in and out of their breathing passages. The pauses in breathing reduce blood oxygen levels and can cause cardiac and vascular damage, increasing a person's risk of cardiovascular disease.

A person with sleep apnea will awaken frequently throughout the night gasping for breath, an action that disrupts sleep. Sleep apnea has also been linked to high blood pressure. Fortunately, snoring and sleep apnea can be treated. Both men and women who snore loudly, especially if there are pauses in their snoring, should consult a health professional to determine if they have sleep apnea.

This chapter includes text excerpted from "What Are Some Myths about Sleep?" National Institutes of Health (NIH), July 9, 2013.

Myth 2: You can "cheat" on the amount of sleep you get.

Despite popular belief, when people are sleep deprived they are not able to regain lost sleep by sleeping more. With inadequate sleep, you accumulate a sleep debt that is impossible to repay as it becomes larger. In addition, long-term sleep deprivation contributes to several conditions involving health, safety, and mental outlook, as well as work performance. Sleep deprivation has been linked to obesity, high blood pressure, negative mood and behavior, decreased worker productivity, and safety issues in the home, on the job, and on the road.

Myth 3: Daytime sleepiness always means a person isn't getting enough sleep.

Excessive daytime sleepiness, characterized by a feeling of extreme drowsiness and the urge to fall asleep quickly, can occur even after you have gotten enough sleep at night. It can be a sign of an underlying medical condition such as sleep apnea or a sleep disorder like narcolepsy. These problems are often treatable. If you have excessive daytime sleepiness after sleeping the recommended 7 to 9 hours, you should speak with your healthcare provider. Daytime sleepiness is dangerous because it can put you at risk for drowsy driving, injury, and illness. It can also impair mental abilities, emotions, and performance.

Myth 4: The older you get, the fewer hours of sleep you need.

Sleep experts recommend 7 to 9 hours of sleep for most adults. While sleep patterns may change as we age, the amount of sleep the body needs does not usually change. Older people may awaken more frequently throughout the night and end up getting less sleep during the overnight hours. However, their need for sleep is not drastically less than that of younger adults. Older people may take more naps during the day because they get less sleep at night.

Part Two

The Causes and Consequences of Sleep Deprivation

Chapter 9

The Problem of
Sleep Deprivation

Insufficient Sleep Is a Public Health Problem

**Continued public health surveillance of sleep quality, dura-
tion, behaviors, and disorders is needed to monitor sleep difficulties and their health impact.**

Sleep is increasingly recognized as important to public health,
with sleep insufficiency linked to motor vehicle crashes, industrial
disasters, and medical and other occupational errors. Unintentionally falling asleep, nodding off while driving, and having difficulty
performing daily tasks because of sleepiness all may contribute to
these hazardous outcomes. Persons experiencing sleep insufficiency
are also more likely to suffer from chronic diseases such as hypertension, diabetes, depression, and obesity, as well as from cancer,
increased mortality, and reduced quality of life and productivity.
Sleep insufficiency may be caused by broad scale societal factors such

This chapter contains text excerpted from the following sources: Text under
the heading "Insufficient Sleep Is a Public Health Problem" is excerpted from
"Insufficient Sleep Is a Public Health Problem," Centers for Disease Control
and Prevention (CDC), September 3, 2015; Text under the heading "One-Third
of American Adults Don't Get Enough Sleep" is excerpted from "1 in 3 Adults
Don't Get Enough Sleep," Centers for Disease Control and Prevention (CDC),
February 16, 2016.

as round-the-clock access to technology and work schedules, but sleep disorders such as insomnia or obstructive sleep apnea also play an important role. An estimated 50-70 million U.S. adults have sleep or wakefulness disorder. Notably, snoring is a major indicator of obstructive sleep apnea.

In recognition of the importance of sleep to the nation's health, CDC surveillance of sleep-related behaviors has increased in recent years. Additionally, the Institute of Medicine encouraged collaboration between CDC and the National Center on Sleep Disorders Research to support development and expansion of adequate surveillance of the U.S. population's sleep patterns and associated outcomes. Two new reports on the prevalence of unhealthy sleep behaviors and self-reported sleep-related difficulties among U.S. adults provide further evidence that insufficient sleep is an important public health concern.

Sleep-Related Unhealthy Behaviors

The Behavioral Risk Factor Surveillance System (BRFSS) survey included a core question regarding perceived insufficient rest or sleep in 2008 (included since 1995 on the Health Related Quality of Life module) and an optional module of four questions on sleep behavior in 2009. Data from the 2009 BRFSS Sleep module were used to assess the prevalence of unhealthy/sleep behaviors by selected sociodemographic factors and geographic variations in 12 states.

The analysis, determined that, among 74,571 adult respondents in 12 states, 35.3% reported <7 hours of sleep during a typical 24-hour period, 48.0% reported snoring, 37.9% reported unintentionally falling asleep during the day at least once in the preceding month, and 4.7% reported nodding off or falling asleep while driving at least once in the preceding month. This is the first CDC surveillance report to include estimates of drowsy driving and unintentionally falling asleep during the day. The National Department of Transportation estimates drowsy driving to be responsible for 1,550 fatalities and 40,000 nonfatal injuries annually in the United States.

Self-Reported Sleep-Related Difficulties among Adults

The National Health and Nutrition Examination Survey (NHANES) introduced the Sleep Disorders Questionnaire in 2005 for participants

16 years of age and older. This analysis was conducted using data from the last two survey cycles (2005–2006 and 2007–2008) to include 10,896 respondents aged ≥20 years. A short sleep duration was found to be more common among adults ages 20–39 years (37.0%) or 40–59 years (40.3%) than among adults aged ≥60 years (32.0%), and among non-Hispanic blacks (53.0%) compared to non-Hispanic whites (34.5%), Mexican-Americans (35.2%), or those of other race/ethnicity (41.7%). Adults who reported sleeping less than the recommended 7–9 hours per night were more likely to have difficulty performing many daily tasks.

How Much Sleep Do We Need? And How Much Sleep Are We Getting?

How much sleep we need varies between individuals but generally changes as we age. The National Institutes of Health (NIH) suggests that school-age children need at least 10 hours of sleep daily, teens need 9-10 hours, and adults need 7-8 hours. According to data from the National Health Interview Survey, nearly 30% of adults reported an average of ≤6 hours of sleep per day in 2005-2007. In 2009, only 31% of high school students reported getting at least 8 hours of sleep on an average school night.

One-Third of American Adults Don't Get Enough Sleep

More than a third of American adults are not getting enough sleep on a regular basis, according to a new study in the Centers for Disease Control and Prevention's (CDC) Morbidity and Mortality Weekly Report. This is the first study to document estimates of self-reported healthy sleep duration (7 or more hours per day) for all 50 states and the District of Columbia.

The American Academy of Sleep Medicine and the Sleep Research Society recommend that adults aged 18–60 years sleep at least 7 hours each night to promote optimal health and well-being. Sleeping less than seven hours per day is associated with an increased risk of developing chronic conditions such as obesity, diabetes, high blood pressure, heart disease, stroke, and frequent mental distress.

"As a nation we are not getting enough sleep," said Wayne Giles, M.D., director of CDC's Division of Population Health. "Lifestyle changes such as going to bed at the same time each night; rising at the same time each morning; and turning off or removing televisions, computers, mobile devices from the bedroom, can help people get the healthy sleep they need."

Prevalence of healthy sleep duration varies by geography, race/ethnicity, employment, marital status

CDC researchers reviewed data from the 2014 Behavioral Risk Factor Surveillance System (BRFSS), a state-based, random-digit–dialed telephone survey conducted collaboratively by state health departments and CDC.

Key Findings:

- Healthy sleep duration was lower among Native Hawaiians/ Pacific Islanders (54 percent), non-Hispanic blacks (54 percent), multiracial non-Hispanics (54 percent) and American Indians/ Alaska Natives (60 percent) compared with non-Hispanic whites (67 percent), Hispanics (66 percent), and Asians (63 percent).

- The prevalence of healthy sleep duration varied among states and ranged from 56 percent in Hawaii to 72 percent in South Dakota.

- A lower proportion of adults reported getting at least seven hours of sleep per day in states clustered in the southeastern region of the United States and the Appalachian Mountains. Previous studies have shown that these regions also have the highest prevalence of obesity and other chronic conditions.

- People who reported they were unable to work or were unemployed had lower healthy sleep duration (51 percent and 60 percent, respectively) than did employed respondents (65 percent). The prevalence of healthy sleep duration was highest among people with a college degree or higher (72 percent).

- The percentage reporting a healthy sleep duration was higher among people who were married (67 percent) compared with those who were never married (62 percent) or divorced, widowed, or separated (56 percent).

Healthy Sleep Tips:

- Healthcare providers should routinely assess patients' sleep patterns and discuss sleep-related problems such as snoring and excessive daytime sleepiness.

- Healthcare providers should also educate patients about the importance of sleep to their health.

- Individuals should make getting enough sleep a priority and practice good sleep habits.

- Employers can consider adjusting work schedules to allow their workers time to get enough sleep.

- Employers can also educate their shift workers about how to improve their sleep.

Chapter 10

People at Risk of Sleep Deprivation

Who Is at Risk for Sleep Deprivation and Deficiency?

Sleep deficiency, which includes sleep deprivation, affects people of all ages, races, and ethnicities. Certain groups of people may be more likely to be sleep deficient. Examples include people who:

- Have limited time available for sleep, such as caregivers or people working long hours or more than one job

- Have schedules that conflict with their internal body clocks, such as shift workers, first responders, teens who have early school schedules, or people who must travel for work

- Make lifestyle choices that prevent them from getting enough sleep, such as taking medicine to stay awake, abusing alcohol or drugs, or not leaving enough time for sleep

This chapter contains text excerpted from the following sources: Text under the heading "Who Is at Risk for Sleep Deprivation and Deficiency?" is excerpted from "Sleep Deprivation and Deficiency," National Heart, Lung, and Blood Institute (NHLBI), February 22, 2012. Reviewed July 2016; Text under the heading "Sleep Disorders and Law Enforcement Officers" is excerpted from "Sleep Disorders and Law Enforcement Officers," National Institute of Justice (NIJ), August 13, 2012. Reviewed July 2016.

- Have undiagnosed or untreated medical problems, such as stress, anxiety, or sleep disorders

- Have medical conditions or take medicines that interfere with sleep

Certain medical conditions have been linked to sleep disorders. These conditions include heart failure, heart disease, obesity, diabetes, high blood pressure, stroke or transient ischemic attack (mini-stroke), depression, and attention-deficit hyperactivity disorder (ADHD).

If you have or have had one of these conditions, ask your doctor whether you might benefit from a sleep study.

What Are the Signs and Symptoms of Problem Sleepiness?

Sleep deficiency can cause you to feel very tired during the day. You may not feel refreshed and alert when you wake up. Sleep deficiency also can interfere with work, school, driving, and social functioning.

How sleepy you feel during the day can help you figure out whether you're having symptoms of problem sleepiness. You might be sleep deficient if you often feel like you could doze off while:

- Sitting and reading or watching TV

- Sitting still in a public place, such as a movie theater, meeting, or classroom

- Riding in a car for an hour without stopping

- Sitting and talking to someone

- Sitting quietly after lunch

- Sitting in traffic for a few minutes

Sleep deficiency can cause problems with learning, focusing, and reacting. You may have trouble making decisions, solving problems, remembering things, controlling your emotions and behavior, and coping with change. You may take longer to finish tasks, have a slower reaction time, and make more mistakes.

The signs and symptoms of sleep deficiency may differ between children and adults. Children who are sleep deficient might be overly active and have problems paying attention. They also might misbehave, and their school performance can suffer.

Sleep-deficient children may feel angry and impulsive, have mood swings, feel sad or depressed, or lack motivation.

You may not notice how sleep deficiency affects your daily routine. A common myth is that people can learn to get by on little sleep with no negative effects. However, research shows that getting enough quality sleep at the right times is vital for mental health, physical health, quality of life, and safety.

To find out whether you're sleep deficient, try keeping a sleep diary for a couple of weeks. Write down how much you sleep each night, how alert and rested you feel in the morning, and how sleepy you feel during the day.

Sleep Disorders and Law Enforcement Officers

Overview

With ever-changing schedules, overtime, and overnight shifts, it is not surprising that some police officers suffer from sleep disorders. Sleep disorders, which are typically associated with poor health, performance and safety outcomes, are twice as prevalent among police officers compared to the general public - and a new study suggests that they remain largely undiagnosed and untreated.

Research on Sleep Disorders

Over an 18-month period, researchers at Brigham and Women's Hospital, a teaching affiliate of Harvard Medical School in Boston, gathered data on sleep disorders, health, and performance from almost 5,000 police officers in North America. The data showed that just over 40 percent of police officers screened positive for sleep disorders— almost double the 15 to 20 percent estimated rate of sleep disorders in the general population.

The most common sleep disorder was obstructive sleep apnea, affecting more than one-third of the officers (34 percent or 1,666 of 4,597 respondents). Moderate to severe insomnia came in second (7 percent or 281 of 4,298 respondents), followed by shift work disorder (defined as "excessive wake time sleepiness and insomnia associated with night work," affecting 5 percent or 269 of 4,597 respondents).

But the potential risks to officers—and the general public—due to fatigue are even more common than these findings suggest. According to the researchers, excessive sleepiness is common among police officers, whether they have sleep disorders or not. In fact, almost half of all participants (46 percent) reported having fallen asleep while driving. Approximately one-quarter (26 percent) reported that this occurs one to two times per month.

Impact on Officer Safety

Officers with sleep disorders had a higher risk of falling asleep while driving, committing an error or safety violation attributable to fatigue, and experiencing uncontrolled anger towards a suspect. These officers were also more likely to report committing a serious administrative error and had a higher rate of absenteeism than those without sleep disorders.

Chapter 11

Why Your Body Needs Sleep

Overview

Poor sleep health is a common problem with 25 percent of U.S. adults reporting insufficient sleep or rest at least 15 out of every 30 days. The public health burden of chronic sleep loss and sleep disorders, coupled with low awareness of poor sleep health among the general population, healthcare professionals, and policymakers, necessitates a well-coordinated strategy to improve sleep-related health.

Why Is Sleep Health Important?

Sleep, like nutrition and physical activity, is a critical determinant of health and well-being. Sleep is a basic requirement for infant, child, and adolescent health and development. Sleep loss and untreated sleep disorders influence basic patterns of behavior that negatively affect family health and interpersonal relationships. Fatigue and sleepiness can reduce productivity and increase the chance for mishaps such as medical errors and motor vehicle or industrial accidents.

This chapter contains text excerpted from the following sources: Text under the heading "Overview" is excerpted from "Sleep Health," Office of Disease Prevention and Health Promotion (ODPHP), U.S. Department of Health and Human Services (HHS), June 30, 2016; Text under the heading "How Is the Body Affected by Sleep Deprivation?" is excerpted from "Sleep: Condition Information," National Institutes of Health (NIH), July 9, 2013.

Adequate sleep is necessary to:

- Fight off infection
- Support the metabolism of sugar to prevent diabetes
- Perform well in school
- Work effectively and safely

Sleep timing and duration affect a number of endocrine, metabolic, and neurological functions that are critical to the maintenance of individual health. If left untreated, sleep disorders and chronic short sleep are associated with an increased risk of:

- Heart disease
- High blood pressure
- Obesity
- Diabetes
- All-cause mortality

Sleep health is a particular concern for individuals with chronic disabilities and disorders such as arthritis, kidney disease, pain, human immunodeficiency virus (HIV), epilepsy, Parkinson disease, and depression. Among older adults, the cognitive and medical consequences of untreated sleep disorders decrease health-related quality of life, contribute to functional limitations and loss of independence, and are associated with an increased risk of death from any cause.

Understanding Sleep Health

The odds of being a short sleeper (defined as someone who sleeps less than 6 hours a night) in the United States have increased significantly over the past 30 years. Competition between sleep schedules, employment, and lifestyle is a recent trend. Intermittent sleep disturbances due to lifestyle choices are associated with temporary fatigue, disorientation, and decreased alertness.

Sleep-disordered breathing (SDB), which includes sleep apnea, is another serious threat to health. SDB is characterized by intermittent airway obstruction or pauses in breathing. People with untreated SDB have 2 to 4 times the risk of heart attack and stroke. Obesity is a significant risk factor for SDB, and weight loss is associated with a decrease in SDB severity.

- **SDB in Children**:

  African American children are at least twice as likely to develop SDB than children of European descent. The risk of SDB during childhood is associated with low socioeconomic status independent of obesity and other risk factors. Left untreated, SDB in children is associated with difficulties in school, metabolic disorders, and future heart disease risk.

- **SDB in Older Adults:**

  SDB may affect 20 to 40 percent of older adults and, if left untreated, is associated with a 2- to 3-fold increased risk of stroke and mortality. Sleep health education and promotion strategies are needed to address disparities in sleep health across age, race, education, and socioeconomic groups. Health education and promotion programs can increase awareness of common sleep disorders, such as insomnia, restless leg syndrome, and SDB. Sleep health education programs in workplaces can promote better work schedule patterns and motivate managers and workers to adopt strategies that reduce risks to health and safety. Without sleep health education, individuals often prioritize other activities over sleep and accept constant sleepiness and sleep disruption as inevitable.

Emerging Issues in Sleep Health

Progress in the following areas will yield more information on sleep health over the coming decade:

- Further evolution of biomedical sleep research
- Quantification of health risks associated with untreated SDB across the lifespan
- Findings from the first U.S.-based phase III SDB treatment trials in children and adults

How Is the Body Affected by Sleep Deprivation?

Sleep deprivation, either from regularly not allowing enough time for sleep or due to a physical or mental problem that prevents restful sleep, produces noticeable symptoms, including the following:

- Feeling drowsy during the day
- Routinely falling asleep within only 5 minutes of lying down in bed for the night

- Experiencing "microsleeps," which are very brief episodes of sleep while being awake

Sleep deprivation can noticeably affect people's performance, including their ability to think clearly, react quickly, and form memories. Sleep deprivation also affects mood, leading to irritability; problems with relationships, especially for children and teenagers; and depression. Sleep deprivation can also increase anxiety.

Sleep is important for overall health, and inadequate sleep is associated with numerous health problems. Research shows that not getting enough sleep, or getting poor-quality sleep, increases the risk of high blood pressure, heart disease, obesity, and diabetes.

Sleep deprivation can also be very dangerous. Sleep-deprived people who were tested using a driving simulator or performing hand-eye coordination tasks did as badly as, or worse than, people who were intoxicated. According to the National Department of Transportation, drowsy driving causes 1,500 deaths and 40,000 nonfatal injuries each year.

Sleep deprivation magnifies the effect of alcohol on the body. A fatigued person who drinks will be more impaired than a well-rested person.

Are There Diseases or Conditions That Disrupt Sleep Patterns?

People experiencing certain conditions, such as pregnancy, some intellectual and developmental disabilities (IDDs), depression, Alzheimer disease, and cancer, may have disrupted sleep patterns.

- **Pregnancy.** Many women who become pregnant find that they develop sleeping problems during pregnancy that they did not have previously. Fatigue is common during pregnancy, for example, especially during the first and third trimesters. Many types of sleep disturbances develop in women who are pregnant, including insomnia, restless legs syndrome, sleep apnea, nocturnal heartburn—which can cause long-term damage to the esophagus—and frequent nighttime urination. Sleep problems during pregnancy are difficult to treat because of possible damage to the developing fetus. As a result, many women must cope with sleeping problems and disrupted sleep throughout their pregnancy.

- **IDDs.** Particularly in children, IDDs are associated with sleeping problems. For example, children with autism spectrum disorders often have sleep disturbances. In addition, children with attention deficit/hyperactivity disorder also have sleep disturbances.

- **Other conditions.** Sleeping problems occur in nearly everyone who has an intellectual disability or mental illness, including people with depression or schizophrenia. Sleeping difficulties are also commonly seen in many other disorders and illnesses, including Alzheimer disease, stroke, cancer, and head injury. Some researchers believe that many of these sleep problems occur because of changes in the brain regions and brain chemicals that control sleep. Another possible cause is medications used to control the symptoms of other conditions (cancer, for example).

How Does Inadequate Sleep Affect Health?

Beyond its short-term effects, inadequate sleep affects overall health in a number of ways. Diabetes, cardiovascular disease, hypertension, obesity, and depression have all been linked to inadequate sleep.

Obesity

Clinical research funded by the NIH shows that a short duration of sleep is associated with excess body weight. All age groups, including children, seem to be affected in the same manner. In addition, analysis of blood samples from people with inadequate sleep has shown metabolic changes that are similar to those seen in obese people. Researchers think that inadequate sleep could lead to changes in the brain's hypothalamus, which regulates appetite and energy expenditure. These changes in the brain may explain how inadequate sleep contributes to weight gain.

Diabetes

Insufficient sleep has been associated with the development of type 2 diabetes. A study funded by the NIH, for example, reported that the duration and quality of sleep can predict a person's levels of hemoglobin A1c, which healthcare providers measure to monitor blood sugar levels.

Cardiovascular Disease

Sleep apnea, a condition in which a person temporarily stops breathing while sleeping, causes an increase in a person's risk for several different cardiovascular conditions, including hypertension, stroke, coronary heart disease, and irregular heartbeat.

High Blood Pressure

Research has found that having even one night of inadequate sleep further increases blood pressure levels in people who already have hypertension. This finding may be one of the factors explaining the increased risk of cardiovascular disease in people who sleep too little.

Mood Disorders

While a single night of inadequate sleep can make you irritable and moody, chronically insufficient sleep can lead to long-term mood disorders. Chronic sleep problems have been linked to depression, anxiety, and mental distress. For example, one study reported that participants who slept only 4.5 hours per night were more stressed, sad, angry, and mentally exhausted than a comparison group with longer sleep.

Extreme sleep deprivation can lead to a psychotic state of mind, with paranoia and hallucinations experienced by people who otherwise seem healthy. In addition, disrupted sleep can trigger manic episodes, including agitation and hyperactivity, in people with manic depression. Manic depression is a mood disorder in which people experience cycles of extreme highs and extreme lows in their mood.

Chapter 12

Why Your Brain Needs Sleep

Chapter Contents

Section 12.1

How Sleep Clears the Brain

This section includes text excerpted from "How Sleep Clears the Brain," National Institutes of Health (NIH), October 28, 2013.

Sleep and Its Impact on the Brain

A mouse study suggests that sleep helps restore the brain by flushing out toxins that build up during waking hours. The results point to a potential new role for sleep in health and disease.

Scientists and philosophers have long wondered why people sleep and how it affects the brain. Sleep is important for storing memories. It also has a restorative function. Lack of sleep impairs reasoning, problem-solving, and attention to detail, among other effects. However, the mechanisms behind these sleep benefits have been unknown.

Dr. Maiken Nedergaard and her colleagues at the University of Rochester Medical Center recently discovered a system that drains waste products from the brain. Cerebrospinal fluid, a clear liquid surrounding the brain and spinal cord, moves through the brain along a series of channels that surround blood vessels. The system is managed by the brain's glial cells, and so the researchers called it the glymphatic system.

The scientists also reported that the glymphatic system can help remove a toxic protein called beta-amyloid from brain tissue. Beta-amyloid is renowned for accumulating in the brains of patients with Alzheimer disease. Other research has shown that brain levels of beta-amyloid decrease during sleep. In their new study, the team tested the idea that sleep might affect beta-amyloid clearance by regulating the glymphatic system. The work was funded by NIH's National Institute of Neurological Disorders and Stroke (NINDS).

The researchers first injected dye into the cerebrospinal fluid of mice and monitored electrical brain activity as they tracked the dye flow through the animals' brains. As reported in the October 18, 2013, edition of Science, the dye barely flowed when the mice were awake. In contrast, when the mice were unconscious—asleep or anesthetized—it flowed rapidly.

Changes in the way fluid moves through the brain between conscious and unconscious states may reflect differences in the space available for movement. To test the idea, the team used a method that measures the volume of the space outside brain cells. They found that this "extracellular" volume increased by 60% in the brain's cortex when the mice were asleep or anesthetized.

The researchers next injected mice with labeled beta-amyloid and measured how long it lasted in their brains when they were asleep and awake. Beta-amyloid disappeared twice as quickly in the brains of mice that were asleep.

Glial cells control flow through the glymphatic system by shrinking and swelling. The hormone noradrenaline, which increases alertness, is known to cause cells to swell. The researchers thus tested whether the hormone might affect the glymphatic system. Treating mice with drugs that block noradrenaline induced a sleep-like state and increased brain fluid flow and extracellular brain volume. This result suggests a molecular connection between the sleep-wake cycle and the brain's cleaning system.

The study raises the possibility that certain neurological disorders might be prevented or treated by manipulating the glymphatic system. "These findings have significant implications for treating 'dirty brain' diseases like Alzheimer's," Nedergaard says. "Understanding precisely how and when the brain activates the glymphatic system and clears waste is a critical first step in efforts to potentially modulate this system and make it work more efficiently."

Section 12.2

Sleep and Memory

This section includes text excerpted from "Sleep On It,"
National Institutes of Health (NIH), April 2013.

How Snoozing Strengthens Memories

When you learn something new, the best way to remember it is to sleep on it. That's because sleeping helps strengthen memories you've formed throughout the day. It also helps to link new memories to earlier ones. You might even come up with creative new ideas while you slumber.

What happens to memories in your brain while you sleep? And how does lack of sleep affect your ability to learn and remember? NIH-funded scientists have been gathering clues about the complex relationship between sleep and memory. Their findings might eventually lead to new approaches to help students learn or help older people hold onto memories as they age.

"We've learned that sleep before learning helps prepare your brain for initial formation of memories," says Dr. Matthew Walker, a sleep scientist at the University of California, Berkeley. "And then, sleep after learning is essential to help save and cement that new information into the architecture of the brain, meaning that you're less likely to forget it."

While you snooze, your brain cycles through different phases of sleep, including light sleep, deep sleep, and rapid eye movement (REM) sleep, when dreaming often occurs. The cycles repeat about every 90 minutes.

The non-REM stages of sleep seem to prime the brain for good learning the next day. If you haven't slept, your ability to learn new things could drop by up to 40%. "You can't pull an all-nighter and still learn effectively," Walker says. Lack of sleep affects a part of the brain called the hippocampus, which is key for making new memories.

You accumulate many memories, moment by moment, while you're awake. Most will be forgotten during the day. "When we first form memories, they're in a very raw and fragile form," says sleep expert Dr. Robert Stickgold of Harvard Medical School.

But when you doze off, "sleep seems to be a privileged time when the brain goes back through recent memories and decides both what to keep and what not to keep," Stickgold explains. "During a night of sleep, some memories are strengthened." Research has shown that memories of certain procedures, like playing a melody on a piano, can actually improve while you sleep.

Memories seem to become more stable in the brain during the deep stages of sleep. After that, REM—the most active stage of sleep—seems to play a role in linking together related memories, sometimes in unexpected ways. That's why a full night of sleep may help with problem-solving. REM sleep also helps you process emotional memories, which can reduce the intensity of emotions.

It's well known that sleep patterns tend to change as we age. Unfortunately, the deep memory-strengthening stages of sleep start to decline in our late 30s. A study by Walker and colleagues found that adults older than 60 had a 70% loss of deep sleep compared to young adults ages 18 to 25. Older adults had a harder time remembering things the next day, and memory impairment was linked to reductions in deep sleep. The researchers are now exploring options for enhancing deep stages of sleep in this older age group.

"While we have limited medical treatments for memory impairment in aging, sleep actually is a potentially treatable target," Walker says. "By restoring sleep, it might be possible to improve memory in older people."

For younger people, especially students, Stickgold offers additional advice. "Realize that the sleep you get the night after you study is at least as important as the sleep you get the night before you study." When it comes to sleep and memory, he says, "you get very little benefit from cutting corners."

Section 12.3

Brain Protein Affects Aging and Sleep

This section includes text excerpted from "Brain Protein Affects Aging and Sleep," National Institutes of Health (NIH), July 15, 2013.

Brain Protein and Its Impact on Aging and Sleep

A new study revealed how an aging-related protein in the brain affects sleep patterns. A better understanding of the connections between aging and sleep may lead to improved methods for treating or preventing certain diseases of aging.

Our sleep/wake cycle is governed by an internal circadian clock that's coordinated by a tiny brain region known as the suprachiasmatic nucleus (SCN). The circadian clock adjusts to several cues in your surroundings, especially light and darkness. Animal studies have shown that disrupting the circadian cycle may trigger health problems, such as obesity and diabetes. In contrast, a stable circadian cycle that includes healthy, consistent sleep is associated with longer lifespans in mice.

Many people develop sleeping problems as they age. Recent studies have linked circadian activity with SIRT1, a protein known to be involved in the aging process. Researchers have been searching for ways to raise SIRT1 activity in hope of warding off age-related diseases. Strategies include calorie restriction and the compound resveratrol, found in grapes and wine.

To further explore the links between SIRT1 and the circadian clock, a research team led by Dr. Leonard Guarente at the Massachusetts Institute of Technology altered SIRT1 levels in the brain tissue of mice. Their study, funded in part by NIH's National Institute on Aging (NIA), appeared in the June 20, 2013, issue of Cell.

The team created genetically engineered mice that produce different amounts of SIRT1 in the brain. They studied groups of mice with normal levels of SIRT1, no SIRT1, and 2 groups with increased SIRT1—either 2 times or 10 times the normal amount. The researchers conducted "jet lag" experiments with the mice by shifting their light/dark cycles and observing their ability to adjust their sleep patterns.

Similar to previous findings, older mice with unaltered SIRT1 levels took much longer to adapt to shifting cycles than younger ones. Young mice lacking SIRT1 took twice as long to adapt as those with normal SIRT1 levels. Increasing SIRT1 levels, in contrast, had a protective effect. Old mice with 10 times the level of SIRT1 were able to adapt their sleep patterns much more quickly than normal SIRT1 mice of the same age.

A genetic analysis found that SIRT1 levels in the SCN affect the expression of genes involved in circadian control. All the circadian genes tested were expressed at significantly lower levels in mice lacking SIRT1. In contrast, the genes were expressed at higher levels in mice with more SIRT1. SIRT1 activated the 2 major circadian regulators, BMAL1 and CLOCK.

SIRT1 levels in the SCN declined with age in the mice—as did BMAL1 and other circadian regulatory proteins. These results suggest that SIRT1 plays a central role in the decline of circadian function as we age.

"What's now emerging is the idea that maintaining the circadian cycle is quite important in health maintenance," says Guarente, "and if it gets broken, there's a penalty to be paid in health and perhaps in aging." Further research will be needed to see whether dietary or other interventions that increase SIRT1 activity can help slow the onset and progression of sleep problems related to aging.

Chapter 13

Drowsy Driving

Chapter Contents

Section 13.1

Why Drowsy Driving Is a Problem?

This section includes text excerpted from "Drowsy Driving," Centers
for Disease Control and Prevention (CDC), February 18, 2016.

Drive Alert and Stay Unhurt

Learn the risks of drowsy driving and how to protect yourself.

Drowsy driving is a major problem in the United States. The risk,
danger, and sometimes tragic results of drowsy driving are alarming.
Drowsy driving is the dangerous combination of driving and sleepiness
or fatigue. This usually happens when a driver has not slept enough,
but it can also happen due to untreated sleep disorders, medications,
drinking alcohol, and shift work.

What Is Drowsy Driving?

Operating a motor vehicle while fatigued or sleepy is commonly
referred to as "drowsy driving."

The Impact of Drowsy Driving

Drowsy driving poses a serious risk not only for one's own health
and safety, but also for the other people on the road.

The National Highway Traffic Safety Administration (NHTSA)
estimates that between 2005 and 2009 drowsy driving was responsible
for an annual average of:

- 83,000 crashes

- 37,000 injury crashes

- 886 fatal crashes (846 fatalities in 2014)

These estimates are conservative, though, and up to 6,000 fatal
crashes each year may be caused by drowsy drivers.

How Often Do Americans Fall Asleep While Driving?

- Approximately 1 out of 25 adults aged 18 years and older surveyed reported that they had fallen asleep while driving in the past 30 days.

- Individuals who snored or slept 6 hours or less per day were more likely to fall asleep while driving.

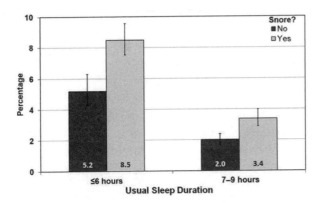

Figure 13.1. *Adults ≥ 18 Years Who Reported Falling Asleep While Driving in Preceding 30 Days*

How Does Sleepiness Affect Driving?

Falling asleep at the wheel is very dangerous, but being sleepy affects your ability to drive safely even if you don't fall asleep. Drowsiness—

- Makes drivers less attentive.

- Slows reaction time.

- Affects a driver's ability to make decisions.

The Warning Signs of Drowsy Driving

- Yawning or blinking frequently.

- Difficulty remembering the past few miles driven.

- Missing your exit.

- Drifting from your lane.

- Hitting a rumble strip.

Who Is More Likely to Drive Drowsy?

- Drivers who do not get enough sleep.
- Commercial drivers who operate vehicles such as tow trucks, tractor trailers, and buses.
- Shift workers (work the night shift or long shifts).
- Drivers with untreated sleep disorders such as one where breathing repeatedly stops and starts (sleep apnea).
- Drivers who use medications that make them sleepy.

How to Prevent Drowsy Driving?

There are four things you should do before taking the wheel to prevent driving while drowsy.

1. Get enough sleep! Most adults need at least 7 hours of sleep a day, while adolescents need at least 8 hours.

2. Develop good sleeping habits such as sticking to a sleep schedule.

3. If you have a sleep disorder or have symptoms of a sleep disorder such as snoring or feeling sleepy during the day, talk to your physician about treatment options.

4. Avoid drinking alcohol or taking medications that make you sleepy. Be sure to check the label on any medications or talk to your pharmacist.

Drowsy Driving Is Similar to Drunk Driving

Your body needs adequate sleep on a daily basis. The more hours of sleep you miss, the harder it is for you to think and perform as well as you would like. Lack of sleep can make you less alert and affect your coordination, judgement, and reaction time while driving. This is known as cognitive impairment.

Studies have shown that going too long without sleep can impair your ability to drive the same way as drinking too much alcohol.

- Being awake for at least 18 hours is the same as someone having a blood content (BAC) of 0.05%.

- Being awake for at least 24 hours is equal to having a blood alcohol content of 0.10%. This is higher than the legal limit (0.08% BAC) in all states.

Additionally, drowsiness increases the effect of even low amounts of alcohol.

Section 13.2

Some Sleep Drugs Can Impair Driving

This section includes text excerpted from "Some Sleep
Drugs Can Impair Driving," U.S. Food and Drug
Administration (FDA), April 11, 2016.

Sleep Drugs

Many people take sedatives to help them sleep. The U.S. Food and
Drug Administration (FDA) is reminding consumers that some drugs
to treat insomnia could make them less able the next morning to perform activities for which they must be fully alert, including driving
a car.

FDA has informed manufacturers that the recommended dose
should be lowered for sleep drugs approved for bedtime use that contain a medicine called zolpidem. FDA is also evaluating the risk of
next-morning impairment in other insomnia medications.

People with insomnia have trouble falling or staying asleep. Zolpidem, which belongs to a class of medications called sedative-hypnotics,
is a common ingredient in widely prescribed sleep medications. Some
sleep drugs contain an extended-release form of zolpidem that stays
in the body longer than the regular form.

FDA is particularly concerned about extended-release forms of
zolpidem. They are sold as generic drugs and under the brand name
Ambien CR. New data show that the morning after use, many people
who take products containing extended-release zolpidem have drug
levels that are high enough to impair driving and other activities. FDA
says that women are especially vulnerable because zolpidem is cleared
from the body more slowly in women than in men.

FDA also found that some medicines containing the immediate-release form of zolpidem can impair driving and other activities the next
morning. They are marketed as generic drugs and under the following
brand names:

- Ambien (oral tablet)

- Edluar (tablet placed under the tongue)

89

- Zolpimist (oral spray)

FDA has informed the manufacturers of products containing zolpidem that the recommended dose for women for both immediate- and extended-release products should be lowered. FDA is also suggesting a lower dose range for men.

Drowsiness is already listed as a side effect in the drug labels of insomnia drugs, along with warnings that patients may still feel drowsy the day after taking these products. However, people with high levels of zolpidem in their blood can be impaired even if they feel wide awake. "All insomnia drugs are potent medications, and they must be used carefully," says Russell Katz, M.D., director of FDA's Division of Neurology Products.

Recommended Doses

FDA has informed manufacturers that changes to the dosage recommendations for the use of zolpidem products should be made:

- For women, dosing should be cut in half, from 10 mg to 5 mg for products containing the regular form of zolpidem (Ambien, Edluar, Zolpimist) and from 12.5 mg to 6.25 mg for zolpidem extended-release products (Ambien CR).

- For men, the lower dose of 5 mg for immediate-release zolpidem and 6.25 mg for extended-release should be considered.

Intermezzo, a more recently approved drug containing zolpidem, is used when middle-of-the-night wakening is followed by difficulty returning to sleep and at least 4 hours remain available for sleep. The recommended dose for Intermezzo remains at 1.75 mg for women and 3.5 mg for men.

FDA is evaluating the risk of next-day impairment with other insomnia drugs, both prescription and over-the-counter (OTC) drugs.

Most Widely Used Sleep Drug

Zolpidem—which has been on the market for nearly 20 years—is by far the most widely used active ingredient in prescription sleep medications, says Ronald Farkas, M.D., Ph.D., a medical team leader in FDA's neurology products division. About 9 million patients received products containing zolpidem from retail pharmacies in 2011.

FDA's Adverse Event Reporting System has logged approximately 700 reports of zolpidem use and impaired driving ability and/or traffic accidents. However, FDA cannot be certain that those incidents are conclusively linked to zolpidem. Many of those reports lacked important information, such as the dose of zolpidem and the time at which it was taken, the time of the accident, and whether alcohol or other drugs had also been used.

"We have had longstanding concern about sleep medications and driving. However, only recently have data from clinical trials and specialized driving simulation studies become available that enabled FDA to better establish the risk of driving impairment and to make new recommendations about dosing," Farkas says.

An Individual Decision

FDA is urging healthcare professionals to caution patients who use these products about the risks of next-morning impairment and its effect on activities, such as driving, that require alertness.

The agency recommends that people who take sleep medications talk to their healthcare professional about ways to take the lowest effective dose. It should not be assumed that OTC sleep medicines are necessarily safer alternatives.

With zolpidem, Farkas notes that people must be aware of how this drug affects them personally. "Even with the new dosing recommendations, it's important to work with your healthcare professional to find the sleep medicine and dose that work best for you," he says.

Patients are asked to contact FDA's MedWatch program if they suffer side effects from the use of zolpidem or another insomnia medication.

Chapter 14

Molecular Ties between Lack of Sleep and Weight Gain

Lack of Sleep and Weight Gain

A poor night's sleep can leave you feeling foggy and drowsy throughout the day. Sleep deprivation has also been associated with higher risks of weight gain and obesity in recent years.

A group led by Drs. Erin Hanlon and Eve Van Cauter at the University of Chicago wanted to better understand how sleep and weight gain interact biologically. They noticed that sleep deprivation has effects in the body similar to activation of the endocannabinoid (eCB) system, a key player in the brain's regulation of appetite and energy levels. Perhaps most well-known for being activated by chemicals found in marijuana, the eCB system affects the brain's motivation and reward circuits and can spark a desire for tasty foods.

The researchers enrolled 14 healthy, non-obese people—11 men and 3 women—who were 18 to 30 years old. The participants were placed on a fixed diet and allowed either a normal 8.5 hours of sleep or a restricted 4.5 hours of sleep for 4 consecutive days. All participants underwent both sleep conditions in a controlled clinical setting, with at

This chapter includes text excerpted from "Molecular Ties between Lack of Sleep and Weight Gain," National Institutes of Health (NIH), March 22, 2016.

93

least 4 weeks in between testing. For both conditions, the researchers collected blood samples from the participants beginning the afternoon following the second night. The study was supported in part by NIH's National Center for Research Resources (NCRR) and National Heart, Lung, and Blood Institute (NHLBI).

When sleep-deprived, participants had eCB levels in the afternoons that were both higher and lasted longer than when they'd had a full night's rest. This occurred around the same time that they reported increases in hunger and appetite.

After dinner on the fourth night, the participants fasted until the next afternoon. They were then allowed to choose their own meals and snacks for the rest of the day. All food was prepared and served in the clinical setting. Under both sleep conditions, people consumed about 90% of their daily calories at their first meal. But when sleep-deprived, they consumed more and unhealthier snacks in between meals. This is when eCB levels were at their highest, suggesting that eCBs were driving hedonic, or pleasurable, eating.

Hanlon explains that if you see junk food and you've had enough sleep, you may be able to control some aspects of your natural response. "But if you're sleep deprived, your hedonic drive for certain foods gets stronger, and your ability to resist them may be impaired. So you are more likely to eat it. Do that again and again, and you pack on the pounds."

The authors noted that though the results are based on a small sample size, they are consistent with evidence from other research. Additional studies are needed to look at how changes in eCB levels and timing are affected by other cues, such as the body's internal clock or meal schedules.

Chapter 15

Impact of School Timing on Children's Sleeping Behavior

Adolescents who do not get enough sleep are more likely to be overweight; not engage in daily physical activity; suffer from depressive symptoms; engage in unhealthy risk behaviors such as drinking, smoking tobacco, and using illicit drugs; and perform poorly in school. However, insufficient sleep is common among high school students, with less than one third of U.S. high school students sleeping at least 8 hours on school nights. In a policy statement published in 2014, the American Academy of Pediatrics (AAP) urged middle and high schools to modify start times as a means to enable students to get adequate sleep and improve their health, safety, academic performance, and quality of life.

AAP recommended that "middle and high schools should aim for a starting time of no earlier than 8:30 a.m.". To assess state-specific distributions of public middle and high school start times and establish a pre-recommendation baseline, CDC and the U.S. Department of Education analyzed data from the 2011–12 Schools and Staffing Survey (SASS). Among an estimated 39,700 public middle, high,

This chapter contains text excerpted from the following sources: Text in this chapter begins with excerpts from "Morbidity and Mortality Weekly Report (MMWR)," Centers for Disease Control and Prevention (CDC), August 7, 2015; Text under the heading "Schools Start Too Early" is excerpted from "Healthy Living," Centers for Disease Control and Prevention (CDC), August 13, 2015.

and combined schools in the United States, the average start time was 8:03 a.m. Overall, only 17.7% of these public schools started school at 8:30 a.m. or later. The percentage of schools with 8:30 a.m. or later start times varied greatly by state, ranging from 0% in Hawaii, Mississippi, and Wyoming to more than three quarters of schools in Alaska (76.8%) and North Dakota (78.5%). A school system start time policy of 8:30 a.m. or later provides teenage students the opportunity to achieve the 8.5–9.5 hours of sleep recommended by AAP and the 8–10 hours recommended by the National Sleep Foundation.

Every few years, the U.S. Department of Education conducts SASS, which provides data on the condition of elementary and secondary education in the United States. SASS consists of several questionnaires, including those tailored to schools, teachers, principals, school districts, and library media centers. SASS is a mail-based survey, with telephone and field follow-up, and uses a stratified probability sample design. For the 2011–12 school year, the sample included about 10,250 traditional public schools and 750 public charter schools, with a unit response rate for public schools of 72.5%. As part of the school questionnaire in the 2011–12 school year, respondents were asked, "At what time do most of the students in this school begin the school day?"

Because AAP recommends school start times of 8:30 a.m. or later for both middle schools and high schools, the analyses in this report include public middle schools, high schools, and schools with combined grades. Average start time (with standard error) and percentage distribution of start times were calculated by school level and state. Results are weighted to reflect the complex sample design and to account for nonresponse and other adjustments.

Among an estimated 39,700 U.S. public middle, high, and combined schools (with an estimated total enrollment of 26.3 million students), the average start time was 8:03 a.m. Forty-two states reported that 75%–100% of their public schools had early start times (before 8:30 a.m.). Overall, only 17.7% of public schools (with an estimated total enrollment of 4.2 million students), started school at 8:30 a.m. or later. The proportion was lowest for high schools (14.4%) and highest for combined schools (23.4%). The percentage of schools that started at 8:30 a.m. or later varied greatly by state, ranging from 0% in Hawaii, Mississippi, and Wyoming to 76.8% in Alaska and 78.5% in North Dakota. North Dakota and Alaska also reported the latest average school start times (8:31 a.m. and 8:33 a.m., respectively), whereas Louisiana reported the earliest average school start time

(7:40 a.m.) and the largest percentage of schools starting before 7:30 a.m. (29.9%).

Schools Start Too Early

Starting School Later Can Help Improve an Adolescent's Health, Academic Performance and Quality of Life.

Most American adolescents start school too early. According to a CDC study that analyzed U.S. Department of Education data from the 2011-2012 school year, less than 1 of 5 middle and high schools began at 8:30 a.m. or later. The American Academy of Pediatrics has recommended that middle and high schools start at 8:30 a.m. or later to allow students the opportunity to get the recommended amount of sleep on school nights, about 8.5-9.5 hours. Insufficient sleep is common among high school students and is associated with several health risks including being overweight, drinking alcohol, smoking tobacco, and using drugs, as well as poor academic performance.

Obtaining adequate sleep is important for achieving optimal health. Among adolescents, insufficient sleep has been associated with adverse risk behaviors, poor health outcomes, and poor academic performance. In view of these negative outcomes, the high prevalence of insufficient sleep among high school students is of substantial public health concern. Healthy People 2020 includes a sleep objective for adolescents: to "increase the proportion of students in grades 9 through 12 who get sufficient sleep (defined as 8 or more hours of sleep on an average school night)." However, the proportion of students who get enough sleep has remained approximately 31% since 2007, the first year that the national Youth Risk Behavior Survey included a question about sleep, meaning that more than two thirds of high school students do not get enough sleep.

Multiple contributors to insufficient sleep in this population might exist. In puberty, biological rhythms commonly shift so that adolescents become sleepy later at night and need to sleep later in the morning. These biological changes are often combined with poor sleep hygiene (including irregular bedtimes and the presence of televisions, computers, or mobile phones in the bedroom). During the school week, the chief determinant of wake times is school start time. The combination of delayed bedtimes and early school start times results in inadequate sleep for a large portion of the adolescent population.

Citing evidence of the benefits of delayed school start times for adolescents, AAP released a policy statement in 2014 that encouraged middle and high schools to modify start times to enable students to get sufficient sleep and subsequently improve their health, safety, academic performance, and quality of life. AAP recommended that schools start at 8:30 a.m. or later, but this was the case in only one in six U.S. public middle and high schools, with substantial variation by state. Because school start times are determined at the district or even individual school level, local stakeholders have the most influence on whether start times change in their communities.

Groups seeking to delay school start times in their district often face resistance. Common barriers to delaying school start times include concerns about increased transportation costs because of changes in bus schedules; potential for traffic congestion for students and faculty; difficulty in scheduling after-school activities, especially athletic programs; and lack of education in some communities about the importance of sleep and school start times. Advocates for delayed start times might benefit from

1. becoming familiar with research about the negative impact of insufficient sleep and early start times on adolescents' health, well-being, and academic performance;

2. identification of persons who might be impacted by the decision to delay start times, including parties involved in transportation and school athletic programs, as well as students, teachers, and school staff; and

3. preparing responses to common arguments against delaying start times. Many school systems have successfully overcome barriers to delay start times.

Among the possible public health interventions for increasing sufficient sleep among adolescents, delaying school start times has the potential for the greatest population impact by changing the environmental context for students in entire school districts. However, a late school start time does not preclude the need for other interventions that have the potential to improve the sleep of adolescents. Healthcare providers who treat adolescents, both in and outside of school settings, should educate patients and parents about the importance of adequate sleep, as well as factors that contribute to insufficient sleep among adolescents.

Parents can help their children practice good sleep hygiene (i.e., habits that help promote good sleep). A regular bedtime and rise time, including on weekends, is recommended for everyone, whether they are children, adolescents, or adults. In addition, adolescents with parent-set bedtimes usually get more sleep than those whose parents do not set bedtimes. Adolescents who are exposed to more light (such as room lighting or from electronics) in the evenings are less likely to get enough sleep. Technology use (e.g., computers, video gaming, or mobile phones) might also contribute to late bedtimes and parents might consider implementing a "media curfew" or removing these technologies from the bedroom. Finally, parents might benefit themselves and their children by setting a good example. Adolescent sleep habits tend to reflect their parents' sleep habits.

Study Results

- Among an estimated 39,700 public middle, high, and combined schools in the United States, the average start time was 8:03 a.m.

- 42 states reported that most (75%-100%) public schools started before 8:30 a.m.

- The percentage of schools starting at 8:30 a.m. or later varied greatly. For example,

  - No schools in Hawaii, Mississippi, and Wyoming started after 8:30 a.m.

  - Most schools in schools in North Dakota (78%) and Alaska (76%) started after 8:30 a.m.

  - Louisiana had the earliest average school start time (7:40 AM) and Alaska had the latest average school start time (8:33 AM).

What Are the Effects of Early School Start Times on Adolescents?

- Adolescents who do not get enough sleep are more likely to

  - Be overweight.

- Not engage in daily physical activity.

- Suffer from depressive symptoms.

- Engage in unhealthy risk behaviors such as drinking, smoking tobacco, and using illicit drugs.

- Perform poorly in school.

- Students who get about 8.5-9.5 hours of sleep each night can improve their health, safety, academic performance, and quality of life.

Everyone Can Play an Important Role

Parents

- Model and encourage habits that help promote good sleep such as

  - Setting a regular bedtime and rise time, including on weekends, is recommended for everyone—children, adolescents, and adults alike.

  - Adolescents with parent-set bedtimes usually get more sleep than those whose parents do not set bedtimes.

  - Dim lighting, adolescents who are exposed to more light (such as room lighting or from electronics) in the evening are less likely to get enough sleep.

  - Implement a "media curfew,-technology use (computers, video gaming, or mobile phones) may also contribute to late bedtimes. Parents should consider banning technology use after a certain time or removing these technologies from the bedroom.

- Contact local school officials about later school start times. Be aware of some commonly mentioned barriers, such as concerns about increased transportation costs and scheduling difficulties.

Healthcare Professionals

- Educate adolescent patients and their parents about the importance of adequate sleep and factors that contribute to insufficient sleep among adolescents.

School Officials

- Learn more about the research connecting sleep and school start times. Good sleep hygiene in combination with later school times will enable adolescents to be healthier and better academic achievers.

Chapter 16

Sleep Deprivation and Learning

The Learning Process and Sleep

Learning, sleep, and memory are interconnected processes that are not yet fully understood. The main function of sleep has generally been thought to be related to learning and memory, and research on humans and animals indicates that both the quality and quantity of sleep can impact those functions. Adequate sleep is required for the body and mind to repair and replenish energy. Sleep deprivation can therefore have a negative impact on the cognitive capacity of the brain. It can hinder spatial learning, along with other functions, such as memory, attention span, and reaction time. It can also take a toll on general health and the immune system, and in extreme cases may even result in hallucinations.

Learning and memory are characterized by three phases: acquisition, consolidation, and recall. During acquisition, the brain is fully alert and gathering new information. Consolidation occurs when a person is at rest, and the brain solidifies the freshly acquired information. The last phase, recall, is the process of retrieving stored information when the person is awake.

"Sleep Deprivation and Learning" @ 2016 Omnigraphics 2016. Reviewed July 2016.

Though it is only during waking hours that acquisition and recall take place, research shows that memory consolidation, through the strengthening of neural connections, occurs during sleep. It is still not clear how this process takes place, but it is hypothesized by many researchers that certain characteristics of brainwaves at different sleep stages aid in the formation of memory.

Sleep researchers take two approaches when studying the effect of sleep on learning and memory. The first explores the various stages of sleep and changes in duration as they affect learning new tasks, and the second analyzes the impact of sleep deprivation on learning.

Sleep Stages and Types of Memory

Every learning situation provides different types of memories to be consolidated into the brain. Scientists, through various studies, are investigating the relationship between the consolidation of these types of memories and the stages of sleep. There is, however, speculation that it is most efficient for the brain to form strong neural connections and pathways during sleep, when there is little new information or external stimuli to process.

Lack of adequate sleep can impact attention and short-term (working) memory, thereby affecting retention of long-term (episodic) memories and also higher cognitive functions, such as reasoning and decision-making. Numerous studies have demonstrated how sleep promotes long-term memory processing, which includes both consolidation of short-term memory into long term memory, and also reconsolidation of existing long-term memories.

Long-term memory can be classified into two main types: procedural memory (the unconscious storage of skills and the way we accomplish tasks) and declarative memory (the storage of facts and events). Recent studies show that REM (Rapid Eye Movement) sleep, which usually occurs during the last two hours of sleep, benefits procedural memory, whereas deep slow-wave sleep (SWS), which occurs before REM sleep, benefits declarative memory. Other aspects that play an important role include motor learning, which seems to be dependent on lighter stages of non-REM sleep, and a few types of visual learning that seem to rely on timing and duration of both SWS and REM sleep. REM sleep has also been shown to aid in the retention of emotionally charged declarative memory.

Impact of Sleep Deprivation on Learning

Scientists are also examining the impact that sleep deprivation has on learning and the formation of new memories. Lack of adequate sleep can be partial (deprivation of either early or late sleep), total (no sleep at all) or selective (deprivation of specific stages of sleep).

Sleep deprivation can lead to poor focus, which makes it difficult to grasp information. It also causes the neurons to over-work, which in turn impairs the brain's ability to coordinate information. As a result, one's ability to recall previously stored information is affected. Furthermore, the interpretation of events and the capacity to make logical decisions may also be impeded.

Without proper rest, the body can feel tired to the extreme point of exhaustion. At such a stage, the muscles can weaken from lack of sleep, the body's organs are not synchronized, and neurons do not function optimally. Poor sleep can also have a negative impact on mood, which may affect the ability to acquire and retain new pieces of information. Although the effects of chronic sleep deprivation are not the same in each individual, it is evident that resting well has a profound impact on learning and memory.

References

1. "Sleep, Learning, and Memory," Division of Sleep Medicine, Harvard Medical School, December 18, 2007.

2. Mastin, Luke. "Why Do We Sleep? Memory Processing and Learning," n.d.

3. Renee. "The Surprising Relationship between Sleep and Learning," Udemy, Inc., January 26, 2012.

Part Three

Sleep Disorders

Chapter 17

What Are Sleep Disorders?

At least 40 million Americans each year suffer from chronic, long-term sleep disorders each year, and an additional 20 million experience occasional sleeping problems. These disorders and the resulting sleep deprivation interfere with work, driving, and social activities. They also account for an estimated $16 billion in medical costs each year, while the indirect costs due to lost productivity and other factors are probably much greater. Doctors have described more than 70 sleep disorders, most of which can be managed effectively once they are correctly diagnosed.

Getting Enough Sleep Is Needed for Both Physical and Mental Health

Sleep is an important part of physical and mental health. While we sleep, the brain and body do a number of important jobs that help us stay in good health and function at our best.

Getting the sleep we need:

- Improves our ability to learn, remember, and solve problems.

This chapter contains text excerpted from the following sources: Text in this chapter begins with excerpts from "Brain Basics: Understanding Sleep," National Institute of Neurological Disorders and Stroke (NINDS), July 25, 2014; Text under the heading "Getting Enough Sleep Is Needed for Both Physical and Mental Health" is excerpted from "Sleep Disorders–Patient Version (PDQ®)," National Cancer Institute (NCI), January 27, 2016.

- Lowers blood pressure and gives the heart and blood vessels the rest they need.

- Helps certain hormones control the following:

  - Growth.

  - The repair of cells and tissues.

  - The immune system (to fight infection).

  - Blood sugar levels (which affect energy).

  - Appetite.

Sleep Has Two Main Phases That Repeat during the Sleeping Period

There are two main phases of sleep and both are needed in order to get "a good night's sleep." The two main phases of sleep are rapid eye movement (REM) and non-rapid eye movement (NREM):

- REM sleep, also known as "dream sleep," is the phase of sleep in which the brain is active.

- NREM is the quiet or restful phase of sleep. It has four stages, from light sleep to deep sleep.

The phases of sleep repeat during the night in a cycle of a non-REM phase followed by a REM phase. Each cycle lasts about 90 minutes and is repeated 4 to 6 times during 7 to 8 hours of sleep.

Sleep Disorders Affect Normal Sleep Patterns

Normal sleep patterns differ from person to person. The amount of sleep you need to feel rested may be less or more than others need. If sleep is interrupted or does not last long enough, the phases of sleep are not completed and the brain cannot finish all the tasks that help restore the body and mind. There are five major types of sleep disorders that affect normal sleep.

1. **Insomnia**: Being unable to fall asleep and stay asleep.

2. **Sleep apnea**: A breathing disorder in which breathing stops for 10 seconds or more during sleep.

3. **Hypersomnia**: Being unable to stay awake during the day.

4. **Circadian rhythm disorders**: Problems with the sleep-wake cycle, making you unable to sleep and wake at the right times.

5. **Parasomnia**: Acting in unusual ways while falling asleep, sleeping, or waking from sleep, such as walking, talking, or eating.

Sleep disorders keep you from having a good night's sleep. This may make it hard for you to stay alert and involved in activities during the day. Sleep disorders can cause problems for cancer patients. You may not be able to remember treatment instructions and may have trouble making decisions. Being well-rested can improve energy and help you cope better with side effects of cancer and treatment.

Sleep problems that go on for a long time may increase the risk of anxiety or depression.

Chapter 18

Breathing Disorders of Sleep

Chapter Contents

Section 18.1

Sleep Apnea

This section contains text excerpted from the following sources:
Text under the heading "What Is Sleep Apnea?" is excerpted from
"NINDS Sleep Apnea Information Page," National Institute of
Neurological Disorders and Stroke (NINDS), October 21, 2015; Text
under the heading "What Is Obstructive Sleep Apnea?" is excerpted
from "Fact Sheet–Sleep Apnea in Aviation," Federal Aviation
Administration (FAA), February 2, 2015; Text under the heading
"Facts about Sleep Apnea" is excerpted from "Facts about Sleep
Apnea," U.S. Department of Veterans Affairs (VA), May 11, 2015.

What Is Sleep Apnea?

Sleep apnea is a common sleep disorder characterized by brief interruptions of breathing during sleep. These episodes usually last 10 seconds
or more and occur repeatedly throughout the night. People with sleep
apnea will partially awaken as they struggle to breathe, but in the morning they will not be aware of the disturbances in their sleep. The most
common type of sleep apnea is obstructive sleep apnea (OSA), caused
by relaxation of soft tissue in the back of the throat that blocks the passage of air. Central sleep apnea (CSA) is caused by irregularities in the
brain's normal signals to breathe. Most people with sleep apnea will have
a combination of both types. The hallmark symptom of the disorder is
excessive daytime sleepiness. Additional symptoms of sleep apnea include
restless sleep, loud snoring (with periods of silence followed by gasps),
falling asleep during the day, morning headaches, trouble concentrating,
irritability, forgetfulness, mood or behavior changes, anxiety, and depression. Not everyone who has these symptoms will have sleep apnea, but
it is recommended that people who are experiencing even a few of these
symptoms visit their doctor for evaluation. Sleep apnea is more likely to
occur in men than women, and in people who are overweight or obese.

Is There Any Treatment?

There are a variety of treatments for sleep apnea, depending
on an individual's medical history and the severity of the disorder.

Most treatment regimens begin with lifestyle changes, such as avoiding alcohol and medications that relax the central nervous system (for example, sedatives and muscle relaxants), losing weight, and quitting smoking. Some people are helped by special pillows or devices that keep them from sleeping on their backs, or oral appliances to keep the airway open during sleep. If these conservative methods are inadequate, doctors often recommend continuous positive airway pressure (CPAP), in which a face mask is attached to a tube and a machine that blows pressurized air into the mask and through the airway to keep it open. Also available are machines that offer variable positive airway pressure (VPAP) and automatic positive airway pressure (APAP). There are also surgical procedures that can be used to remove tissue and widen the airway. Some individuals may need a combination of therapies to successfully treat their sleep apnea.

What Is the Prognosis?

Untreated, sleep apnea can be life threatening. Excessive daytime sleepiness can cause people to fall asleep at inappropriate times, such as while driving. Sleep apnea also appears to put individuals at risk for stroke and transient ischemic attacks (TIAs, also known as "ministrokes"), and is associated with coronary heart disease, heart failure, irregular heartbeat, heart attack, and high blood pressure. Although there is no cure for sleep apnea, recent studies show that successful treatment can reduce the risk of heart and blood pressure problems.

What Is Obstructive Sleep Apnea?

OSA affects a person's upper airway in the area of the larynx (voice box) and the back of the throat. This area is normally held open to allow normal breathing by the surrounding muscles. When an individual is asleep, these muscles become slack, and the open area becomes smaller. In some individuals, this area becomes so small that breathing and resulting normal oxygenation of the blood is impaired. The person may actually choke. This causes some degree of arousal from normal sleep levels which the individual may or may not be aware of. These people do not get restorative sleep, and wake feeling tired.

OSA has significant safety implications because it can cause excessive daytime sleepiness, personality disturbances, cardiac dysrhythmias, myocardial infarction, stroke, sudden cardiac death, and hypertension, and cognitive impairment such as decreased memory, attention, planning, problem-solving and multi-tasking.

How Is OSA Treated?

Though several types of treatment are available depending on the severity of OSA, the most effective treatment involves the use of a continuous positive airway pressure (CPAP) or Automatic Positive Airway Pressure device that is worn while sleeping. In fact, there are currently 4,917 FAA-certificated pilots who are being treated for sleep apnea and are flying with a special issuance medical certificate.

Facts about Sleep Apnea

Sleep apnea is a common disorder in which there are one or more pauses in breathing, or shallow breaths while you sleep. These pauses can last from a few seconds to several minutes and can occur 30 times or more an hour. Typically, normal breathing resumes with a loud snort or choking sound.

Sleep apnea causes the airway to collapse or become blocked during sleep. It is more common in people who are overweight and children with enlarged tonsil tissues, but can affect anyone.

Here are some common myths and facts to help you determine if you or a loved one should see a doctor for a proper diagnosis and treatment.

Myth: Sleep apnea is just a fancy diagnosis for snoring.

Fact: Snoring can be a sign of sleep apnea. Then again, it might just be an annoying sound that your bed partner makes throughout the night because the muscles in his or her throat relax too much.

Myth: People with sleep apnea know they have it because they're jolted awake when their breathing stops.

Fact: Most people are unaware they have sleep apnea because they are sleeping when symptoms occur. (Bed partners, pay attention.)

Myth: Sleep apnea is no big deal.

Fact: Unfortunately, sleep apnea is chronic and doesn't allow the body to get the deep sleep it needs to function at its optimum during waking hours. Left untreated, it increases the risk of serious illnesses such as high blood pressure, heart attack, stroke, and heart failure. It is a chronic condition that requires long-term management.

Myth: People who are old or overweight get sleep apnea.

Fact: Sleep apnea can affect people of all ages and sizes. However, people who are overweight may be able to reduce symptoms by shedding pounds.

Myth: Alcohol is a good remedy.

Fact: Sorry, a nightcap may make you drowsy, but it does not promote good quality sleep. Instead, it relaxes the muscles in the back of the throat, blocking the airway. Sleeping pills have the same effect.

Fact: Effective treatments could include lifestyle changes, specially fitted mouthpieces, or breathing devices such as the CPAP, or continuous positive airway pressure machine, which blows a steady stream of air into the airway during sleep. Some people get relief by sleeping on their sides to keep the throat open. Surgery to remove tonsils should be the last straw and is not effective for everyone.

Section 18.2

Snoring

This section includes text excerpted from "Snoring," © 1995–2016. The Nemours Foundation/KidsHealth®. Reprinted with permission.

Snoozing or Snoring?

Snoring is a fairly common problem that can happen to anyone—young or old. Snoring happens when a person can't move air freely through his or her nose and mouth during sleep. That annoying sound is caused by certain structures in the mouth and throat—the tongue, upper throat, soft palate, uvula, as well as big tonsils and adenoids—vibrating against each other.

People usually find out they snore from the people who live with them. Kids may find out they snore from a brother or sister or from a friend who sleeps over. Snoring keeps other people awake and probably doesn't let the snoring person get top quality rest, either.

What Makes You Snore?

People snore for many reasons. Here are some of the most common:

- Seasonal allergies can make some people's noses stuffy and cause them to snore.

- Blocked nasal passages or airways (due to a cold or sinus infection) can cause a rattling snore.

- A deviated septum is when the septum (the tissue and cartilage separating the two nostrils in your nose) is crooked. Some people with a very deviated septum have — surgery to straighten it out. This also helps them breathe better — not just stop snoring.

- Enlarged or swollen tonsils or adenoids may cause a person to snore. Tonsils and adenoids (adenoids are glands located inside of your head, near the inner parts of your nasal passages) help trap harmful bacteria, but they can become very big and swollen all of the time. Many kids who snore have this problem.

- Drinking alcohol can relax the tongue and throat muscles too much, which partially blocks air movement as someone is breathing and can contribute to snoring noises.

- Being overweight can cause narrowing of the air passages. Many people who are very overweight snore.

Snoring is also one symptom of a serious sleep disorder known as sleep apnea. When a person has sleep apnea, his or her breathing is irregular during sleep. Typically, someone with sleep apnea will actually stop breathing for short amounts of time 30 to 300 times a night! It can be a big problem if the person doesn't get enough oxygen.

People with this disorder often wake up with bad headaches and feel exhausted all day long. They may be very drowsy and have difficulty staying awake while having a conversation or even while driving. Kids affected by sleep apnea may be irritable and have difficulty concentrating, particularly in school and with homework.

Snoring Solutions

According to the U.S. government's patent office (this is where you go to register an idea or invention), hundreds of anti-snoring devices are on the market. Some of them startle you awake when they sense you are snoring. Unfortunately, they may only work because they keep you awake!

Those small white strips some football players wear across their noses that kind of look like a bandage are another anti-snoring device. Football players wear them during the game to breathe easier while running a play or making a tackle. Some people wear these breathing strips to try to stop snoring.

Other snoring solutions include tilting the top of a bed upward a few inches, changing sleeping positions (from the back to a side), and not eating a heavy meal (or for an adult, not drinking alcohol) before bedtime. These kinds of "cures" may work only for someone who snores occasionally and lightly—or they may not work at all.

If you can't stop snoring or the snoring becomes heavy, it's a good idea to see a doctor. He or she might tell you how to keep your nasal passages clear and will check your tonsils and adenoids to be sure they aren't enlarged and don't have to be removed.

Some people need to lose weight, change their diets, or develop regular sleeping patterns to stop snoring. It may be helpful to remove allergy triggers (stuffed animals, pets, and feather/down pillows and comforters) from the person's bedroom. The doctor might also suggest medications for allergies or congestion due to a cold.

If someone might have sleep apnea, the doctor will order a test to monitor the person during sleep. This is usually done in a sleep center (a medical building that has equipment to monitor breathing during sleep). The person is attached to machines that check heart rate, oxygen and carbon dioxide levels, eye movement, chest wall movement, and the flow of air through the nose. The doctor can then tell if the person has a disorder like sleep apnea. The best thing about the test is that it doesn't hurt at all. After all, you sleep right through it!

Once doctors know what's wrong, a person can be treated for it, usually with lifestyle changes, sometimes medicines, or even surgery, if necessary.

Solving a snoring problem lets everyone breathe and sleep a little easier!

Chapter 19

Circadian Rhythm Disorders

What Are Circadian Rhythm Disorders?

Circadian rhythm sleep disorders are problems when our internal sleep-wake timing does not match our outside environment.

We all have a master internal time clock in our brain. This internal time clock regulates a number of systems in of our body including temperature and hormone levels. However, the primary job of this internal time clock is to control our sleep-wake times.

Typically, our brain will "set" our internal time clock with environmental cues. Light exposure is the most important way brains calibrate the internal time clock with the outside environment. There is even a direct pathway for light to travel from our eyes to the part of our brain with the internal time clock. Other cues include meals and exercise.

Examples of how our time clock can become mismatched with the environment include:

- Our internal time clock just wants to be a morning person or an evening person even with light exposure and environmental cues (advanced sleep-wake phase and delayed sleep-wake phase)

This chapter contains text excerpted from the following sources: Text under the heading "What Are Circadian Rhythm Disorders?" is excerpted from "Circadian Rhythm Disorder," U.S. Department of Veterans Affairs (VA), September 16, 2015; Text under the heading "The Problem of Jet Lag" is excerpted from "Travelers' Health," Centers for Disease Control and Prevention (CDC), April 21, 2013; Text under the heading "Risk for Travelers" is excerpted from "The Pre-Travel Consultation," Centers for Disease Control and Prevention (CDC), July 10, 2015.

- We cannot time calibrate our internal time clock to light; for example, if we are blind and cannot see light or if we are working the night shift where there is less light (non-24 hour sleep-wake rhythm disorder and shift work disorder)

- We travel to a different time zone and our internal time clock does not have time to adjust to the new environment (jet lag disorder)

What Are the Types of Circadian Rhythm Sleep Disorders?

As hinted above, some common types of circadian rhythm sleep disorders are:

- Advanced sleep-wake phase disorder

- Delayed sleep-wake phase disorder

- Non-24 hour sleep-wake disorder

- Shift work disorder

- Jet lag disorder

Advanced Sleep-Wake Phase Disorder: These are the "morning people" who wake up between 2 am and 5 am and want to go to sleep between 6 pm and 9 pm. The person's time is "advanced" since they regularly go to sleep and wake up several hours earlier than most people in their environment. If allowed to go to bed the preferred time on a regular basis, the person with advanced sleep-wake disorder will have a very stable sleep pattern. Advanced sleep-wake phase disorder tends to increase with age.

Delayed Sleep-Wake Phase Disorder: These are the "evening people" who tend to stay awake until 1 am or later and wake up in the late morning or afternoon. The person's time is "delayed" since they regularly go to sleep and wake up more than two hours later than most people. Again, if allowed to go to bed at the preferred late time on a regular basis, the sleep pattern for people with delayed sleep-wake phase disorder is stable. Delayed sleep-wake phase disorder tends to be more common in adolescents and young adults.

Non-24 hour Sleep-Wake Disorder: Our brain's internal time clock actually runs slightly longer than 24 hours. On a daily basis, we synchronize our time clock to the 24 hour-day primarily through light exposure. If the brain receives no light cues from the environment, the internal time clock will continue to be more than 24 hours. Sleep-wake times will slightly shift later every day. Total blindness is the most important predisposition to a non-24 hour sleep-wake disorder.

Shift Work Disorder: Shift work disorder occurs when scheduled work hours are during a person's normal sleep period. The internal time clock will expect to be asleep during the scheduled work time. Sleepiness during the work shift is common. It can be a struggle to stay awake during the shift. Once off work, the internal time clock will expect to be awake during the time allotted for sleep. Falling asleep then may be a struggle and a person may wake up frequently during the night.

Jet Lag Disorder: Jet lag occurs when long travel by airplane quickly brings someone to another time zone. When the person arrives in the new time zone, their internal time clock sleep-wake times are misaligned with the environment. Jet lag tends to be worse with more time zones crossed. Eastward travel tends to be more difficult adjusting to than westward travel. Fortunately, jet lag is a temporary condition. As the brain takes in the new environmental cues, it can adjust the internal time clock to the new area.

What Can I Do for a Circadian Rhythm Sleep-Wake Disorder?

Treatment for the disorder depends on the type of circadian rhythm sleep disorder and how much it affects a person's quality of life.

Some lifestyle changes that can be tried at home include:

- Regular sleep-wake times

- Avoid naps

- Regular exercise

- Avoid caffeine or smoking prior to bedtime

- Avoid stimulating activities before bedtime

- For delayed sleep-wake phase disorder, avoiding light in the evening hours (including TVs and computer screens)

- For advanced sleep-wake phase disorder, increasing light in the evenings by keeping the lights on or spending more time outdoors

The Problem of Jet Lag

Jet lag can be a problem for travelers who are crossing several time zones. Although it is not a serious condition, jet lag can make it hard for you to enjoy your vacation for the first few days. For business travelers, who may be expected to travel long distances and start work immediately after arrival, jet lag can affect mood, ability to concentrate, and physical and mental performance. Fortunately, you can take steps to minimize the effects of jet lag.

Before Travel

- Exercise, eat a healthful diet, and get plenty of rest.
- A few days before you leave, start going to bed an hour or two later than usual (before traveling west) or earlier than usual (before traveling east) to shift your body's clock.
- Break up a long trip with a short stop in the middle, if possible.

During Travel

- Avoid large meals, alcohol, and caffeine.
- Drink plenty of water.
- On long flights, get up and walk around periodically.
- Sleep on the plane, if you can.

After You Arrive

- Don't make any important decisions the first day.
- Eat meals at the appropriate local time.
- Spend time in the sun.
- Drink plenty of water, and avoid excess alcohol or caffeine.
- If you are sleepy during the day, take short naps (20–30 minutes) so you can still sleep at night.
- Talk to your doctor about taking medicine to help you sleep at night.

What You Need to Know

Circadian rhythm is the internal biological clock that regulates body functions based on our wake/sleep cycle. It can be disrupted by changes in sleep pattern. Aircrew members may experience circadian rhythm disruption (specifically "jet lag") as they work. Here you can learn more about circadian rhythm disruption, why it occurs, possible health effects, and how crewmembers can reduce the effects of circadian disruption.

Risk for Travelers

Eastward travel is associated with difficulty falling asleep at the destination bedtime and difficulty arising in the morning. Westward travel is associated with early evening sleepiness and predawn awakening at the travel destination. Travelers flying within the same time zone typically experience the fewest problems, such as nonspecific travel fatigue. Crossing more time zones or traveling eastward generally increases the time required for adaptation. After eastward flights, jet lag lasts for the number of days roughly equal to two-thirds the number of time zones crossed; after westward flights, the number of days is roughly half the number of time zones.

Individual responses to crossing time zones and ability to adapt to a new time zone vary. Increased age may contribute to a longer recovery period. The intensity and duration of jet lag are related to the number of time zones crossed, the direction of travel, the ability to sleep while traveling, the availability and intensity of local circadian time cues at the destination, and individual differences in phase tolerance

Clinical Presentation

Jet-lagged travelers may experience the following symptoms:

- Poor sleep, including delayed sleep onset (after eastward flight), early awakening (after westward flight), and fractionated sleep (after flights in either direction)

- Poor performance in physical and mental tasks during the new daytime

- Negative subjective changes such as fatigue, headache, irritability, stress, inability to concentrate, and depression

- Gastrointestinal disturbances and decreased interest in and enjoyment of meals

Prevention

Travelers can minimize jet lag by doing the following before travel:

- Exercise, eat a healthful diet, and get plenty of rest.
- Begin to reset the body clock by shifting the timing of sleep to 1–2 hours later for a few days before traveling westward and shifting the timing of sleep to 1–2 hours earlier for a few days before traveling eastward. It can also be helpful to shift mealtimes to hours that coincide with these changes.
- Seek exposure to bright light in the evening if traveling westward, in the morning if traveling eastward. Mobile apps, such as Jet Lag Rooster and Entrain, are available to help travelers calculate and adhere to a light/dark schedule.
- Break up a long journey with a stopover, if possible.

Travelers should do the following during travel:

- Avoid large meals, alcohol, and caffeine.
- Drink plenty of water to remain hydrated.
- Move around on the plane to promote mental and physical acuity, as well as protect against deep vein thrombosis.
- Wear comfortable shoes and clothing.
- Sleep, if possible, during long flights.

Travelers should do the following on arrival at the destination:

- Avoid situations requiring critical decision making, such as important meetings, for the first day after arrival.
- Adapt to the local schedule as soon as possible.
- Depending on the number of time zones crossed, people with diabetes may need to adjust their insulin schedule during travel and on arrival at their destination. Providers should work with their patients to arrange schedule changes before travel.
- Optimize exposure to sunlight after arrival from either direction. Exposure to bright light in the morning moves the stage of circadian rhythm forward, while exposure to light in the evening delays the stage and encourages later sleep.
- Eat meals appropriate to the local time, drink plenty of water, and avoid excess caffeine or alcohol. Eat a balanced diet, including carbohydrates.

- Take short naps (20–30 minutes) to increase energy but not undermine nighttime sleep.

The use of the nutritional supplement melatonin is controversial for preventing jet lag. Some clinicians advocate the use of 0.5–5.0 mg of melatonin during the first few days of travel, and data suggest its efficacy. However, its production is not regulated by the U.S. Food and Drug Administration (FDA), and contaminants have been found in commercially available products. Current information also does not support the use of special diets to ameliorate jet lag.

Treatment

The 2008 American Academy of Sleep Medicine recommendations include the following:

- Remain on home time if the travel period is ≤2 days.

- Promote sleep with hypnotic medication, although the effects of hypnotics on daytime symptoms of jet lag have not been well studied.

- Nonaddictive sedative hypnotics (non-benzodiazepines), such as zolpidem, have been shown in some studies to promote longer periods of high-quality sleep. If a benzodiazepine is preferred, a short-acting one, such as temazepam, is recommended to minimize oversedation the following day. Because alcohol intake is often high during international travel, the risk of interaction with hypnotics should be emphasized with patients.

- If necessary, promote daytime alertness with a stimulant such as caffeine in limited quantities. Avoid caffeine after midday.

- Take short naps (20–30 minutes), shower, and spend time in the afternoon sun.

Chapter 20

Congenital Central Hypoventilation Syndrome

Overview of Congenital Central Hypoventilation Syndrome

Congenital central hypoventilation syndrome (CCHS) is a disorder that affects breathing. People with this disorder take shallow breaths (hypoventilate), especially during sleep, resulting in a shortage of oxygen and a buildup of carbon dioxide in the blood. Ordinarily, the part of the nervous system that controls involuntary body processes (autonomic nervous system) would react to such an imbalance by stimulating the individual to breathe more deeply or wake up. This reaction is impaired in people with CCHS, and they must be supported with a machine to help them breathe (mechanical ventilation) or a device that stimulates a normal breathing pattern (diaphragm pacemaker). Some affected individuals need this support 24 hours a day, while others need it only at night.

Symptoms of CCHS usually become apparent shortly after birth. Affected infants hypoventilate upon falling asleep and exhibit a bluish appearance of the skin or lips (cyanosis). Cyanosis is caused by lack of oxygen in the blood. In some milder cases, CCHS may be

This chapter includes text excerpted from "Congenital Central Hypoventilation Syndrome," Genetics Home Reference (GHR), National Institutes of Health (NIH), June 21, 2016.

diagnosed later in life. In addition to the breathing problem, people with this disorder may have difficulty regulating their heart rate and blood pressure, for example in response to exercise or changes in body position. They may have abnormalities in the nerves that control the digestive tract (Hirschsprung disease), resulting in severe constipation, intestinal blockage, and enlargement of the colon. They are also at increased risk of developing certain tumors of the nervous system called neuroblastomas, ganglioneuromas, and ganglioneuroblastomas. Some affected individuals develop learning difficulties or other neurological problems, which may be worsened by oxygen deprivation if treatment to support their breathing is not completely effective.

Individuals with CCHS usually have eye abnormalities, including a decreased response of the pupils to light. They also have decreased perception of pain, low body temperature, and occasional episodes of profuse sweating.

People with CCHS, especially children, may have a characteristic appearance with a short, wide, somewhat flattened face often described as "box-shaped." Life expectancy and the extent of any cognitive disabilities depend on the severity of the disorder, timing of the diagnosis, and the success of treatment.

Frequency

CCHS is a relatively rare disorder. Approximately 1,000 individuals with this condition have been identified. Researchers believe that some cases of sudden infant death syndrome (SIDS) or sudden unexplained death in children may be caused by undiagnosed CCHS.

Genetic Changes

Mutations in the *PHOX2B* gene cause CCHS. The *PHOX2B* gene provides instructions for making a protein that acts early in development to help promote the formation of nerve cells (neurons) and regulate the process by which the neurons mature to carry out specific functions (differentiation). The protein is active in the neural crest, which is a group of cells in the early embryo that give rise to many tissues and organs. Neural crest cells migrate to form parts of the autonomic nervous system, many tissues in the face and skull, and other tissue and cell types.

Mutations are believed to interfere with the *PHOX2B* protein's role in promoting neuron formation and differentiation, especially in the autonomic nervous system, resulting in the problems regulating breathing and other body functions that occur in CCHS.

Inheritance Pattern

This condition is inherited in an autosomal dominant pattern, which means one copy of the altered gene in each cell is sufficient to cause the disorder.

More than 90 percent of cases of CCHS result from new mutations in the *PHOX2B* gene. These cases occur in people with no history of the disorder in their family. Occasionally an affected person inherits the mutation from one affected parent. The number of such cases has been increasing as better treatment has allowed more affected individuals to live into adulthood.

About 5 to 10 percent of affected individuals inherit the mutation from a seemingly unaffected parent with somatic mosaicism. Somatic mosaicism means that some of the body's cells have a *PHOX2B* gene mutation, and others do not. A parent with mosaicism for a *PHOX2B* gene mutation may not show any signs or symptoms of CCHS.

Chapter 21

Excessive Sleeping

Chapter Contents

Section 21.1

Hypersomnia

This section includes text excerpted from "NINDS Hypersomnia
Information Page," National Institute of Neurological
Disorders and Stroke (NINDS), November 11, 2015.

What Is Hypersomnia?

Hypersomnia is characterized by recurrent episodes of excessive daytime sleepiness or prolonged nighttime sleep. Different from feeling tired due to lack of or interrupted sleep at night, persons with hypersomnia are compelled to nap repeatedly during the day, often at inappropriate times such as at work, during a meal, or in conversation. These daytime naps usually provide no relief from symptoms. Patients often have difficulty waking from a long sleep, and may feel disoriented. Other symptoms may include anxiety, increased irritation, decreased energy, restlessness, slow thinking, slow speech, loss of appetite, hallucinations, and memory difficulty. Some patients lose the ability to function in family, social, occupational, or other settings. Hypersomnia may be caused by another sleep disorder (such as narcolepsy or sleep apnea), dysfunction of the autonomic nervous system, or drug or alcohol abuse. In some cases it results from a physical problem, such as a tumor, head trauma, or injury to the central nervous system. Certain medications, or medicine withdrawal, may also cause hypersomnia. Medical conditions including multiple sclerosis, depression, encephalitis, epilepsy, or obesity may contribute to the disorder. Some people appear to have a genetic predisposition to hypersomnia; in others, there is no known cause. Typically, hypersomnia is first recognized in adolescence or young adulthood.

Is There Any Treatment?

Treatment is symptomatic in nature. Stimulants, such as amphetamine, methylphenidate, and modafinil, may be prescribed. Other drugs used to treat hypersomnia include clonidine, levodopa, bromocriptine, antidepressants, and monoamine oxidase inhibitors. Changes in behavior (for example avoiding night work and social activities that delay bed time) and diet may offer some relief. Patients should avoid alcohol and caffeine.

What Is the Prognosis?

The prognosis for persons with hypersomnia depends on the cause of the disorder. While the disorder itself is not life threatening, it can have serious consequences, such as automobile accidents caused by falling asleep while driving. The attacks usually continue indefinitely.

What Research Is Being Done?

The National Institute of Neurological Disorders and Stroke (NINDS) supports and conducts research on sleep disorders such as hypersomnia. The goal of this research is to increase scientific understanding of the condition, find improved methods of diagnosing and treating it, and discover ways to prevent it.

Section 21.2

Kleine-Levin Syndrome

This section includes text excerpted from "NINDS Kleine-Levin Syndrome Information Page," National Institute of Neurological Disorders and Stroke (NINDS), July 25, 2014.

What Is Kleine-Levin Syndrome?

Kleine-Levin syndrome is a rare disorder that primarily affects adolescent males (approximately 70 percent of those with Kleine-Levin syndrome are male). It is characterized by recurring but reversible periods of excessive sleep (up to 20 hours per day). Symptoms occur as "episodes," typically lasting a few days to a few weeks. Episode onset is often abrupt, and may be associated with flu-like symptoms. Excessive food intake, irritability, childishness, disorientation, hallucinations, and an abnormally uninhibited sex drive may be observed during episodes. Mood can be depressed as a consequence, but not a cause, of the

135

disorder. Affected individuals are completely normal between episodes, although they may not be able to remember afterwards everything that happened during the episode. It may be weeks or more before symptoms reappear. Symptoms may be related to malfunction of the hypothalamus and thalamus, parts of the brain that govern appetite and sleep.

Is There Any Treatment?

There is no definitive treatment for Kleine-Levin syndrome and watchful waiting at home, rather than pharmacotherapy, is most often advised. Stimulant pills, including amphetamines, methylphenidate, and modafinil, are used to treat sleepiness but may increase irritability and will not improve cognitive abnormalities. Because of similarities between Kleine-Levin syndrome and certain mood disorders, lithium and carbamazepine may be prescribed and, in some cases, have been shown to prevent further episodes. This disorder should be differentiated from cyclic re-occurrence of sleepiness during the premenstrual period in teen-aged girls, which may be controlled with birth control pills. It also should be differentiated from encephalopathy, recurrent depression, or psychosis.

What Is the Prognosis?

Episodes eventually decrease in frequency and intensity over the course of eight to 12 years.

What Research Is Being Done?

National Institute of Neurological Disorders and Stroke (NINDS) supports a broad range of clinical and basic research on diseases causing sleep disorders in an effort to clarify the mechanisms of these conditions and to develop better treatments for them.

Chapter 22

Fatal Familial Insomnia

Fatal familial insomnia (FFI) is an inherited prion disease that affects the brain and other parts of the nervous system. Prion diseases, also known as transmissible spongiform encephalopathies (TSE), are a group of rare neurodegenerative conditions that occur when abnormal proteins clump together and accumulate in the brain, leading to tissue damage. The first symptoms of FFI usually begin in mid-life and may include insomnia that worsens over time and vivid dreams when sleep is achieved. These symptoms may be followed by high blood pressure; episodes of hyperventilation; excessive tearing; and/or sexual and urinary tract dysfunction. As the disease progresses, most affected people develop ataxia. FFI usually leads to death within a few months to a few years. Genetic prion diseases are inherited in an autosomal dominant manner and may be caused by mutations in the PRNP gene. Treatment aims at alleviating symptoms when possible.

What Are the Signs and Symptoms of Fatal Familial Insomnia?

The first signs and symptoms of fatal familial insomnia (FFI) generally develop in midlife (40s to 50s) and may include insomnia that worsens over time and vivid dreams when sleep is achieved. As the

This chapter includes text excerpted from "Fatal Familial Insomnia," Genetic and Rare Diseases Information Center (GARD), December 16, 2014.

disease progresses and disturbs the autonomic nervous system (the part of the nervous system that controls involuntary actions), affected people may experience

- Elevated blood pressure
- Episodes of hyperventilation
- Excessive tearing
- Sexual and/or urinary tract dysfunction
- Change in basal body temperature
- Decreased ability to gaze upwards
- Jerky eye movements
- Double vision
- Dysarthria

Many people also develop ataxia (the inability to coordinate movements) which is characterized by a jerky, unsteady, to-and-fro motion of the middle of the body (trunk); an unsteady gait (walking style); and/or uncoordinated movements of the arms and legs. Advancing disease leads to more severe insomnia, worsening ataxia, and confusion. Ultimately, FFI is fatal within a few months to a few years after the development of symptoms.

What Causes Fatal Familial Insomnia?

Fatal familial insomnia (FFI) is caused by a specific change (mutation) in the *PRNP* gene. *PRNP* encodes the prion protein. Although the exact function of this protein is unknown, scientists suspect that it plays an important role in the brain. Mutations in the *PRNP* gene result in an abnormal form of the protein that clumps together and accumulates in the brain. This leads to the destruction of neurons (brain cells) and creates tiny holes in the brain, which give the brain a "sponge-like" appearance when viewed under a microscope. The progressive loss of neurons leads to the many signs and symptoms of FFI.

How Is Fatal Familial Insomnia Inherited?

Fatal familial insomnia (FFI) is inherited in an autosomal dominant manner. This means that to be affected, a person only needs a change (mutation) in one copy of the responsible gene in each cell. In some cases, an affected person inherits the mutation from an affected parent. Other cases may result from new (de novo) mutations in the gene. These cases occur in people with no history of the disorder in their family. A person with FFI has a 50% chance with each pregnancy of passing along the altered gene to his or her child.

Is Genetic Testing Available for Fatal Familial Insomnia?

Yes, genetic testing is available for PRNP, the gene known to cause fatal familial insomnia (FFI). Carrier testing for at-risk relatives and prenatal testing are possible if the disease-causing mutation in the family is known.

The Genetic Testing Registry (GTR) is a centralized online resource for information about genetic tests. The intended audience for the GTR is healthcare providers and researchers. Patients and consumers with specific questions about a genetic test should contact a healthcare provider or a genetics professional.

How Is Fatal Familial Insomnia Diagnosed?

A diagnosis of genetic prion disease is typically made based on a combination of the following:

- Various, adult-onset neurologic signs and symptoms

- Neuropathologic findings (diagnosis made by examining cells and tissues of the brain under a microscope)

- A family history consistent with autosomal dominant inheritance

- *PRNP* disease-causing mutation

The *PRNP* gene is the only gene in which changes (mutations) are known to cause genetic prion diseases, including fatal familial insomnia. Finding a mutation in this gene is necessary to confirm a diagnosis in a person with symptoms. Testing of the *PRNP* gene may not detect all disease-causing mutations, so if a mutation is not found, a person may still have the disease. Other studies such as EEG, brain imaging, or examining cerebrospinal fluid may be helpful in supporting a diagnosis, but none of these can diagnose a genetic prion disease on its own.

How Might Fatal Familial Insomnia Be Treated?

There is currently no cure for fatal familial insomnia or treatment that can slow the disease progression. Management is based on alleviating symptoms and making affected people as comfortable as possible. A number of potential therapies are under current development, some of which have shown promising results in animal studies.

What Is the Long-Term Outlook for People with Fatal Familial Insomnia?

The long-term outlook (prognosis) for people with fatal familial insomnia (FFI) is poor. There is currently no cure for the condition or treatment to slow the disease progression. After the onset of symptoms, FFI is usually fatal within 12 to 16 months, with a range of a few months to five years.

Chapter 23

Insomnia

Adults around the globe struggle to achieve an appropriate duration and quality of sleep. Sleep difficulties are one of the most common complaints for adults in primary care. These difficulties, associated with a decline in overall health status and perception of poor health, can have negative personal and social consequences.

In the literature, the term insomnia can describe a symptom and/or a disorder and definitions used are not consistent. Individuals with insomnia report higher levels of anxiety, physical pain and discomfort, and cognitive deficiencies than those without sleep problems. Insomnia may be associated with long-term health consequences such as increased morbidity, respiratory disease, rheumatic disease, cardiovascular disease, cerebrovascular conditions, and diabetes.

Estimates of the annual costs of insomnia in the United States range between $30 and $107 billion. These include direct costs of $12–$14 billion for expenses such as medical appointments, over-the-counter sleep aids, and prescription medication. The remainder includes indirect costs such as lost productivity due to absenteeism and presenteeism (attending work while sick, fatigued), reduced quality of life, and accidents and injuries.

Insomnia involves dissatisfaction with sleep quantity or quality. It is associated with one or more of the following subjective

This chapter includes text excerpted from "Treatment of Insomnia Disorder," Agency for Healthcare Research and Quality (AHRQ), April 3, 2014.

complaint(s): difficulty with sleep initiation, difficulty maintaining sleep, or early morning waking with inability to return to sleep. For an insomnia disorder diagnosis according to the *American Psychiatric Association's Diagnostic and Statistical Manual*, Fifth Edition (DSM-5), these symptoms must cause clinically significant distress or impairment(s) in functioning (social, occupational, educational, academic, behavioral or other) and occur despite adequate opportunity for sleep on at least 3 nights per week for at least three months. Additionally, the diagnosis requires that symptoms not be better explained by other sleep disorders or occur exclusively during the course of another sleep-wake disorder (narcolepsy, breathing-related sleep disorder, circadian rhythm disorder); not be attributable to the physiological effects of a substance; and not be explained by coexisting mental disorders or medical conditions. Dysfunction that can accompany insomnia disorder includes fatigue, poor cognitive function, mood disturbance, and distress or interference with personal functioning.

Prevalence

Prevalence estimates of insomnia vary by how the condition is defined. Estimates range from nearly 33 percent in an international sample of primary care patients to 17 percent of U.S. adults reporting "regularly having insomnia or trouble sleeping in the past 12 months" to 6–10 percent of adults meeting established diagnostic criteria. Previous diagnostic criteria for insomnia did not specify a minimum timeframe for sleep difficulties; chronic insomnia was used to describe cases that lasted from weeks to months, and insomnia was considered chronic in 40–70 percent of cases.

Older adults and women have higher prevalence of insomnia and about half of insomnia cases coexist with a psychiatric diagnosis. Aging is often accompanied by changes in sleep patterns (disrupted sleep, frequent waking, early waking) that can lead to insomnia. Women are 1.4 times more likely than men to suffer from insomnia.

Despite the condition's prevalence, patients may not discuss insomnia with primary care or general mental health providers, who may have little training in identifying and treating the disorder. Additionally, the use of established diagnostic criteria in these settings is not known, and failure to use standard diagnostic criteria could lead to inappropriate treatment and/or delayed diagnosis of other medical or sleep disorders. For treatments to be effective, an accurate diagnosis must first be made.

Diagnosing

Sleep medicine clinics diagnose insomnia according to criteria established by the International Classification of Sleep Disorders (ICSD) to diagnose insomnia. The *Diagnostic and Statistical Manual of Mental Disorders* (DSM) diagnostic criteria is also frequently used in the United States and geared towards primary care and general mental health providers. Diagnostic criteria continue to evolve with advances in practice and research. Both criteria recognize sleep-related complaint(s) despite adequate opportunity for sleep combined with distress or dysfunction created by the sleep difficulty. Until recently, diagnostic criteria classified insomnia as primary or comorbid, depending on the absence or presence of other conditions. However, the most recent criteria describe in DSM-5 uses "insomnia disorder" and removed the distinction between primary and comorbid insomnia. The distinction had questionable relevance in clinical practice, and revisions reflect this understanding by suggesting a diagnosis of insomnia disorder for patients who meet diagnostic criteria, despite any coexisting conditions.

Other sleep-wake disorders can co-occur with insomnia and/or present with similar symptoms. As required by the DSM-5 insomnia disorder criteria, providers should rule out or diagnose these sleep-wake disorders in order to select an appropriate course of treatment. For example, circadian rhythm disorder involves a discrepancy between circadian rhythms and sleep-wake cycles and often presents with sleepiness. Other sleep disorders should also be considered during evaluation of sleep complaints, including breathing-related sleep disorders, restless legs syndrome, narcolepsy, and parasomnias. Insomnia disorder diagnosis is contingent upon ruling out other sleep, medical, or mental health disorders that explain the sleep problems.

Treatment

Individuals suffering from sleep problems tend to seek treatment when symptoms become bothersome (e.g., distress, fatigue, daytime functioning, cognitive impairment). Once insomnia disorder is accurately diagnosed, many treatments are available. These include over-the-counter medications and supplements, education on sleep hygiene and recommended lifestyle changes, behavioral and psychological interventions, prescription medications, and complementary and alternative (CAM) treatments.

Insomnia is often treated with prescription medication. Several prescription medications are U.S. Food and Drug Administration (FDA) approved for the treatment of insomnia (doxepin, triazolam, estazolam, temazepam, flurazepam, quazepam, zaleplon, zolpidem, eszopiclone, ramelteon). Several other prescription medications from various drug classes (e.g., antidepressants, antipsychotics) are used off-label.

American Academy of Sleep Medicine (AASM) guidelines describe treatment goals, including reduction of sleep and waking symptoms and improvement in daytime functioning. These guidelines stress the importance of identifying and treating coexisting conditions. Various treatment options described in the guidelines include psychological and behavioral interventions, drugs, and combined approaches. AASM practice parameters state that psychological and behavioral interventions are effective and recommended for primary chronic insomnia and secondary insomnia (ICSD-II criteria) in adults. Recommendations were supported by the highest quality evidence. Support for short-term use of pharmacological interventions was based on consensus. However, an updated review of evidence synthesis and recommendations on these interventions is underway. Combined or stepped care models have more recently been used in treatment (initiating one intervention followed by another modality) studied. Combination therapy specifies the timing of certain intervention components. The stepped care model has been described in terms of how limited CBT therapies could be used. These approaches are promising because they are designed to maximize treatment benefits while minimizing harms while assisting in efficient delivery of services at the level appropriate for the patient.

Treatment options are not limited to psychological and behavioral therapies and pharmacologic interventions. Efficacy research has been conducted on a variety of CAM approaches (Chinese herbal medicine, acupuncture, reflexology, Suanzaoren decoction, etc.). Unfortunately, methodological limitations have prevented conclusive evidence synthesis for these treatments.

The evaluation of treatments for insomnia disorder may need to specifically address certain subpopulations (the elderly, adults with coexisting conditions prevalent among insomnia patients). Older age and coexisting conditions may complicate treatment, especially when drug interventions are used. The prevalence of insomnia is particularly high among individuals with existing psychiatric and chronic pain disorders. Treatments may differ in these groups due to their enhanced susceptibility to medication harms, use of medications, and other potential confounders.

Insomnia treatment goals include meaningful improvements in sleep and associated distress and/or dysfunction. Improvements in sleep can be measured in a variety of ways. Because patient complaints can encompass specific symptoms such as sleep-onset latency, number of awakenings, wake after sleep onset, and total sleep time, these are often measured to assess efficacy or effectiveness. Sleep efficiency (total sleep time/total time in bed) is a broader sleep measure that may capture the net effect of specific sleep symptoms. Assessing improvements in specific sleep symptoms or in sleep efficiency can be measured objectively or subjectively. Sleep parameters are objectively measured with polysomnography (measuring sleep continuity parameters, sleep time spent in each stage) or actigraphy (measuring body movements). Subjective sleep symptoms that may cause significant distress are typically collected using sleep diaries. Despite discrepancies between objective and subjective measures of sleep parameters, the subjective measures are considered more valuable because they are patient-centered outcomes.

Sleep quality, subjectively measured in a variety of ways, is also an important measure. Additionally, a number of questionnaires have been developed to assess sleep and the impact on distress/dysfunction. Unfortunately, many currently available sleep symptom questionnaires were developed to identify poor sleepers and are not adequately sensitive to detect clinically meaningful treatment effects. Two important questionnaires that measure both constructs include the Pittsburgh Sleep Quality Index (PSQI) and the Insomnia Impact (ISI). Ideally, valid and reliable questionnaires that measure both constructs simultaneously; have the sensitivity to detect changes resulting from treatment; and measured and analyzed using clinically meaningful improvements would be valuable in demonstrating efficacy and effectiveness.

Insomnia has been shown to have a negative impact on emotional status and quality of life. Treatments can potentially improve secondary patient-centered outcomes such as mood and well-being, quality of life, and productivity.

Chapter 24

Sleep-Related Movement Disorders

Chapter Contents

147

Section 24.1

Periodic Limb Movement Disorder

"Periodic Limb Movement Disorder," © 2016 Omnigraphics.
Reviewed July 2016.

Periodic limb movement disorder (PLMD) is a type of sleep disorder in which patients experience repetitive, rhythmic jerking or twitching movements in the legs or other limbs during sleep. The movements typically occur in a regular pattern every 20 to 40 seconds. Episodes most commonly take place in the early part of the night and last for less than an hour. Although the patient is usually not aware of them, the movements often disrupt sleep, resulting in such symptoms as daytime drowsiness and memory or attention problems.

PLMD is often confused with restless leg syndrome. In this condition, patients experience uncomfortable sensations in their legs while awake that create an irresistible urge to move the affected limbs. Although approximately 80 percent of people with restless leg syndrome also have PLMD, PLMD is considered a separate condition and does not appear to increase the risk of restless leg syndrome.

Symptoms

The main symptom of PLMD is tightening or flexing of muscles in the lower legs—including the big toe, foot, ankle, knee, or hip—during sleep. Although PLMD can also affect the arms or occur while awake, this is uncommon. The movements are usually concentrated during non-Rapid Eye Movement (REM) sleep in the first half of the night. Each movement typically lasts around 2 seconds, and they tend to recur every 20 to 40 seconds, although the pattern can vary from night to night. The movements can range from slight twitches to strenuous kicks.

Most people with PLMD are unaware of the movements and only learn about them from another person who shares the same bed. For some patients, however, the repetitive movements can disrupt sleep and cause such symptoms as not feeling well rested after a good night's sleep, feeling tired or falling asleep during the day, having trouble remembering or paying attention, or becoming depressed.

Causes and Risk Factors

Researchers have not uncovered the cause of primary PLMD, although some believe that it may be linked to abnormalities in the regulation of nerve impulses from the brain to the limbs. PLMD affects males and females equally, and it can affect people of any age. The incidence of PLMD increases with age, however, and affects 34 percent of people over the age of 60.

Secondary PLMD is caused by underlying medical conditions, including the following:

- diabetes
- iron deficiency anemia
- spinal cord injury
- restless leg syndrome
- sleep apnea
- narcolepsy
- REM sleep behavior disorder
- sleep-related eating disorder
- multiple-system atrophy

Certain types of medications have also been found to increase the risk or worsen symptoms of PLMD, including antidepressants such as amitriptyline (Elavil) and lithium; dopamine-receptor antagonists like Haldol; and withdrawal from sedatives like Valium.

Diagnosis

Diagnosis of PLMD begins with a visit to a sleep specialist. Patients are typically asked to keep a sleep diary for several weeks, to evaluate their sleep using a rating system such as the Epworth Sleepiness Scale, and to provide a complete medical history, including any medications taken. In most cases, patients will then undergo an overnight sleep study, during which a polysomnogram keeps track of brain activity, heartbeat, breathing, and limb movement. In addition to diagnosing PLMD and other sleep disorders, the sleep specialist can help identify other potential causes of sleep problems, such as medical conditions, medications, substance abuse, or mental health disorders.

Other medical tests can be used to detect underlying causes of PLMD, such as diabetes, anemia, or metabolic disorders. Doctors may take blood samples to check hormone levels, organ function, and blood chemistry. They may also look for infections or traces of drugs that can contribute to secondary PLMD. If no underlying cause can be found, the patient may be referred to a neurologist to rule out nervous system disorders and confirm the diagnosis of PLMD.

Treatment

Many people with PLMD do not experience symptoms or require treatment. When sleep disruption makes treatment necessary, however, there are several medications available to help reduce the movements or help the patient sleep through them. Some of the medications commonly prescribed to treat PLMD include:

- Benzodiazepines like clonazepam (Klonopin), which suppress muscle contractions;

- Anticonvulsant agents like gabapentin (Neurontin), which also reduce muscle contractions;

- Dopaminergic agents like levodopa/carbidopa (Sinemet) and pergolide (Permax), which increase the levels of the neurotransmitter dopamine in the brain and are also used to treat restless leg syndrome and Parkinson disease;

- GABA agonists like baclofen (Lioresal), which inhibit the release of neurotransmitters in the brain that stimulate muscle contractions.

References

1. "Periodic Limb Movement Disorder," WebMD, 2016.

2. "Sleep Education: Periodic Limb Movements," American Academy of Sleep Medicine, 2014.

Section 24.2

Restless Legs Syndrome

This section includes text excerpted from "Restless Legs Syndrome," Genetic Home Reference (GHR), National Institutes of Health (NIH), April 20, 2016.

Overview

Restless legs syndrome is a neurological condition that causes an irresistible urge to move the legs. The movement is triggered by strange or uncomfortable feelings, often described as crawling, pulling, or itching, deep within both legs. The feelings usually occur while the affected person is sitting or lying down and are worse at night. Movement, such as kicking, stretching, rubbing, or pacing, make the discomfort go away, at least temporarily. The unpleasant feelings and the resulting need to move the legs often make it difficult for an affected person to fall asleep or stay asleep.

Signs and Symptoms

The signs and symptoms of restless legs syndrome range from mild to severe; people with mild cases may experience symptoms a few times a month, while those with more severe cases may have symptoms every night. In severe cases, the uncomfortable feelings can affect the arms or other parts of the body in addition to the legs.

Many people with restless legs syndrome also experience uncontrollable, repetitive leg movements that occur while they are sleeping or while relaxed or drowsy. When these movements occur during sleep, they are called periodic limb movements of sleep (PLMS); when they occur while a person is awake, they are called periodic limb movements of wakefulness (PLMW). It is unclear whether PLMS and PLMW are features of restless legs syndrome itself or represent similar, but separate, conditions.

Restless legs syndrome and PLMS can affect the quality and amount of sleep. As a result of these conditions, affected individuals may have difficulty concentrating during the day, and some develop mood swings, depression, or other health problems.

Researchers have described early-onset and late-onset forms of restless legs syndrome. The early-onset form begins before age 45, and sometimes as early as childhood. The signs and symptoms of this form usually worsen slowly with time. The late-onset form begins after age 45, and its signs and symptoms tend to worsen more rapidly.

Frequency

Restless legs syndrome is one of the most common sleep and movement disorders. It affects an estimated 5 to 10 percent of adults and 2 to 4 percent of children in the United States. For unknown reasons, the disorder affects women more often than men. The prevalence of restless legs syndrome increases with age.

Genetic Changes

Restless legs syndrome likely results from a combination of genetic and environmental factors, many of which are unknown.

Studies suggest that restless legs syndrome is related to a shortage (deficiency) of iron in certain parts of the brain. Iron is involved in several critical activities in brain cells, including the production of a chemical messenger (neurotransmitter) called dopamine. Among its many functions, dopamine triggers signals within the nervous system that help the brain control physical movement. Researchers believe that malfunction of the dopamine signaling system may underlie the abnormal movements in people with restless legs syndrome. However, it is unclear how iron deficiency is related to abnormal dopamine signaling, or how these changes in the brain lead to the particular signs and symptoms of the condition.

Variations in several genes have been studied as risk factors for restless legs syndrome. Most of these genes are thought to be involved in the development of nerve cells (neurons) before birth. It is unclear whether any of the genes play roles in brain iron levels or in dopamine signaling. Variations in known genes appear to account for only a small percentage of the risk of developing restless legs syndrome. Changes in other genes, which have not been identified, probably also contribute to this complex disorder. Researchers suspect that the early-onset form of restless legs syndrome is more likely than the late-onset form to have a genetic basis.

Nongenetic factors are also thought to play a role in restless legs syndrome. For example, several other disorders increase the risk of developing the condition. These include a life-threatening failure of kidney function called end-stage renal disease, diabetes mellitus, multiple sclerosis, rheumatoid arthritis, and Parkinson disease. People with low iron levels associated with a shortage of red blood cells (anemia) and women who are pregnant are also more likely to develop restless legs syndrome. In these cases, the condition usually improves or goes away when iron levels increase or after the woman gives birth.

Restless legs syndrome can be triggered by medications, including certain drugs used to treat nausea, depression and other mental health disorders, colds and allergies, heart problems, and high blood pressure. Use of caffeine, nicotine, or alcohol can also trigger restless legs syndrome or make the signs and symptoms worse. In these cases, the condition usually improves or goes away once a person stops using these medications or substances.

Inheritance Pattern

The inheritance pattern of restless legs syndrome is usually unclear because many genetic and environmental factors can be involved. The disorder often runs in families: 40 to 90 percent of affected individuals report having at least one affected first-degree relative, such as a parent or sibling, and many families have multiple affected family members. Studies suggest that the early-onset form of the disorder is more likely to run in families than the late-onset form.

In some affected families, restless legs syndrome appears to have an autosomal dominant pattern of inheritance. Autosomal dominant inheritance suggests that one copy of an altered gene in each cell is sufficient to cause the disorder. However, the genetic changes associated with restless legs syndrome in these families have not been identified.

Chapter 25

Narcolepsy

What Is Narcolepsy?

Narcolepsy is a chronic brain disorder that involves poor control of sleep-wake cycles. People with narcolepsy experience periods of extreme daytime sleepiness and sudden, irresistible bouts of sleep that can strike at any time. These "sleep attacks" usually last a few seconds to several minutes.

Narcolepsy can greatly affect daily activities. People may unwillingly fall asleep while at work or at school, when having a conversation, playing a game, eating a meal, or, most dangerously, when driving or operating other types of machinery. In addition to daytime sleepiness, other major symptoms may include cataplexy (a sudden loss of voluntary muscle tone while awake that makes a person go limp or unable to move), vivid dream-like images or hallucinations, as well as total paralysis just before falling asleep or just after waking-up.

Contrary to common beliefs, people with narcolepsy do not spend a substantially greater proportion of their time asleep during a 24-hour period than do normal sleepers. In addition to daytime drowsiness and uncontrollable sleep episodes, most individuals also experience poor sleep quality that can involve frequent waking during night time sleep, and other sleep disorders.

For most adults, a normal night's sleep lasts about 8 hours and is composed of four to six separate sleep cycles. A sleep cycle is defined

This chapter includes text excerpted from "Narcolepsy Fact Sheet," National Institute of Neurological Disorders and Stroke (NINDS), April 6, 2016.

by a segment of non-rapid eye movement (NREM) sleep followed by a period of rapid eye movement (REM) sleep. The NREM segment can be further divided into increasingly deeper stages of sleep according to the size and frequency of brain waves. REM sleep is accompanied by bursts of rapid eye movement along with sharply heightened brain activity and temporary paralysis of the muscles that control posture and body movement. When subjects are awakened, they report that they were "having a dream" more often if they had been in REM sleep than if they had been in NREM sleep. Transitions from NREM to REM sleep are controlled by interactions among groups of neurons (nerve cells) located in different parts of the brain.

For normal sleepers a typical sleep cycle is about 100 to 110 minutes long, beginning with NREM sleep and transitioning to REM sleep after 80 to 100 minutes. People with narcolepsy frequently enter REM sleep within a few minutes of falling asleep.

Who Gets Narcolepsy?

Narcolepsy affects both males and female equally and appears throughout the world. Symptoms often start in childhood or adolescence, but can occur later in life. The condition is life-long. Narcolepsy is not rare, but it is an underrecognized and underdiagnosed condition. Narcolepsy with cataplexy is estimated to affect about one in every 3,000 Americans. More cases without cataplexy are also likely to exist.

What Are the Symptoms?

People with narcolepsy experience various types of day- and nighttime sleep problems that are associated with REM sleep disturbances that tend to begin subtly and may change dramatically over time. The most common major symptom, other than excessive daytime sleepiness (EDS), is cataplexy, which occurs in about 70 percent of all people with narcolepsy. Sleep paralysis and hallucinations are somewhat less common. Only 10 to 25 percent of affected individuals, however, display all four of these major symptoms during the course of their illness.

Excessive Daytime Sleepiness (EDS)

EDS, the symptom most consistently experienced by almost all individuals with narcolepsy, is usually the first to become clinically apparent. Generally, EDS interferes with normal activities on a daily basis, whether or not individuals had sufficient sleep at night. People with EDS describe it as a persistent sense of mental cloudiness, a lack of energy, a depressed mood, or extreme exhaustion. Some people experience memory lapses, and many have great difficulty maintaining their concentration while at school, work, or home. People tend to awaken from such unavoidable sleeps feeling refreshed and finding that their drowsiness and fatigue subsides for an hour or two.

Involuntary sleep episodes are sometimes very brief, lasting no more than seconds at a time. As many as 40 percent of people with narcolepsy are prone to automatic behavior during such "microsleeps." Automatic behavior involves performing a task during a short period of sleep but without any apparent interruption. During these episodes, people are usually engaged in habitual, essentially "second nature" activities such as taking notes in class, typing, or driving. They cannot recall their actions, and their performance is almost always impaired. Their handwriting may, for example, degenerate into an illegible scrawl, or they may store items in bizarre locations and then forget where they placed them. If an episode occurs while driving, individuals may get lost or have an accident.

EDS, the most common of all narcoleptic symptoms, can be the result of a wide range of medical conditions, including other sleep disorders such as sleep apnea, various viral or bacterial infections, mood disorders such as depression, and chronic illnesses such as anemia, congestive heart failure, and rheumatoid arthritis that disrupt normal sleep patterns. Some medications can also lead to EDS, as can consumption of caffeine, alcohol, and nicotine. Finally, sleep deprivation has become one of the most common causes of EDS among Americans.

Cataplexy

Cataplexy is a sudden loss of muscle tone while the person is awake that leads to feelings of weakness and a loss of voluntary muscle control. Attacks can occur at any time during the waking period, with individuals usually experiencing their first episodes several weeks or months after the onset of EDS. But in about 10 percent of all cases, cataplexy is the first symptom to appear and can be misdiagnosed as a seizure disorder. Cataplectic attacks vary in duration and severity. The loss of muscle tone can be barely perceptible, involving no more than a momentary sense of slight weakness in a limited number of muscles, such as mild drooping of the eyelids. The most severe attacks result in a complete loss of tone in all voluntary muscles, leading to physical collapse during which individuals are unable to move, speak, or keep their eyes open. But even during the most severe episodes, people remain fully conscious, a characteristic that distinguishes cataplexy from seizure disorders. Although cataplexy can occur spontaneously, it is more often triggered by sudden, strong emotions such as fear, anger, stress, excitement, or humor. Laughter is reportedly the most common trigger.

The loss of muscle tone during a cataplectic episode resembles the interruption of muscle activity that naturally occurs during REM sleep. A group of neurons in the brain stem halts activity during REM sleep, inhibiting muscle movement. Using an animal model, scientists have learned that this same group of neurons becomes inactive during cataplectic attacks, a discovery that provides a clue to at least one of the neurological abnormalities contributing to human narcoleptic symptoms.

Sleep Paralysis

The temporary inability to move or speak while falling asleep or waking is similar to REM-induced inhibitions of voluntary muscle activity. This natural inhibition usually goes unnoticed by people who experience normal sleep because it occurs only when they are fully asleep and entering the REM stage at the appropriate time in the sleep cycle. The attacks usually last a few seconds or minutes. Experiencing sleep paralysis resembles undergoing a cataplectic attack affecting the entire body. As with cataplexy, people remain fully conscious. Even when severe, cataplexy and sleep paralysis do not result in permanent dysfunction—after episodes end, people rapidly recover their full capacity to move and speak.

Hallucinations

Hallucinations can accompany sleep paralysis and occur when people are falling asleep, waking, or during sleep. Referred to as hypnagogic hallucinations when occurring during sleep onset and as hypnopompic hallucinations when occurring during waking, these images are unusually vivid, seem real, and can be frightening. Most often, the content is primarily visual, but any of the other senses can be involved.

Disrupted Nocturnal Sleep

While individuals with narcolepsy have no difficulties falling asleep at night, most experience difficulties staying asleep. Sleep may be disrupted by insomnia, vivid dreaming, sleep talking, acting out while dreaming, and periodic leg movements.

Obesity

After developing narcolepsy, many individuals suddenly gain weight, a side effect that can be prevented by active treatment.

When Do Symptoms Appear?

In most cases, symptoms first appear when people are between the ages of 7 and 25. In rare cases, however, narcolepsy may appear at younger age or in older adults. If left undiagnosed and untreated, early onset narcolepsy can interfere with psychological, social, and cognitive function and development and can undermine academic and social activities.

What Causes Narcolepsy?

Narcolepsy may have several causes. Most people with narcolepsy have low levels of the neurotransmitter hypocretin, which promotes wakefulness. Neurotransmitters are chemicals that neurons produce to communicate with each other and to regulate biological processes.

Most cases of narcolepsy are sporadic, meaning the disorder occurs in individuals with no known family history of the disorder. But clusters in families sometimes occur—up to 10 percent of individuals diagnosed with narcolepsy with cataplexy report having a close relative with the same symptoms. In extremely rare cases, narcolepsy is caused by a genetic defect that prevents normal production of hypocretin molecules. While close relatives of people with narcolepsy have a statistically higher risk of developing the disorder than do members of the general population, that risk remains low when compared to diseases that are purely genetic in origin.

When cataplexy is present, the cause is most often the discrete loss of brain cells that produce hypocretin. Although the reason for such cell loss remains unknown, it appears to be autoimmune in nature (an autoimmune disorder is when the body's immune system mistakenly attacks healthy cells or tissue). That is, the body's immune system selectively attacks hypocretin-containing brain cells.

Other factors appear to play important roles in the development of narcolepsy. Some rare cases are known to result from traumatic injuries to parts of the brain involved in REM sleep or from tumor growth and other disease processes in the same regions. Infections, exposure to toxins, dietary factors, stress, hormonal changes such as those occurring during puberty or menopause, and alterations in a person's sleep schedule are just a few of the many factors that may exert direct or indirect effects on the brain, thereby possibly contributing to disease development.

How Is Narcolepsy Diagnosed?

A clinical examination and exhaustive medical history are essential for diagnosis and treatment. Your doctor may ask you to keep a sleep journal noting the times of sleep and symptoms over a one-to-two-week period. Although none of the major symptoms is exclusive to narcolepsy, cataplexy is the most specific symptom and is rarely present outside of narcolepsy.

A physical exam can rule out or identify a condition that may be causing the symptoms. A battery of specialized tests, which can be performed in a sleep disorders clinic, is usually required before a diagnosis can be confirmed.

Two tests in particular are essential in confirming a diagnosis of narcolepsy: the polysomnogram (PSG) and the multiple sleep latency test (MSLT). The PSG is an overnight test that takes continuous multiple measurements while the individual is asleep to document abnormalities in the sleep cycle. It records heart and respiratory rates, electrical activity in the brain using electroencephalography, and nerve activity in muscles through electromyography. A PSG can help reveal whether REM sleep occurs at abnormal times in the sleep cycle and can rule out the possibility that an individual's symptoms result from another condition.

The MSLT is performed during the day to measure a person's tendency to fall asleep and to determine whether isolated elements of REM sleep intrude at inappropriate times during the waking hours. The sleep latency test measures the amount of time it takes for a person to fall asleep. As part of the test, an individual is asked to take four or five short naps usually scheduled 2 hours apart over the course of a day. Because sleep latency periods are normally 12 minutes or longer, a latency period of 8 minutes or less suggests a disorder of excessive daytime sleepiness. However, a sleep latency of 8 minutes or less can be due to many conditions other than narcolepsy. The MSLT also measures heart and respiratory rates, records nerve activity in muscles, and pinpoints the occurrence of abnormally timed REM episodes through EEG recordings. If a person enters REM sleep either at the beginning or within a few minutes of sleep onset during at least two of the scheduled naps, this is considered an indication of narcolepsy. Other reasons for REM sleep on the MSLT must be ruled out, such as the effects of medication and disrupted sleep from sleep apnea or an irregular work-rest schedule.

In some cases, human leukocyte antigen (HLA) typing (a marker of viral infection) may be helpful. Most HLA-associated disorders are autoimmune in nature. Certain alleles (genetic information found on a specific location on specific chromosomes) located on chromosome 6 are strongly associated with narcolepsy-cataplexy. To definitively identify a lack of hypocretin as the cause of narcolepsy, a sample of the cerebrospinal fluid (CSF) is removed by using a lumbar puncture and the level of hypocretin-1 is measured. When no other serious medical condition is present, low CSF hypocretin-1 can establish hypocretin deficiency as the cause of narcolepsy.

When cataplexy is not present, diagnosis must be made after excluding other possible causes of daytime sleepiness and fatigue, along with a positive MSLT.

What Treatments Are Available?

Narcolepsy cannot yet be cured, but some of the symptoms can be treated with medicines and lifestyle changes. When cataplexy is present, the loss of hypocretin is believed to be irreversible and life-long. But EDS and cataplexy can be controlled in most individuals with drug treatment. Modafinil and sodium oxybate are two drugs that have been approved by the U.S. Food and Drug Administration (FDA) for the treatment of narcolepsy.

Doctors prescribe central nervous system alerting agents such as modafinil and amphetamine-like stimulants such as methylphenidate to alleviate EDS and reduce the incidence of sleep attacks. For most people these medications are generally quite effective at reducing daytime drowsiness and improving levels of alertness. However, use of these medications may be associated with several undesirable side effects and must be carefully monitored. Common side effects include irritability and nervousness, shakiness, disturbances in heart rhythm, stomach upset, nighttime sleep disruption, and anorexia. Individuals may also develop tolerance with long-term use, leading to the need for increased dosages to maintain effectiveness. In addition, doctors should be careful when prescribing these drugs and people should be careful using them because the potential for abuse is high with any amphetamine.

Two classes of antidepressant drugs have proved effective in controlling cataplexy in many individuals: tricyclics (including imipramine, desipramine, clomipramine, and protriptyline) and selective serotonin and noradrenergic reuptake inhibitors (including venlafaxine, fluoxetine, and atomoxetine). In general, antidepressants produce fewer adverse effects than do amphetamines. But troublesome side effects still occur in some individuals, including impotence, high blood pressure, and heart rhythm irregularities.

In addition to central nervous system alerting agents and antidepressants, sodium oxybate or gamma hydroxybutyrate, also known as GHB or Xyrem®, can be used to treat narcolepsy. Sodium oxybate is a strong sedative that must be taken during the night. Sodium oxybate induces sleep and reduces the symptoms of daytime sleepiness and cataplexy. Due to safety concerns associated with the use of this drug, the distribution of sodium oxybate is tightly restricted.

What Behavioral Strategies Help People Cope with Symptoms?

The available medications do not enable all people with narcolepsy to consistently maintain a fully normal state of alertness. Drug therapy should accompany various behavioral strategies according to the needs of the affected individual.

Many individuals take short, regularly scheduled naps at times when they tend to feel sleepiest.

Improving the quality of nighttime sleep can combat EDS and help relieve persistent feelings of fatigue. Among the most important common-sense measures people can take to enhance sleep quality are:

- maintain a regular sleep schedule—go to bed and wake up at the same time every day

- avoid alcohol and caffeine-containing beverages for several hours before bedtime

- avoid large, heavy meals just before bedtime

- avoid smoking, especially at night

- maintain a comfortable, adequately warmed bedroom environment, and

- engage in relaxing activities such as a warm bath before bedtime.

Exercising for at least 20 minutes per day at least 4 or 5 hours before bedtime also improves sleep quality and can help people with narcolepsy avoid gaining excess weight.

Safety precautions, particularly when driving, are particularly important for all persons with narcolepsy. EDS and cataplexy can lead to serious injury or death if left uncontrolled. Suddenly falling asleep or losing muscle control can transform actions that are ordinarily safe, such as walking down a long flight of stairs, into hazards. People with untreated narcoleptic symptoms are involved in automobile accidents roughly 10 times more frequently than the general population. However, accident rates are normal among individuals who have received appropriate medication.

Chapter 26

Parasomnias

What Are Parasomnias?

Parasomnias are "odd" actions that we do, or unpleasant events that we experience while asleep or while partially asleep. Almost everyone has a nightmare. A nightmare is considered a parasomnia since it is an unpleasant event that occurs while we are asleep.

The term parasomnia is much broader than just nightmares, however. Other common parasomnia events include:

- REM Behavior Disorder (RBD)
- Sleep paralysis
- Sleepwalking
- Confusional arousals

What Are Common Parasomnias?

Typically parasomnias are classified by whether they occur during the rapid eye movement (REM) sleep or the non-REM sleep. The REM sleep parasomnias tend to present as traits of wakefulness while in REM sleep, or as traits of REM sleep while awake. The non-REM sleep parasomnias tend to present as a middle ground where the patient is doing activities but is not fully awake.

This chapter includes text excerpted from "Parasomnia," U.S. Department of Veterans Affairs (VA), August 14, 2015.

REM Behavior Disorder (RBD)–Most dreaming occurs in REM sleep. Normally in REM sleep, most of our body muscles are paralyzed to prevent us from acting out our dreams. In REM Behavior Disorder (RBD) a person does not have this protective paralysis during REM sleep. A person therefore might "act out" their dream. Since dreams may involve violence and protecting oneself, a person acting out their dream may injure themselves or their bed partner. The person will usually recall the dream, but not realize that they were moving in real life.

Sleep Paralysis and Sleep Hallucinations–REM sleep is usually associated with dreams and the body paralyzing most of the muscles so dreams do not get acted out. Sometimes the REM-related paralysis or dream images can occur when falling asleep or when waking up from sleep. Sleep paralysis and sleep hallucinations can occur together or alone. The person is fully aware of what is happening. Events can be very scary. An event will usually last seconds to minutes and fortunately end on its own.

Sleepwalking–In sleepwalking, the person is just awake enough to be active but is still asleep so unaware of the activities. Sometimes disorders like sleepwalking are called "disorders of arousal" since the person is in a mixed state of awareness (not fully asleep or awake). Sleepwalking disorders can range from sitting up in bed to complex behaviors such as driving a car. Sleepwalkers are unaware of their surroundings so can fall down or put themselves in danger. Despite the myths, it is not dangerous to wake up a sleepwalker. However the person will not typically have recall of the sleepwalking event and may be confused or disoriented.

Confusional Arousals–We all have experienced that strange and confused feeling when we first wake up. Confusional arousal is a sleep disorder that causes a person to act that way for a prolonged period. Episodes usually start when someone is abruptly woken up. The person does not wake up completely and so remains in a foggy state of mind. The person with a confusional arousal may have difficulty understanding situations around them, react slowly to commands or react aggressively as a first response to others.

What Can I Do for Parasomnias?

Many people with parasomnias see an improvement by improving their sleep habits. Some sleep healthy sleep tips include:

- Ensure you are getting enough sleep

- Keep a regular schedule of going to bed and waking up
- Avoid alcohol or other sedatives at night that might make it hard for you to completely wake up
- Avoid caffeine or smoking
- Keep the bedroom quiet to avoid getting disturbed

We need to make sure that persons suffering from parasomnias remain safe. Some tips for bedroom safety with a parasomnia include:

- Avoiding large objects that can fall by the bedside
- Make sure there are no objects on the floor that can be tripped over
- Close and lock bedroom doors and windows to ensure a person cannot go outside
- Consider an alarm or bell on the door
- Close shades over windows in case they are hit to protect a person from glass
- Remove potentially dangerous objects and weapons in the bedroom
- Avoid significant elevation. No bunk beds. Consider mattresses on the ground, and ground floor bedrooms.

Part Four

Other Health Problems That Often Affect Sleep

Chapter 27

The Link between Alzheimer Disease and Sleep

Aging and Sleeplessness

Studies confirm what many people already know: Sleep gets worse with age. Middle-aged and older adults often sleep less deeply, wake more frequently at night, or awake too early in the morning. Could these problems be related to risk of cognitive decline or Alzheimer disease?

Scientists are beginning to probe the complex relationship between the brain changes involved in poor sleep and those in very early-stage Alzheimer disease. It's an intriguing area of research, given that both risk for disturbed sleep and Alzheimer disease increase with age.

"Nearly 60 percent of older adults have some kind of chronic sleep disturbance," said Phyllis Zee, Ph.D., a sleep expert at Northwestern University's Feinberg School of Medicine, Chicago.

It's long been known that people with Alzheimer disease often have sleep problems—getting their days and nights mixed up, for example. Now scientists are probing the link between sleep and Alzheimer

This chapter includes text excerpted from "Does Poor Sleep Raise Risk for Alzheimer's Disease?" National Institute on Aging (NIA), February 29, 2016.

disease earlier in the disease process and in cognitively normal adults. They wonder if improving sleep with existing treatments might help memory and other cognitive functions—and perhaps delay or prevent Alzheimer disease.

Which Comes First, Poor Sleep or Alzheimer Disease?

The chicken-and-egg question is whether Alzheimer disease-related brain changes lead to poor sleep, or whether poor sleep somehow contributes to Alzheimer disease. Scientists believe the answer may be both.

"We're gaining new insights, primarily in animal studies, about a possible bidirectional relationship between sleep and Alzheimer disease," said Mack Mackiewicz, Ph.D., who oversees sleep research for National Institute on Aging's (NIA) Division of Neuroscience. Findings show that brain activity induced by poor sleep may influence Alzheimer disease-related brain changes, which begin years before memory loss and other disease symptoms appear.

NIA-funded scientists are studying the biological underpinnings of this relationship in animals and humans to better understand how these changes occur. Although evidence points to certain sleep problems as a risk factor for Alzheimer disease, "it is not known whether improving sleep will reduce the likelihood of developing Alzheimer disease," Dr. Mackiewicz said. He adds, "There is no scientific evidence that sleep medications or other sleep treatments will reduce risk for Alzheimer disease."

Effects of Good and Bad Sleep

At any age, getting a good night's sleep serves a number of important functions for our bodies and brains. Although our bodies rest during sleep, our brains are active. The process is not totally understood, but researchers think that sleep might benefit the brain—and the whole body—by removing metabolic waste that accumulates in the brain during wakefulness. In addition, it has been shown that some memories are consolidated, moving from short-term to long-term storage during periods of deep sleep. Other sleep stages may also influence memory and memory consolidation, research shows.

Disturbed sleep—whether due to illness, pain, anxiety, depression, or a sleep disorder—can lead to trouble concentrating, remembering, and learning. A return to normal sleep patterns usually eases these problems. But in older people, disturbed sleep may have more dire and long-lasting consequences.

Scientists long believed that the initial buildup of the beta-amyloid protein in the brain, an early biological sign of Alzheimer disease, causes disturbed sleep, Dr. Mackiewicz said. Recently, though, evidence suggests the opposite may also occur—disturbed sleep in cognitively normal older adults contributes to the risk of cognitive decline and Alzheimer disease.

For example, in a study of older men free of dementia, poor sleep, including greater nighttime wakefulness, was associated with cognitive decline over a period of more than 3 years. Sleep was assessed through participants' reports and a device worn on the wrist that tracks movements during sleep.

Sleep disorders such as sleep apnea may pose an even greater risk of cognitive impairment. In a 5-year study of older women, those with sleep-disordered breathing (SDB)—repeated arousals from sleep due to breathing disruptions, as happens in sleep apnea—had a nearly twofold increase in risk for mild cognitive impairment (a precursor to Alzheimer disease in some people) or dementia.

In addition, certain types of poor sleep seem to be associated with risk of cognitive impairment, according to Kristine Yaffe, M.D., of the University of California, San Francisco. These include hypoxia (low oxygen levels that can be caused by sleep disorders) and difficulty in falling or staying asleep.

What's the Connection between Sleep and Alzheimer Disease?

Evidence of a link between sleep and risk of Alzheimer disease has led to investigations to explain the brain activity that underlies this connection in humans. Some recent studies suggest that poor sleep contributes to abnormal levels of beta-amyloid protein in the brain, which in turn leads to the amyloid plaques found in the Alzheimer disease brain. These plaques might then affect sleep-related brain regions, further disrupting sleep.

Studies in laboratory animals show a direct link between sleep and Alzheimer disease. One study in mice, led by researchers at Washington University, St. Louis, showed that beta-amyloid levels naturally rose during wakefulness and fell during sleep. Mice deprived of sleep for 21 days showed significantly greater beta-amyloid plaques than those that slept normally. Increasing sleep had the opposite effect—it reduced the amyloid load.

A subsequent study, also by Washington University researchers, showed that when Alzheimer disease mice were treated with antibodies, beta-amyloid deposits decreased and sleep returned to normal. Mice that received a placebo saline solution continued to sleep poorly. The results suggest that sleep disruption could be a sign of Alzheimer disease beginning in the brain, but not necessarily its cause.

Studies in humans have also addressed the relationship between sleep and biomarkers of Alzheimer disease. One study found that in cognitively normal older adults, poor sleep quality (more time awake at night and more daytime naps) was associated with lower beta-amyloid levels in cerebrospinal fluid, a preclinical sign of Alzheimer. Another study, by researchers at NIA and Johns Hopkins University,

Baltimore, found that healthy older adults who reported short sleep duration and poor sleep quality had more beta-amyloid in the brain than those without such sleep problems.

Emerging Insights—Stay Tuned

How exactly do poor sleep and Alzheimer disease influence each other? Research so far suggests a few possible mechanisms:

- Orexin, a molecule that regulates wakefulness and other functions, has been found to affect beta-amyloid levels in mice.

- Chronic hypoxia, insufficient oxygen in blood or tissue that is a feature of sleep apnea, increased the level of harmful beta-amyloid in brain tissue of mice.

- Reduced slow-wave sleep leads to increased neuronal activity.

Other factors may also be involved. For example, it has been shown in laboratory animals that the glymphatic system, the brain's waste removal system, removes beta-amyloid during sleep. A recent mouse study suggests that sleeping in different positions impacts waste removal from the brain. Sleeping on the side cleared beta-amyloid more efficiently than sleeping on the back or belly, researchers found. They pointed to the glymphatic system as a possible pathway for intervention.

Further biological and epidemiological studies and clinical trials should cast more light on the mechanisms behind the sleep-Alzheimer connection, and whether treating poor sleep might help delay or prevent cognitive decline in older adults.

"Sleep is something we can fix, and people with sleep problems should consult a doctor so that they can function at their best," Dr. Mackiewicz said. As for Alzheimer disease, for now, he said, improving sleep is "not the same as preventing Alzheimer disease. Researchers are committed to a achieving a better understanding of this complex dynamic in hopes of making a difference in the lives of older adults."

Chapter 28

Cancer Patients and Sleep Disorders

Sleep Disorders Are More Common in People with Cancer

While sleep disorders affect a small number of healthy people, as many as half of patients with cancer have problems sleeping. The sleep disorders most likely to affect patients with cancer are insomnia and an abnormal sleep-wake cycle.

There are many reasons a cancer patient may have trouble sleeping, including:

- Physical changes caused by the cancer or surgery.
- Side effects of drugs or other treatments.
- Being in the hospital.
- Stress about having cancer.
- Health problems not related to the cancer.

Tumors May Cause Sleep Problems

For patients with tumors, the tumor may cause the following problems that make it hard to sleep:

- Pressure from the tumor on nearby areas of the body

This chapter includes text excerpted from "Sleep Disorders–Patient Version (PDQ®)," National Cancer Institute (NCI), January 27, 2016.

- Gastrointestinal problems (nausea, constipation, diarrhea, being unable to control your bowels)

- Bladder problems (irritation, being unable to control urine flow)

- Pain

- Fever

- Cough

- Trouble breathing

- Itching

- Feeling very tired

Certain Drugs or Treatments May Affect Sleep

Common cancer treatments and drugs can affect normal sleep patterns. How well a cancer patient sleeps may be affected by:

- Hormone therapy

- Corticosteroids

- Sedatives and tranquilizers

- Antidepressants

- Anticonvulsants

Long-term use of certain drugs may cause insomnia. Stopping or decreasing the use of certain drugs can also affect normal sleep. Other side effects of drugs and treatments that may affect the sleep-wake cycle include the following:

- Pain

- Anxiety

- Night sweats or hot flashes

- Gastrointestinal problems such as nausea, constipation, diarrhea, and being unable to control the bowels

- Bladder problems, such as irritation or being unable to control urine

- Breathing problems

Being in the Hospital May Make It Harder to Sleep

Getting a normal night's sleep in the hospital is difficult. The following may affect how well a patient sleeps:

- Hospital environment–Patients may be bothered by an uncomfortable bed, pillow, or room temperature; noise; or sharing a room with a stranger.

- Hospital routine–Sleep may be interrupted when doctors and nurses come in to check on you or give you drugs, other treatments, or exams

Getting sleep during a hospital stay may also be affected by anxiety and the patient's age.

Stress Caused by Learning the Cancer Diagnosis Often Causes Sleeping Problems

Stress, anxiety, and depression are common reactions to learning you have cancer, receiving treatments, and being in the hospital. These are common causes of insomnia.

Other Health Problems Not Related to Cancer May Cause a Sleep Disorder

Cancer patients can have sleep disorders that are caused by other health problems. Conditions such as snoring, headaches and daytime seizures increase the chance of having a sleep disorder.

Chapter 29

Mental Health and Sleep

Chapter Contents

Section 29.1

Generalized Anxiety Disorder (GAD) and Sleep

This section includes text excerpted from "Generalized Anxiety Disorder (GAD): When Worry Gets Out of Control," National Institute of Mental Health (NIMH), 2013.

Are you extremely worried about everything in your life, even if there is little or no reason to worry? Are you very anxious about just getting through the day? Are you afraid that everything will always go badly?

If so, you may have an anxiety disorder called generalized anxiety disorder (GAD).

What Is GAD?

All of us worry about things like health, money, or family problems. But people with GAD are extremely worried about these or other things, even when there is little or no reason to worry about them. They are very anxious about just getting through the day. They think things will always go badly. At times, worrying keeps people with GAD from doing everyday tasks.

GAD develops slowly. It often starts during the teen years or young adulthood. Symptoms may get better or worse at different times, and often are worse during times of stress.

People with GAD may visit a doctor many times before they find out they have this disorder. They ask their doctors to help them with headaches or trouble falling asleep, which can accompany GAD but they don't always get the help they need right away. It may take doctors some time to be sure that a person has GAD instead of something else.

What Causes GAD?

GAD sometimes runs in families, but no one knows for sure why some people have it, while others don't. Researchers have found that several parts of the brain are involved in fear and anxiety. Research suggests that the extreme worries of GAD may be a way for a person to avoid or ignore some deeper concern. If the person deals with this concern, then the worries of GAD would also disappear. By learning more about fear and anxiety in the brain, scientists may be able to create better treatments. Researchers are also looking for ways in which stress and environmental factors may play a role.

What Are the Signs and Symptoms of GAD?

A person with GAD may:

- Worry very much about everyday things
- Have trouble controlling their constant worries
- Know that they worry much more than they should
- Have trouble relaxing
- Have a hard time concentrating
- Be easily startled
- Have trouble falling asleep or staying asleep
- Feel tired all the time
- Have headaches, muscle aches, stomach aches, or unexplained pains
- Have a hard time swallowing
- Tremble or twitch
- Be irritable, sweat a lot, and feel light-headed or out of breath
- Have to go to the bathroom a lot.

How Is GAD Treated?

First, talk to your doctor about your symptoms. Your doctor should do an exam to make sure that an unrelated physical problem isn't causing the symptoms. The doctor may refer you to a mental health specialist.

GAD is generally treated with psychotherapy, medication, or both.

- **Psychotherapy**. A type of psychotherapy called cognitive behavioral therapy (CBT) is especially useful for treating GAD. It teaches a person different ways of thinking, behaving, and reacting to situations that help him or her feel less anxious and worried.

- **Medication**. Doctors also may prescribe medication to help treat GAD. Two types of medications are commonly used to treat GAD—anti-anxiety medications and antidepressants. Anti-anxiety medications are powerful and there are different types. These side effects are usually not severe for most people, especially if the dose starts off low and is increased slowly over time.

Antidepressants are used to treat depression, but they also are helpful for GAD. They may take several weeks to start working. These medications may cause side effects such as headache, nausea, or difficulty sleeping. These side effects are usually not a problem for most people, especially if the dose starts off low and is increased slowly over time. **Talk to your doctor about any side effects you may have**.

It's important to know that although antidepressants can be safe and effective for many people, they may be risky for some, especially children, teens, and young adults. A "black box"—the most serious type of warning that a prescription drug can have—has been added to the labels of antidepressant medications. These labels warn people that antidepressants may cause some people to have suicidal thoughts or make suicide attempts. Anyone taking antidepressants should be monitored closely, especially when they first start treatment.

Some people do better with CBT, while others do better with medication. Still others do best with a combination of the two. Talk with your doctor about the best treatment for you.

Section 29.2

Depression and Sleep

This section includes text excerpted from "Depression," National Institute of Mental Health (NIMH), May 2016.

The relationship between sleep and depression is complex. While sleep disturbance has long been held to be an important symptom of depression, recent research has indicated that depressive symptoms may decrease once sleep apnea has been effectively treated and sufficient sleep restored. The interrelatedness of sleep and depression suggests it is important that the sleep sufficiency of persons with depression be assessed and that symptoms of depression be monitored among persons with a sleep disorder.

What Is Depression?

Depression (major depressive disorder or clinical depression) is a common but serious mood disorder. It causes severe symptoms that affect how you feel, think, and handle daily activities, such as sleeping, eating, or working. To be diagnosed with depression, the symptoms must be present for at least two weeks.

Some forms of depression are slightly different, or they may develop under unique circumstances, such as:

- **Persistent depressive disorder** (also called dysthymia) is a depressed mood that lasts for at least two years. A person diagnosed with persistent depressive disorder may have episodes of major depression along with periods of less severe symptoms, but symptoms must last for two years to be considered persistent depressive disorder.

- **Perinatal depression** is much more serious than the "baby blues" (relatively mild depressive and anxiety symptoms that typically clear within two weeks after delivery) that many women experience after giving birth. Women with perinatal depression experience full-blown major depression during pregnancy or after delivery (postpartum depression). The feelings of extreme sadness, anxiety, and exhaustion that accompany perinatal depression may make it difficult for these new mothers to complete daily care activities for themselves and/or for their babies.

- **Psychotic depression** occurs when a person has severe depression plus some form of psychosis, such as having disturbing false fixed beliefs (delusions) or hearing or seeing upsetting things that others cannot hear or see (hallucinations). The psychotic symptoms typically have a depressive "theme," such as delusions of guilt, poverty, or illness.

- **Seasonal affective disorder** is characterized by the onset of depression during the winter months, when there is less natural sunlight. This depression generally lifts during spring and summer. Winter depression, typically accompanied by social withdrawal, increased sleep, and weight gain, predictably returns every year in seasonal affective disorder.

• **Bipolar disorder** is different from depression, but it is included in this list is because someone with bipolar disorder experiences episodes of extremely low moods that meet the criteria for major depression (called "bipolar depression"). But a person with bipolar disorder also experiences extreme high–euphoric or irritable–moods called "mania" or a less severe form called "hypomania."

Examples of other types of depressive disorders newly added to the diagnostic classification of DSM-5 include disruptive mood dysregulation disorder (diagnosed in children and adolescents) and premenstrual dysphoric disorder (PMDD).

Signs and Symptoms

If you have been experiencing some of the following signs and symptoms most of the day, nearly every day, for at least two weeks, you may be suffering from depression:

• Persistent sad, anxious, or "empty" mood

• Feelings of hopelessness, or pessimism

• Irritability

• Feelings of guilt, worthlessness, or helplessness

• Loss of interest or pleasure in hobbies and activities

• Decreased energy or fatigue

• Moving or talking more slowly

• Feeling restless or having trouble sitting still

• Difficulty concentrating, remembering, or making decisions

• Difficulty sleeping, early-morning awakening, or oversleeping

• Appetite and/or weight changes

• Thoughts of death or suicide, or suicide attempts

• Aches or pains, headaches, cramps, or digestive problems without a clear physical cause and/or that do not ease even with treatment

Not everyone who is depressed experiences every symptom. Some people experience only a few symptoms while others may experience many. Several persistent symptoms in addition to low mood are required for a diagnosis of major depression, but people with only a few–but distressing–symptoms may benefit from treatment of their "subsyndromal" depression. The severity and frequency of symptoms and how long they last will vary depending on the individual and his or her particular illness. Symptoms may also vary depending on the stage of the illness.

Risk Factors

Depression is one of the most common mental disorders in the United States. Current research suggests that depression is caused by a combination of genetic, biological, environmental, and psychological factors.

Depression can happen at any age, but often begins in adulthood. Depression is now recognized as occurring in children and adolescents, although it sometimes presents with more prominent irritability than low mood. Many chronic mood and anxiety disorders in adults begin as high levels of anxiety in children.

Depression, especially in midlife or older adults, can co-occur with other serious medical illnesses, such as diabetes, cancer, heart disease, and Parkinson disease. These conditions are often worse when depression is present. Sometimes medications taken for these physical illnesses may cause side effects that contribute to depression. A doctor experienced in treating these complicated illnesses can help work out the best treatment strategy.

Risk factors include:

- Personal or family history of depression

- Major life changes, trauma, or stress

- Certain physical illnesses and medications

Treatment and Therapies

Depression, even the most severe cases, can be treated. The earlier that treatment can begin, the more effective it is. Depression is usually treated with medications, psychotherapy, or a combination of the two. If these treatments do not reduce symptoms, electroconvulsive therapy (ECT) and other brain stimulation therapies may be options to explore.

Section 29.3

Posttraumatic Stress Disorder and Sleep

This section contains text excerpted from the following sources:
Text in this section begins with excerpts from "Sleep and PTSD,"
U.S. Department of Veterans Affairs (VA), August 13, 2015; Text
under the heading "Prevalence of Sleep Problems in Veterans
with PTSD" is excerpted from "Sleep Problems in Veterans
with PTSD," U.S. Department of Veterans Affairs (VA),
February 23, 2016..

Many people have trouble sleeping sometimes. This is even more likely, though, if you have PTSD. Trouble sleeping and nightmares are two symptoms of PTSD.

Why Do People with PTSD Have Sleep Problems?

They may be "on alert." Many people with PTSD may feel they need to be on guard or "on the lookout," to protect himself or herself from danger. It is difficult to have restful sleep when you feel the need to be always alert. You might have trouble falling asleep, or you might wake up easily in the night if you hear any noise.

They may worry or have negative thoughts. Your thoughts can make it difficult to fall asleep. People with PTSD often worry about general problems or worry that they are in danger. If you often have trouble getting to sleep, you may start to worry that you won't be able to fall asleep. These thoughts can keep you awake.

They may use drugs or alcohol. Some people with PTSD use drugs or alcohol to help them cope with their symptoms. In fact, using too much alcohol can get in the way of restful sleep. Alcohol changes the quality of your sleep and makes it less refreshing. This is true of many drugs as well.

They may have bad dreams or nightmares. Nightmares are common for people with PTSD. Nightmares can wake you up in the middle of the night, making your sleep less restful. If you have frequent nightmares, you may find it difficult to fall asleep because you are afraid you might have a nightmare.

They may have medical problems. There are medical problems that are commonly found in people with PTSD, such as chronic pain, stomach problems, and pelvic-area problems in women. These physical problems can make going to sleep difficult.

What Can You Do If You Have Problems?

There are a number of things you can do to make it more likely that you will sleep well:

Change Your Sleeping Area

Too much noise, light, or activity in your bedroom can make sleeping harder. Creating a quiet, comfortable sleeping area can help. Here are some things you can do to sleep better:

- Use your bedroom only for sleeping and sex

- Move the TV and radio out of your bedroom

- Keep your bedroom quiet, dark, and cool. Use curtains or blinds to block out light. Consider using soothing music or a "white noise" machine to block out noise

Keep a Bedtime Routine and Sleep Schedule

Having a bedtime routine and a set wake-up time will help your body get used to a sleeping schedule. You may want to ask others in your household to help you with your routine.

- Don't do stressful or energizing things within two hours of going to bed

- Create a relaxing bedtime routine. You might want to take a warm shower or bath, listen to soothing music, or drink a cup of tea with no caffeine in it

- Use a sleep mask and earplugs, if light and noise bother you

- Try to get up at the same time every morning, even if you feel tired. That will help to set your sleep schedule over time, and you will be more likely to fall asleep easily when bedtime comes. On weekends do not to sleep more than an hour past your regular wake-up time

Try to Relax If You Can't Sleep

- Imagine yourself in a peaceful, pleasant scene. Focus on the details and feelings of being in a place that is relaxing

- Get up and do a quiet activity, such as reading, until you feel sleepy

Watch your activities during the day

Your daytime habits and activities can affect how well you sleep. Here are some tips:

- Exercise during the day. Don't exercise within two hours of going to bed, though, because it may be harder to fall asleep

- Get outside during daylight hours. Spending time in sunlight helps to reset your body's sleep and wake cycles

- Cut out or limit what you drink or eat that has caffeine in it, such as coffee, tea, cola, and chocolate

- Don't drink alcohol before bedtime. Alcohol can cause you to wake up more often during the night

- Don't smoke or use tobacco, especially in the evening. Nicotine can keep you awake

- Don't take naps during the day, especially close to bedtime

- Don't drink any liquids after 6 p.m. if you wake up often because you have to go to the bathroom

- Don't take medicine that may keep you awake, or make you feel hyper or energized right before bed. Your doctor can tell you if your medicine may do this and if you can take it earlier in the day

Talk to your doctor

If you can't sleep because you are in pain or have an injury, you often feel anxious at night, or you often have bad dreams or nightmares, talk to your doctor.

There are a number of medications that are helpful for sleep problems in PTSD. Depending on your sleep symptoms and other factors, your doctor may prescribe some medication for you. There are also other skills you can learn to help improve your sleep.

Prevalence of Sleep Problems in Veterans with PTSD

PTSD is unique among mental health disorders in that sleep problems are mentioned twice among its diagnostic criteria in DSM-5: the presence of insomnia qualifying as a symptom of an alteration in arousal and reactivity and the presence of frequent nightmares as an intrusion symptom. Insomnia is reported to occur in 90-100% of Vietnam era Veterans with PTSD. Insomnia was also the most commonly reported PTSD symptom in a survey of Veterans from Afghanistan and Iraq (OEF/OIF). In the Millennium Cohort Study, 92% of active duty personnel with PTSD, compared to 28% of those without PTSD, reported clinically significant levels of insomnia.

It has been argued that sleep problems, rather than being just symptoms of PTSD, are a hallmark of the disorder. In support of this viewpoint, insomnia occurring in the acute aftermath of a traumatic event is a significant risk factor for the later development of PTSD in civilian and active duty populations. Studies also indicate that insomnia often persists following PTSD-focused treatments such as Prolonged Exposure or Cognitive Processing Therapy. Even when PTSD-focused treatment has been associated with statistically significant improvements in sleep, effect sizes are small and not clinically significant.

There are fewer data on the prevalence of chronic nightmares with PTSD. In the National Vietnam Veterans Readjustment Study, 52% of combat Veterans with PTSD reported significant nightmares. In a second study in the general community, 71% of individuals with PTSD endorsed nightmares; and, compared to civilians with PTSD, the nightmares of Veterans were more likely to be a replay of their trauma(s). Posttraumatic nightmares are independently associated with daytime distress, and impaired functioning. Nightmares frequently do not improve with trauma-focused treatment although the degree of improvement is larger for nightmares than for insomnia in general.

Treatment of Sleep Problems in PTSD

There are two primary approaches to treating sleep problems in PTSD, pharmacology (i.e., sleep medications) and psychotherapy. To date, little is known about the efficacy of using both approaches concurrently. The preferred treatment approach, when available, is cognitive behavioral therapy.

Chapter 30

Multiple Sclerosis and Sleep Disorders

Common Sleep Disorders and MS

Sleep plays an important role in your physical health and well-being. Sleep supports healthy brain functioning, is involved in the healing and repair of your heart and blood vessels, regulates mood, reduces stress, and even helps your immune system defend your body against foreign or harmful substances. The average adult needs 7-9 hours of sleep each day to function well. Yet, many people do not get adequate amounts of sleep. People with MS often say they sleep poorly at night and are fatigued in the daytime. In the general population the three most common sleep problems reported are insomnia, sleep apnea, and restless leg syndrome (RLS). Recent research suggests that people with MS have these problems even more often.

Insomnia is characterized by problems getting to sleep or staying asleep, or waking up too early. Insomnia can have multiple causes and is a significant problem at some point for almost half of people with MS. Insomnia can be caused by nighttime MS symptoms that disrupt sleep, such as pain, muscle spasms, and urinary frequency. Medications, including some antidepressants (SSRIs), stimulants used to treat daytime fatigue, and corticosteroids used to treat MS exacerbations can also contribute to insomnia. Depression, which is common with

This chapter includes text excerpted from "Where There's a Will, There's Way," U.S. Department of Veterans Affairs (VA), 2015.

193

MS, is also associated with insomnia. Although occasional self medication of insomnia with over-the-counter sleep medications containing antihistamines can help, if you use them often they'll probably stop working and will also make you sleepy or foggy during the day. Many approaches can be effective for treating insomnia including adjusting your current medication regimen, addressing MS symptoms that are contributing to poor sleep, using non-medication cognitive behavioral therapy approaches, and, in resistant cases, using prescribed sleep enhancing medications.

Sleep apnea affects at least 1 in 5 Americans, and probably an even greater proportion of people with MS. Sleep apnea is characterized by repeatedly stopping breathing during sleep. The frequent pauses in breathing can cause fragmented sleep as well as low blood oxygen levels. Untreated, sleep apnea is associated with poor daytime functioning, mood and memory problems and, if severe, cardiovascular disorders such as heart disease and stroke. Sleep apnea may also worsen fatigue, poor energy, and daytime tiredness common in people with MS. Treatment of sleep apnea can reduce these symptoms which may have been attributed solely to MS.

Restless leg syndrome (RLS) is characterized by an uncomfortable urge to move your legs or, more rarely, other body areas. This urge is temporarily relieved by moving your legs. RLS symptoms are generally worst in the evening or at night. RLS is three times more common in people with MS than in the general population. RLS may affect up to 1/3 of individuals with MS and is more common in those who are older, have had MS for longer, have primary progressive MS, and have greater disability. The exact cause of RLS is not known, but RLS appears to be linked with iron metabolism in the brain. Checking for low iron levels with a blood test, and replacing iron when low, can improve symptoms. Decreasing the intake of caffeine, nicotine, and alcohol, massaging your legs, and taking warm baths before bedtime may decrease RLS symptoms. When these interventions fail, medications to treat RLS symptoms are available.

In summary, sleep problems such as insomnia, sleep apnea, and RLS are common in individuals with MS. These sleep problems may be troublesome on their own and may contribute to daytime fatigue, poorer quality of life, and may be associated with greater disability. Fortunately, treatments are available for the most common sleep problems so if you have poor quality, unrefreshing sleep, it is important that you discuss your symptoms with your provider. Good sleep practices such as keeping a regular bedtime and wake time, protecting your sleep time from other activities, setting up your bedroom only for sleep, and limiting caffeinated beverages can also help. While symptoms may not completely resolve with treatment, substantial improvements in daytime functioning and an improved sense of well-being are possible.

Chapter 31

Nocturia: When the Need to Urinate Interrupts Sleep

Nocturia

Nocturia, also known as nocturnal polyuria or frequent nighttime urination, is a problem that affects an estimated 33 percent of adults. Normally, hormones signal the bladder to produce less urine at night, so most people can sleep for 6 to 8 hours without needing to get up to use the bathroom. Waking up once per night to empty the bladder is considered normal as well. People with nocturia, on the other hand, produce excessive amounts of urine and are regularly awakened several times per night by the need to urinate.

Waking up multiple times each night to use the bathroom can lead to chronic sleep deprivation. Since the incidence of nocturia increases with age, the majority of people affected are over the age of 60. Nocturia often appears as a symptom of underlying medical conditions, such as an enlarged prostate, diabetes, heart failure, or bladder problems. Nocturia should not be confused with enuresis—also known as bed-wetting—a condition in which urine is passed unintentionally

"Nocturia: When the Need to Urinate Interrupts Sleep," © 2016 Omnigraphics. Reviewed July 2016.

during sleep. Nocturia also differs from urinary incontinence, in which patients experience a lack of voluntary control over urination in the daytime.

Causes of Nocturia

The main causes of nocturia are excessive urine production and reduced bladder capacity. Many different factors and conditions can contribute to nocturia, including the following:

- Age

  Elderly people are more prone to nocturia because the bladder gradually loses elasticity over time. In addition, levels of the hormones that signal the bladder to reduce urine production at night tend to decline with age. Nocturia commonly affects older men who have an enlarged prostate, which can press on the urethra and prevent the bladder from emptying completely, but it affects older women as well.

- Diabetes

  Poorly controlled diabetes leads to sugar in the urine, which stimulates the production of additional urine.

- Congestive heart failure and other circulatory problems

  When the heart cannot adequately pump blood through the body, fluid tends to build up in the legs (edema). Lying down at night reduces the burden on the heart and improves circulation, causing the fluid to fill the bladder.

- Pregnancy

  The growing fetus takes up space usually occupied by the bladder and restricts its capacity to hold fluids.

- Lower urinary tract conditions

  Infections of the urinary tract or kidneys can cause nocturia by irritating the bladder and decreasing its capacity to hold urine. Conditions like cystitis can result in an overactive bladder. Bladder obstructions can prevent the full elimination of urine, which may increase the frequency of urination at night.

- Constipation

  Excessive waste in the bowels or intestines can put pressure on the bladder.

- Medications

   Certain drugs, such as diuretics, increase the production of urine. Other examples include cardiac glycosides, demeclocycline, lithium, methoxyflurane, phenytoin, and propoxyphene. It is important to consult a doctor before stopping any prescribed medication, however, even if it causes nocturia as a side effect.

- Diet

   Consuming excessive fluids before bedtime can contribute to nocturia. Alcohol and caffeinated beverages, in particular, act as diuretics to increase urine production.

- Sleep disorders

   Obstructive sleep apnea and other sleep disorders can disrupt the normal reduction in urine output at night.

- Neurological disorders

   Conditions that affect the transmission of signals and hormones from the brain to the bladder—such as multiple sclerosis, Parkinson disease, or spinal cord injury—can result in nocturia.

Symptoms and Diagnosis

Many experts consider nocturia to be a symptom rather than a health condition. As a result, doctors usually place an emphasis on diagnosing the underlying medical causes of frequent and excessive nighttime urination that disrupts sleep. To evaluate a patient with nocturia, medical practitioners generally collect detailed information about the problem as well as the patient's overall health. The patient may be asked to keep a record of their bladder activity for several days, including the amount of fluid consumed, the frequency of urination during the day and at night, the amount of urine output, and any leaking of urine or wetting the bed. The patient will also be asked about any medications they take regularly, how much alcohol and caffeine they consume each day, and any discomfort they may experience during urination. The doctor may order a urinalysis to evaluate kidney function and check for a urinary tract infection.

Prevention and Treatment

Since nocturia is usually a symptom, most methods of treatment address the underlying medical conditions that contribute to frequent nighttime urination. Several of these conditions—such as enlarged prostate or overactive bladder—can be managed with the help of medications. A number of lifestyle modifications can also help reduce urine production at night and prevent people from needing to get up to use the bathroom. Some of the recommended methods of prevention and treatment for nocturia include the following:

- Avoid consuming fluids in the evening (but be sure that total fluid intake is adequate during the day)

- Eliminate or reduce consumption of caffeinated beverages and alcohol

- Take an afternoon nap to improve circulatory function and drain fluids from the extremities consistently throughout the day

- Wear compression stockings or elevate the legs to reduce fluid accumulation

- Perform Kegel exercises to strengthen the pelvic muscles and improve bladder control (these exercises are particularly helpful for pregnant women and for men with an enlarged prostate)

- Take diuretic medications in the late afternoon—six hours before bedtime—so that their therapeutic effects are completed before nighttime

- Eliminate urinary tract infections with antibiotic medications

- Treat enlarged prostate with medications such as tamsulosin (Flomax), finasteride, or dutasteride

- Control an unstable or overactive bladder with anticholinergic medications such as oxybutynin, tolterodine, or solifenacin

- Reduce urine production at night with medications such as desmopressin (DDAVP)

References

1. Marchione, Victor. "Nocturia: Frequent Urination at Night," Doctors Health Press, 2016.

2. "Nocturia," Cleveland Clinic, 2016.

3. "Nocturia (Night-time Urination)," NetDoctor, October 4, 2012.

Chapter 32

Pain Disorders That Impact Sleep

Chapter Contents

Section 32.1

Pain and Sleep: An Overview

Pain is the leading cause of insomnia. People who experience chronic pain—which includes about 15% of the overall U.S. population and half of all elderly people—often have trouble falling asleep and staying asleep. In fact, about 65% of people with chronic pain report having disrupted sleep or non-restorative sleep, resulting in an average deficit of 42 minutes between the amount of sleep they need and the amount they actually get. Shorter sleep duration and poorer sleep quality, in turn, exacerbate chronic pain and interfere with activities, work, mood, relationships, and other aspects of daily life.

How Pain Impacts Sleep

People who experience chronic pain often have trouble falling asleep. Most people prepare for sleep by eliminating distractions and trying to relax. This process may include preparing the covers and pillows, turning off the lights, quieting noises in the bedroom, and making themselves comfortable. For people with chronic pain, however, distractions may serve as a pain management tool. As long as they are able to focus on working, socializing, preparing meals, performing household tasks, reading, watching television, or engaging in recreational activities, their perception of pain tends to decrease. When they eliminate distractions and try to fall asleep, however, their brain tends to focus on the pain. Their level of stress and experience of pain may increase with the amount of time it takes them to fall asleep.

People dealing with pain also tend to have trouble sleeping through the night. Research has shown, for instance, that people with chronic back pain experience a number of microarousals—or changes from a deeper to a lighter stage of sleep—per hour each night. Such disruptions to the normal stages of sleep lead to frequent awakenings during the night and less restorative sleep. The poor quality of sleep means that people with chronic pain do not feel rested and refreshed in the morning. As a result, they often experience drowsiness, diminished energy, depressed mood, and increased pain throughout the day.

In some cases, people with pain also have other medical problems that disrupt sleep, such as restless leg syndrome or nocturnal leg cramps. People with restless leg syndrome experience an uncomfortable tingling or tickling sensation in their legs at night. This sensation creates an uncontrollable urge to move the legs, which can result in involuntary kicking or jerking motions during sleep. The symptoms of restless leg syndrome can contribute to problems falling asleep or staying asleep. They are sometimes relieved through massage, hot baths before bedtime, daily exercise, or eliminating caffeine or nicotine. They can also be treated with prescription medications.

Nocturnal leg cramps are sudden, painful muscle spasms that tend to occur during sleep or during the process of falling asleep. They may affect the feet, calves, or thighs and last between a few seconds and several minutes. Dehydration is the most common cause of muscle cramps, so staying well hydrated during the day can help prevent them from occurring. Overuse of the leg muscles is another factor that sometimes contributes to nocturnal cramping. Stretching before bedtime often helps with this problem. Deficiencies in calcium, magnesium, or potassium may also cause muscle cramps, so supplementing intake of these minerals in the diet may also prove helpful.

Improving Pain and Sleep

When pain impacts sleep, it is important to treat both problems together with a multidisciplinary approach. Since chronic pain and insomnia reinforce each other in a vicious cycle, treatments aimed at improving pain may also help improve sleep, while treatments aimed at improving sleep may also help improve pain. Many behavioral and psychological approaches are available to treat both pain and sleep issues.

Practices and habits that can lead to better quality sleep are known as "sleep hygiene." In many cases, people who experience chronic pain develop bad habits and poor sleep hygiene over time. Some of the practices that have proven safe and effective in improving sleep include the following:

- Develop a regular routine to help the body get into a consistent, healthy sleep-wake cycle. Try to go to bed at the same time every night and wake up at the same time each morning. Chronic pain sufferers sometimes try to compensate for having trouble falling asleep by sleeping late the next morning, but this practice disrupts the sleep-wake pattern.

- Avoid taking naps during the day, which can make insomnia worse in the long run by disrupting the sleep-wake cycle.

- Do not go to bed unless sleepy. Instead, spend some time engaging in relaxing activities like listening to music, reading a book, or meditating.

- Get out of bed if sleep does not come within 30 minutes. Trying to fall asleep for hours on end only increases anxiety levels and turns the bedroom into a stressful place. Instead, get up and return to a relaxing activity until a feeling of drowsiness occurs.

- Develop bedtime rituals to aid in relaxation and train the body to fall asleep. Suggestions include taking a warm bath or shower, listening to music, reading a book, or having a light snack.

- Avoid caffeine, nicotine, and alcohol before bedtime. Research has shown that these substances can be disruptive to a good night's sleep.

- Exercise at least four to six hours before bedtime. Although regular exercise can help ease chronic pain and promote good sleep, vigorous exercise within a few hours of bedtime can disrupt sleep.

- Create a comfortable, pleasant, relaxing sleep environment. People with chronic pain tend to be highly sensitive to environmental factors, such as light, noise, temperature, mattresses, and bedding. As a result, choosing comfortable bedding, making sure the temperature is neither too hot nor too cold, and eliminating sources of distracting noise or light can make a big difference in helping them get a good night's sleep.

- Try alternative techniques such as meditation, yoga, deep breathing, deep muscle relaxation, or hypnosis to aid in chronic pain management and relaxation. These techniques can help people reduce stress, decrease the perception of pain, and improve sleep.

If these approaches are not effective in improving sleep, chronic pain sufferers should consult a doctor. A variety of medications are available to help address sleep problems. Before taking any sleep medication, however, patients must be sure to tell the doctor about any other medications they may be taking for chronic pain or other medical conditions.

References

1. "Chronic Pain and Insomnia: Breaking the Cycle," Drugs and Usage, December 23, 2015.

2. "Pain and Sleep," National Sleep Foundation, 2016.

3. Silberman, Stephanie. "What's Really Causing Your Sleepless Nights?" *Huffington Post,* July 21, 2011.

Section 32.2

Fibromyalgia and Sleep Problems

This section includes text excerpted from "What Is Fibromyalgia?" National Institute of Arthritis and Musculoskeletal and Skin Diseases (NIAMS), November 2014.

What Is Fibromyalgia?

Fibromyalgia is a disorder that causes muscle pain and fatigue (feeling tired).

People with fibromyalgia have pain and tenderness throughout the body.

People with fibromyalgia may also have other symptoms, such as:

- Trouble sleeping

- Morning stiffness

- Headaches

- Painful menstrual periods

- Tingling or numbness in hands and feet

- Problems with thinking and memory (sometimes called "fibro fog").

A person may have two or more chronic pain conditions at the same time. Such conditions can include chronic fatigue syndrome, endometriosis, fibromyalgia, inflammatory bowel disease, interstitial cystitis, temporomandibular joint dysfunction, and vulvodynia. It is not known whether these disorders share a common cause.

What Causes Fibromyalgia?

- The causes of fibromyalgia are unknown. There may be a number of factors involved. Fibromyalgia has been linked to:
- Stressful or traumatic events, such as car accidents
- Repetitive injuries
- Illness
- Certain diseases.

Fibromyalgia can also occur on its own.

Some scientists think that a gene or genes might be involved in fibromyalgia. The genes could make a person react strongly to things that other people would not find painful.

Who Is Affected by Fibromyalgia?

Scientists estimate that fibromyalgia affects 5 million Americans 18 or older. Between 80 and 90 percent of people diagnosed with fibromyalgia are women. However, men and children also can have the disorder. Most people are diagnosed during middle age.

People with certain other diseases may be more likely to have fibromyalgia. These diseases include:

- Rheumatoid arthritis
- Systemic lupus erythematosus (commonly called lupus)
- Ankylosing spondylitis (spinal arthritis).

Women who have a family member with fibromyalgia may be more likely to have fibromyalgia themselves.

How Is Fibromyalgia Treated?

Fibromyalgia can be hard to treat. It's important to find a doctor who is familiar with the disorder and its treatment. Many family physicians, general internists, or rheumatologists can treat fibromyalgia. Rheumatologists are doctors who specialize in arthritis and other conditions that affect the joints or soft tissues.

Fibromyalgia treatment often requires a team approach. The team may include your doctor, a physical therapist, and possibly other healthcare providers. A pain or rheumatology clinic can be a good place to get treatment.

What Can I Do to Try to Feel Better?

There are many things you can do to feel better, including:

- Taking medicines as prescribed
- Getting enough sleep
- Exercising
- Eating well
- Making work changes if necessary.

What Research Is Being Done on Fibromyalgia?

The NIAMS sponsors research to help understand fibromyalgia and find better ways to diagnose, treat, and prevent it. Researchers are studying:

- Why people with fibromyalgia have increased sensitivity to pain.
- Medicines and behavioral treatments.
- Whether there is a gene or genes that make a person more likely to have fibromyalgia.
- The use of imaging methods, such as magnetic resonance imaging (MRI), to better understand fibromyalgia.
- Inflammation in the body and its relationship to fibromyalgia.
- Nondrug therapies to help reduce pain.
- Methods to improve sleep in people with fibromyalgia.

Section 32.3

Headaches and Sleep

This section includes text excerpted from "Headache:
Hope Through Research," National Institute of Neurological
Disorders and Stroke (NINDS), June 30, 2016.

You're sitting at your desk, working on a difficult task, when it suddenly feels as if a belt or vice is being tightened around the top of your head. Or you have periodic headaches that occur with nausea and increased sensitivity to light or sound. Maybe you are involved in a routine, non-stressful task when you're struck by head or neck pain. Perhaps you have daily head pain that just won't go away.

Sound familiar? If so, you've suffered one of the many symptoms of headache that can occur on their own or as part of another disease or health condition.

Anyone can experience a headache. Nearly 2 out of 3 children will have a headache by age 15. More than 9 in 10 adults will experience a headache sometime in their life. Headaches are the most frequent neurological condition and our most common form of pain, yet relatively little is known about what causes them.

Certain types of headache run in families. Episodes of headache may ease or even disappear for a time and recur later in life. It's even possible to have more than one type of headache at the same time.

Headaches can range in frequency and severity of pain. Some individuals may experience headaches once or twice a year, while others may experience headaches more than 15 days a month. Headaches are called chronic in nature when they occur more than 14 days a month. Some headaches may last for weeks at a time. Pain can range from mild to disabling and may be accompanied by symptoms such as nausea or increased sensitivity to noise or light, depending on the type of headache.

Headache is a major reason cited for days missed at work or school as well as visits to the doctor. Headaches cost the U.S. billions of dollars a year in direct costs and lost productivity. Indirect costs are difficult to determine, such as the potential impact of severe chronic headaches in children and how they might interference in academic progress or social engagement.

Without proper treatment, headaches can be severe and interfere with daily activities. For children in their formative years, headaches can be very disruptive.

Headache and Sleep Disorders

Headaches are often a secondary symptom of a sleep disorder but may also contribute to sleep disorders. For example, tension-type headache is regularly seen in persons with insomnia or sleep-wake cycle disorders. Nearly three-fourths of individuals who suffer from narcolepsy complain of either migraine or cluster headache. Migraines and cluster headaches appear to be related to the number of and transition between rapid eye movement (REM) and other sleep periods an individual has during sleep. Hypnic headache awakens individuals mainly at night but may also interrupt daytime naps. Reduced oxygen levels in people with sleep apnea may trigger early morning headaches.

Getting the proper amount of sleep can ease headache pain. Generally, too little or too much sleep can precipitate headaches, as can overuse of sleep medicines. Daytime naps often reduce deep sleep at night and can produce headaches in some adults. Some sleep disorders and secondary headache are treated using antidepressants. Check with a doctor before using over-the-counter medicines to ease sleep-associated headaches.

Chapter 33

Parkinson Disease and Sleep

What Is Parkinson Disease?

Parkinson disease (PD) is a degenerative disorder of the central nervous system that belongs to a group of conditions called movement disorders. It is both chronic, meaning it persists over a long period of time, and progressive, meaning its symptoms grow worse over time. As nerve cells (neurons) in parts of the brain become impaired or die, people may begin to notice problems with movement, tremor, stiffness in the limbs or the trunk of the body, or impaired balance. As these symptoms become more pronounced, people may have difficulty walking, talking, or completing other simple tasks.

What Causes the Disease?

Parkinson disease occurs when nerve cells, or neurons, in the brain die or become impaired. Although many brain areas are affected, the most common symptoms result from the loss of neurons in an area near the base of the brain called the *substantia nigra*. Normally, the neurons in this area produce an important brain chemical known as *dopamine*. Dopamine is a chemical messenger responsible for transmitting signals between the substantia nigra and the next "relay station" of the brain, *the corpus striatum*, to produce smooth, purposeful

This chapter includes text excerpted from "Parkinson Disease: Hope through Research," National Institute of Neurological Disorders and Stroke (NINDS), April 21, 2016.

movement. Loss of dopamine results in abnormal nerve firing patterns within the brain that cause impaired movement. Studies have shown that most people with Parkinson have lost 60 to 80 percent or more of the dopamine-producing cells in the substantia nigra by the time symptoms appear, and that people with PD also have loss of the nerve endings that produce the *neurotransmitter* norepinephrine. Norepinephrine, which is closely related to dopamine, is the main chemical messenger of the sympathetic nervous system, the part of the nervous system that controls many automatic functions of the body, such as pulse and blood pressure. The loss of norepinephrine might explain several of the non-motor features seen in PD, including fatigue and abnormalities of blood pressure regulation.

The affected brain cells of people with PD contain Lewy bodies— deposits of the protein alpha-synuclein. Researchers do not yet know why Lewy bodies form or what role they play in the disease. Some research suggests that the cell's protein disposal system may fail in people with PD, causing proteins to build up to harmful levels and trigger cell death. Additional studies have found evidence that clumps of protein that develop inside brain cells of people with PD may contribute to the death of neurons. Some researchers speculate that the protein buildup in Lewy bodies is part of an unsuccessful attempt to protect the cell from the toxicity of smaller aggregates, or collections, of synuclein.

Who Gets Parkinson Disease?

Estimates suggest that about 50,000 Americans are diagnosed with PD each year, although some estimates are much higher. Getting an accurate count of the number of cases is difficult because many people in the early stages of the disease may assume their symptoms are the result of normal aging and do not seek medical attention. Diagnosis is sometimes complicated by the fact that other conditions may produce symptoms of PD and there is no definitive test for the disease. People with PD may sometimes be told by their doctors that they have other disorders, and people with PD-like diseases may be incorrectly diagnosed as having PD.

PD affects about 50 percent more men than women, and the reasons for this discrepancy are unclear. While PD occurs in people throughout the world, a number of studies have found a higher incidence in developed countries. Other studies have found an increased risk in people who live in rural areas with increased pesticide use. However, those apparent risks are not fully characterized.

One clear risk factor for PD is age. The average age of onset is 60 years, and the incidence rises significantly with advancing age. However, about 5 to 10 percent of people with PD have "early-onset" disease that begins before the age of 50. Some early-onset cases are linked to specific gene mutations such as parkin. People with one or more close relatives who have PD have an increased risk of developing the disease themselves, but the total risk is still about 2 to 5 percent unless the family has a known gene mutation for the disease. An estimated 15 to 25 percent of people with PD have a known relative with the disease.

In very rare cases, parkinsonian symptoms may appear in people before the age of 20. This condition is called juvenile parkinsonism. It often begins with *dystonia* and *bradykinesia*, and the symptoms often improve with levodopa medication.

Parkinson Disease and Sleep problems

Sleep problems are common in PD and include difficulty staying asleep at night, restless sleep, nightmares and emotional dreams, and drowsiness or sudden sleep onset during the day. Another common problem is "REM behavior disorder," in which people act out their dreams, potentially resulting in injury to themselves or their bed partners. The medications used to treat PD may contribute to some of these sleep issues. Many of these problems respond to specific therapies.

Parkinsonism Resulting from Neurological Disorders

- **Arteriosclerotic parkinsonism**. Sometimes known as pseudoparkinsonism, vascular parkinsonism, or atherosclerotic parkinsonism, arteriosclerotic parkinsonism involves damage to the brain due to multiple strokes. Tremor is rare in this type of parkinsonism, while dementia and difficulties with gait are common. Antiparkinsonian drugs are of little help to people with this form of parkinsonism.

- **Post-traumatic parkinsonism**. Also known as post-traumatic encephalopathy or "punch-drunk syndrome," parkinsonian symptoms can develop after a severe head injury or frequent head trauma associated with boxing or other activities. This type of trauma can also cause a form of dementia called chronic traumatic encephalopathy.

- **Essential tremor**. Sometimes called benign essential tremor or familial tremor, this common condition tends to run in families and progresses slowly over time. The tremor is usually equal in both hands and increases when the hands are moving. It may involve the head but usually spares the legs. Essential tremor is not the same as Parkinson disease and does not usually lead to it, although in some cases the two conditions may overlap in one person. People with essential tremor have no other parkinsonian features. Essential tremor does not respond to levodopa or to most other PD drugs, but there are medications to treat it.

- **Normal pressure hydrocephalus**. Normal pressure hydrocephalus (NPH) is an abnormal increase of cerebrospinal fluid (CSF) in the brain's ventricles, or cavities. This causes the ventricles to enlarge, putting pressure on the brain. Symptoms include problems with walking, impaired bladder control leading to increased urinary frequency or incontinence, and progressive mental impairment and dementia. The person may also have a general slowing of movements or may complain that his or her feet feel "stuck." These symptoms may sometimes be mistaken for PD. They do not respond to Parkinson medications. Brain scans, intracranial pressure monitoring, and other tests can help to diagnose NPH. NPH can sometimes be treated by surgically implanting a CSF shunt that drains excess cerebrospinal fluid into the abdomen, where it is absorbed.

- **Parkinsonism accompanying other conditions**. Parkinsonian symptoms appear in individuals with other, clearly distinct neurological disorders such as Wilson disease, Huntington disease, Alzheimer disease, spinocerebellar ataxias, and Creutzfeldt-Jakob disease. Each of these disorders has specific features that help to distinguish it from PD.

How Is Parkinson Disease Diagnosed?

There are currently no blood or laboratory tests that diagnose sporadic PD. Therefore the diagnosis is based on medical history and a neurological examination. In some cases PD can be difficult to diagnose accurately early on in the course of the disease. Early signs and symptoms of PD may sometimes be dismissed as the effects of normal aging. Doctors may sometimes request brain scans or laboratory tests in order to rule out other disorders. However, computed tomography (CT) and magnetic resonance imaging (MRI) brain scans of people with PD usually appear normal. Since many other diseases have similar features but require different treatments, making a precise diagnosis is important so that people can receive the proper treatment.

What Is the Prognosis?

The average life expectancy of a person with PD is generally the same as for people who do not have the disease. Fortunately, there are many treatment options available for people with PD. However, in the late stages, PD may no longer respond to medications and can become associated with serious complications such as choking, pneumonia, and falls.

PD is a slowly progressive disorder. It is not possible to predict what course the disease will take for an individual person. One commonly used scale neurologists use for describing how the symptoms of PD have progressed in a patient is the Hoehn and Yahr scale.

Hoehn and Yahr Staging of Parkinson Disease

Stage one–symptoms on one side of the body only.

Stage two–symptoms on both sides of the body. No impairment of balance.

Stage three–balance impairment. Mild to moderate disease. Physically independent.

Stage four–severe disability, but still able to walk or stand unassisted.

Stage five–wheelchair-bound or bedridden unless assisted.

Another commonly used scale is the Movement Disorders Society-Unified Parkinson Disease Rating Scale (MDS-UPDRS). This four-part scale measures motor movement in PD: non-motor experiences of daily living, motor experiences of daily living, motor examination, and motor complications. Both the Hoehn and Yahr scale and the MDS-UPDRS are used to describe how individuals are faring and to help assess treatment response.

How Is the Disease Treated?

At present, there is no cure for PD, but medications or surgery can often provide improvement in the motor symptoms.

Drug Therapy

Medications for PD fall into three categories. The first category includes drugs that increase the level of dopamine in the brain. The most common drugs for PD are dopamine precursors—substances such as levodopa that cross the blood-brain barrier and are then changed into dopamine. Other drugs mimic dopamine or prevent or slow its breakdown.

The second category of PD drugs affects other neurotransmitters in the body in order to ease some of the symptoms of the disease. For example, *anticholinergic drugs* interfere with production or uptake of the neurotransmitter acetylcholine. These can be effective in reducing tremors.

The third category of drugs prescribed for PD includes medications that help control the non-motor symptoms of the disease, that is, the symptoms that don't affect movement. For example, people with PD-related depression may be prescribed antidepressants.

- **Levodopa/Carbidopa.** The cornerstone of therapy for PD is the drug levodopa (also called L-dopa). Nerve cells can use levodopa to make dopamine and replenish the brain's reduced supply. People cannot simply take dopamine pills because dopamine does not easily pass through the blood-brain barrier. (The blood-brain barrier is a protective lining of cells inside blood vessels that regulate the transport of oxygen, glucose, and other substances in the brain.) Usually, people are given levodopa combined with another substance called carbidopa. When added to levodopa, carbidopa prevents the conversion of levodopa into dopamine except for in the brain; this stops or diminishes the side effects due to dopamine in the bloodstream. Levodopa/carbidopa is often very successful at reducing or eliminating the tremors and other motor symptoms of PD during the early stages of the disease. It allows the majority of people with PD to extend the period of time in which they can lead active, productive lives.

Although levodopa/carbidopa helps most people with PD, not all symptoms respond equally to the drug. Levodopa usually helps most with bradykinesia and rigidity. Problems with balance may not respond. People often see noticeable improvement in their symptoms after starting levodopa/carbidopa therapy. However, they may need to increase the dose gradually for maximum benefit. Levodopa is often so effective that some people may not show symptoms during the early stages of the disease as long as they take the medicine. But levodopa is not a cure. Although it can reduce the symptoms of PD, it does not replace lost nerve cells and it does not stop the progression of the disease.

Levodopa/carbidopa can have a variety of side effects. The most common initial side effects include nausea, low blood pressure, and restlessness. The nausea and vomiting caused by levodopa are greatly reduced by the right combination of levodopa and carbidopa. The drug also can cause drowsiness or sudden sleep onset, which can make driving and other activities dangerous. Long-term use of levodopa sometimes causes hallucinations and psychosis.

Dyskinesias, or involuntary movements such twisting and writhing, commonly develop in people who take levodopa over an extended period. These movements may be either mild or severe. Some doctors start younger individuals with PD on drugs that act directly like dopamine itself and add levodopa later in the course of the disease. The dosage of levodopa is sometimes reduced in order to lessen these drug-induced movements. The drug amantadine may help control dyskinesias but if dyskinesias are severe, surgical treatment such as deep brain stimulation may be considered.

Other difficulties may be encountered later in the disease course. People with PD may begin to notice more pronounced symptoms before their first dose of medication in the morning and between doses as the period of effectiveness after each dose begins to shorten, called the wearing-off effect. People experience sudden, unpredictable "off periods," where the medications do not seem to be working. One approach to alleviating these side effects is to take levodopa more often and in smaller amounts. People with PD should never stop taking levodopa without their physician's input, because rapidly withdrawing the drug can have potentially serious side effects.

In addition to levodopa/carbidopa, there are other available treatments:

- **Dopamine agonists**. These drugs, which include apomorphine, pramipexole, ropinirole, and rotigotine, mimic the role of dopamine in the brain. They can be given alone or with levodopa. They are somewhat less effective than levodopa in treating PD symptoms, but work for longer periods of time. Many of the potential side effects are similar to those associated with the use of levodopa, including drowsiness, sudden sleep onset, hallucinations, confusion, dyskinesias, edema (swelling due to excess fluid in body tissues), nightmares, and vomiting. In rare cases, they can cause an uncontrollable desire to gamble, hypersexuality, or compulsive shopping.

- **MAO-B inhibitors**. These drugs inhibit the enzyme monoamine oxidase B, or MAO-B, which breaks down dopamine in the brain. MAO-B inhibitors cause dopamine to accumulate in surviving nerve cells and reduce the symptoms of PD. Studies supported by the NINDS have shown that selegiline (also called deprenyl) can delay the need for levodopa therapy by up to a year or more. When selegiline is given with levodopa, it appears to enhance and prolong the response to levodopa and thus may reduce wearing-off. Selegiline is usually well-tolerated, although side effects may include nausea, orthostatic hypotension, or insomnia. It should not be taken with the antidepressant fluoxetine or the sedative meperidine, because combining selegiline with these drugs can be harmful. The drug rasagiline is used in treating the motor symptoms of PD with or without levodopa. Whether rasagiline slows progression of PD is still controversial.

- **COMT inhibitors.** COMT stands for catechol-O-methyltransferase, another enzyme that breaks down dopamine. The drug entacapone and tolcapone prolong the effects of levodopa by preventing the breakdown of dopamine. COMT inhibitors can decrease the duration of "off periods" of one's dose of levodopa. The most common side effect is diarrhea. The drugs cause nausea, sleep disturbances, dizziness, urine discoloration, abdominal pain, low blood pressure, or hallucinations. In a few rare cases, tolcapone has caused severe liver disease, and people taking tolcapone need regular monitoring of their liver function.

- **Amantadine.** This antiviral drug can help reduce symptoms of PD and levodopa-induced dyskinesia. It is often used alone in the early stages of the disease. It may also be used with an anticholinergic drug or levodopa. After several months, amantadine's effectiveness wears off in up to half of the people taking it. Amantadine's side effects may include insomnia, mottled skin, edema, agitation, or hallucinations. Researchers are not certain how amantadine works in PD, but it may increase the effects of dopamine.

- **Anticholinergics.** These drugs, which include trihexyphenidyl, benztropine, and ethopropazine, decrease the activity of the neurotransmitter acetylcholine and can be particularly effective for tremor. Side effects may include dry mouth, constipation, urinary retention, hallucinations, memory loss, blurred vision, and confusion.

When recommending a course of treatment, a doctor will assess how much the symptoms disrupt the person's life and then tailor therapy to the person's particular condition. Since no two people will react the same way to a given drug, it may take time and patience to get the dose just right. Even then, symptoms may not be completely alleviated.

Table 33.1. Medications to Treat the Motor Symptoms of Parkinson Disease

Category	Generic	Brand name
Drugs that increase brain levels of dopamine	Levodopa/carbidopa	Parcopa, Sinemet
Drugs that mimic dopamine (dopamine agonists)	Apomorphine	Apokyn
	Pramipexole	Mirapex
	Ropinirole	Requip
	Rotigotine	Neupro
Drugs that inhibit dopamine breakdown (MAO-B inhibitors)	Rasagiline	Azilect
	Selegiline (deprenyl)	Eldepryl, Zelapar
Drugs that inhibit dopamine breakdown (COMT inhibitors)	Entacapone	Comtan
	Tolcapone	Tasmar
Drugs that decrease the action of acetylcholine (anticholinergics)	Benztropine	Cogentin
	Ethopropazine	Parsidol
	Trihexyphenidyl	Artane
Drugs with an unknown mechanism of action for PD	Amantadine	Symmetrek

Surgery

Before the discovery of levodopa, surgery was an option for treating PD. Studies in the past few decades have led to great improvements in surgical techniques, and surgery is again considered for people with PD for whom drug therapy is no longer sufficient.

Pallidotomy and Thalamotomy. The earliest types of surgery for PD involved selectively destroying specific parts of the brain that contribute to PD symptoms. Surgical techniques have been refined and can be very effective for the motor symptoms of PD. The most common lesion surgery is called *pallidotomy*. In this procedure, a surgeon selectively destroys a portion of the brain called the globus pallidus. Pallidotomy can improve symptoms of tremor, rigidity, and bradykinesia, possibly by interrupting the connections between the globus pallidus and the striatum or thalamus. Some studies have also found that pallidotomy can improve gait and balance and reduce the amount of levodopa people require, thus reducing drug-induced dyskinesias. Another procedure, called *thalamotomy*, involves surgically destroying part of the thalamus; this approach is useful primarily to reduce tremor.

Because these procedures cause permanent destruction of small amounts of brain tissue, they have largely been replaced by deep *brain stimulation* for treatment of PD. However, a new method using focused ultrasound from outside the head is being tested because it creates lesions without the need for surgery.

Deep Brain Stimulation. Deep brain stimulation, or DBS, uses an electrode surgically implanted into part of the brain, typically the subthalamic nucleus or the globus pallidus. Similar to a cardiac pacemaker, a pulse generator (battery pack) that is implanted in the chest area under the collarbone sends finely controlled electrical signals to the electrode(s) via a wire placed under the skin. When turned on using an external wand, the pulse generator and electrodes painlessly stimulate the brain in a way that helps to block signals that cause many of the motor symptoms of PD. DBS is approved by the U.S. Food and Drug Administration and is widely used as a treatment for PD.

DBS can be used on one or both sides of the brain. If it is used on just one side, it will affect symptoms on the opposite side of the body. DBS is primarily used to stimulate one of three brain regions: the subthalamic nucleus, the globus pallidus interna, or the thalamus. Stimulation of either the globus pallidus or the subthalamic nucleus can reduce tremor, bradykinesia, and rigidity. Stimulation of the thalamus is useful primarily for reducing tremor.

People who initially responded well to treatment with levodopa tend to respond well to DBS. While the motor function benefits of DBS can be substantial, it usually does not help with speech problems, "freezing," posture, balance, anxiety, depression, or dementia.

One advantage of DBS compared to pallidotomy and thalamotomy is that the electrical current can be turned off using a handheld device. The pulse generator also can be externally programmed.

Individuals must return to the medical center frequently for several months after DBS surgery in order to have the stimulation adjusted very carefully to give the best results. After a few months, the number of medical visits usually decreases significantly, though individuals may occasionally need to return to the center to have their stimulator checked. Currently, the battery for the pulse generator must be surgically replaced every three to five years. DBS does not stop PD from progressing, and some problems may gradually return. DBS is not a good option for everyone. It is generally appropriate for people with levodopa-responsive PD who have developed dyskinesias or other disabling "off" symptoms despite drug therapy. It is not generally an option for people with memory problems, hallucinations, severe depression, poor health, or a poor response to levodopa. DBS has not been demonstrated to be of benefit for "atypical" parkinsonian syndromes such as multiple system atrophy, progressive supranuclear palsy, or post-traumatic parkinsonism, which also do not improve with Parkinson medications.

As with any brain surgery, DBS has potential complications, including stroke or brain hemorrhage. These complications are rare, however. There is also a risk of infection, which may require antibiotics or even replacement of parts of the DBS system.

Complementary and Supportive Therapies

A wide variety of complementary and supportive therapies may be used for PD. Among these therapies are standard physical, occupational, and speech therapy techniques, which can help with such problems as gait and voice disorders, tremors and rigidity, and cognitive decline. Other types of supportive therapies include:

- **Diet**. At this time there are no specific vitamins, minerals, or other nutrients that have any proven therapeutic value in PD. An NINDS clinical study of the dietary supplement coenzyme Q10 was stopped in 2011 when results from an interim analysis showed active treatment with the supplement was unlikely to demonstrate a statistically significant difference than from a placebo. The NINDS and other components of the National Institutes of Health are funding research to determine if caffeine, antioxidants, and other dietary factors may be beneficial for preventing or treating PD. While there is currently no proof that any specific dietary factor is beneficial, a normal, healthy diet can promote overall well-being for people with PD just as it would for anyone else. Eating a fiber-rich diet and drinking plenty of fluids also can help alleviate constipation. A high protein diet, however, may limit levodopa's absorption, highlighting the importance of the timing of medications.

- **Exercise**. Exercise can help people with PD improve their mobility and flexibility. Some doctors prescribe physical therapy or muscle-strengthening exercises to tone muscles and to put underused and rigid muscles through a full range of motion. The effects of exercise on disease progression are not known, but it may improve body strength so that the person is less disabled. Exercises also improve balance, helping people minimize gait problems, and can strengthen certain muscles so that people can speak and swallow better. Exercise can improve emotional well-being and general physical activity, such as walking, gardening, swimming, calisthenics, and using exercise machines, can have other benefit. An NINDS-funded clinical trial demonstrated the benefit of tai chi exercise compared to resistance or stretching exercises. People with PD should always check with their doctors before beginning a new exercise program

Part Five

Preventing, Diagnosing, and Treating Sleep Disorders

Chapter 34

Sleep Hygiene: Tips for Better Sleep

The promotion of regular sleep is known as *sleep hygiene*. The following is a list of sleep hygiene tips which can be used to improve sleep.

National Sleep Foundation Recommendations

- Go to bed at the same time each night and rise at the same time each morning.

- Make sure your bedroom is a quiet, dark, and relaxing environment, which is neither too hot or too cold.

- Make sure your bed is comfortable and use it only for sleeping and not for other activities, such as reading, watching TV, or listening to music. Remove all TVs, computers, and other "gadgets" from the bedroom.

- Avoid large meals before bedtime.

This chapter contains text excerpted from the following sources: Text in this chapter begins with excerpts from "Sleep Hygiene Tips," Centers for Disease Control and Prevention (CDC), December 10, 2014; Text under the heading "Getting Enough Sleep" is excerpted from "Getting Enough Sleep," Office on Women's Health (OWH), April 15, 2014.

Getting Enough Sleep

What's up with sleep? It may seem like a waste of time when you've got so much going on. But sleep can help you do better in school, stress less, and generally be more pleasant to have around. Sound good? Now consider some possible effects of *not* getting enough sleep:

- Feeling angry or depressed
- Having trouble learning, remembering, and thinking clearly
- Having more accidents, including when driving or using machines
- Getting sick more often
- Feeling less motivated
- Possibly gaining weight
- Having lower self-esteem

Tips for Better Sleep

- **Go to bed and wake up at the same time every day**—even on the weekends!
- **Exercise regularly**. Don't exercise at the expense of sleep, though.
- **Don't eat a lot close to bedtime**. Food can give you a burst of energy.
- **Avoid bright lights right before bed**, including the ones that come from the TV or the computer. Sleep in a dark room. Darkness tells your body it's time for sleep.
- **Sleep in a slightly cool room**. If you can't control the temperature, try using fewer blankets or dressing lightly.
- **Follow a bedtime routine**. If you do the same things each night before bed, your body will know it's time for sleep. Take a warm bath or shower. Or drink a glass of milk.
- **Wake up to bright light**. Light tells your body it's time to get up.
- **Listen to your body**. If you're feeling tired, go to sleep. If you can't fall asleep within 20 minutes of going to bed, get up and do something else until you feel sleepy.

- **Avoid caffeine**. That means cutting back on coffee, soda, chocolate, and energy drinks—or at least trying not to have any in the afternoon.

- **Don't nap for longer than an hour** or take naps too close to bedtime.

- **Don't stay up all night studying**. Try doing some each night instead. If you pull an all-nighter, you may be too tired to do well on your test.

- **Set aside time to relax for about an hour before bed**. If your tasks have you worried, write them down to get them off your mind.

- **Remove computers, phones, and other gadgets**. Put your cell phone out of your room so you won't be tempted to use it, and so texts and calls won't wake you.

If these tips don't help, tell your parents or guardians. You also might talk to your doctor or nurse.

How Much Is Enough?

Experts say most teens need a little more than nine hours of sleep each night. Only a tiny number get that much, though. Here are some ways to see if you are getting enough sleep:

- Do you have trouble getting up in the morning?

- Do you have trouble focusing?

- Do you sometimes fall asleep during class?

If you answered yes to these questions, try using the tips above for getting better sleep.

Also keep in mind that good sleep isn't just about the number of hours you're in bed. If you wake up a lot in the night, snore, or have headaches, you may not be getting enough quality sleep to keep you fresh and healthy.

Chapter 35

Identifying Common Sleep Disrupters

Chapter Contents

Section 35.1

Common Causes of Disturbed Sleep

This section includes text excerpted from "Your Guide
to Healthy Sleep," National Heart, Lung, and Blood
Institute (NHLBI), August 2011. Reviewed July 2016.

What Disrupts Sleep?

Many factors can prevent a good night's sleep. These factors range
from well-known stimulants, such as coffee, to certain pain relievers,
decongestants, and other culprits. Many people depend on the caffeine
in coffee, cola, or tea to wake them up in the morning or to keep them
awake. Caffeine is thought to block the cell receptors that adenosine
(a substance in the brain) uses to trigger its sleep inducing signals. In
this way, caffeine fools the body into thinking it isn't tired. It can take
as long as 6–8 hours for the effects of caffeine to wear off completely.
Thus, drinking a cup of coffee in the late afternoon may prevent your
falling asleep at night.

Nicotine is another stimulant that can keep you awake. Nicotine
also leads to lighter than normal sleep, and heavy smokers tend to
wake up too early because of nicotine withdrawal. Although alcohol
is a sedative that makes it easier to fall asleep, it prevents deep sleep
and REM sleep, allowing only the lighter stages of sleep. People who
drink alcohol also tend to wake up in the middle of the night when the
effects of an alcoholic "nightcap" wear off.

Certain commonly used prescription and over-the-counter medicines contain ingredients that can keep you awake. These ingredients
include decongestants and steroids. Many medicines taken to relieve
headaches contain caffeine. Heart and blood pressure medications
known as beta blockers can make it difficult to fall asleep and cause
more awakenings during the night. People who have chronic asthma
or bronchitis also have more problems falling asleep and staying asleep
than healthy people, either because of their breathing difficulties or
because of the medicines they take. Other chronic painful or uncomfortable conditions—such as arthritis, congestive heart failure, and
sickle cell anemia—can disrupt sleep, too.

A number of psychological disorders—including schizophrenia, bipolar disorder, and anxiety disorders—are well known for disrupting sleep. Depression often leads to insomnia, and insomnia can cause depression. Some of these psychological disorders are more likely to disrupt REM sleep. Psychological stress also takes its toll on sleep, making it more difficult to fall asleep or stay asleep. People who feel stressed also tend to spend less time in deep sleep and REM sleep. Many people report having difficulties sleeping if, for example, they have recently lost a loved one, are going through a divorce, or are under stress at work.

Menstrual cycle hormones can affect how well women sleep. Progesterone is known to induce sleep and circulates in greater concentrations in the second half of the menstrual cycle. For this reason, women may sleep better during this phase of their menstrual cycle. On the other hand, many women report trouble sleeping the night before their menstrual flow starts. This sleep disruption may be related to the abrupt drop in progesterone levels that occurs just before menstruation. Women in their late forties and early fifties, however, report more difficulties sleeping (insomnia) than younger women. These difficulties may be linked to menopause, when they have lower concentrations of progesterone. Hot flashes in women of this age also may cause sleep disruption and difficulties.

Certain lifestyle factors also may deprive a person of needed sleep. Large meals or vigorous exercise just before bedtime can make it harder to fall asleep. While vigorous exercise in the evening may delay sleep onset for various reasons, exercise in the daytime is associated with improved nighttime sleep.

If you aren't getting enough sleep or aren't falling asleep early enough, you may be over scheduling activities that can prevent you from getting the quiet relaxation time you need to prepare for sleep. Most people report that it's easier to fall asleep if they have time to wind down into a less active state before sleeping. Relaxing in a hot bath or having a hot, caffeine-free beverage before bedtime may help. In addition, your body temperature drops after a hot bath in a way that mimics, in part, what happens as you fall asleep. Probably for both these reasons, many people report that they fall asleep more easily after a hot bath.

Your sleeping environment also can affect your sleep. Clear your bedroom of any potential sleep distractions, such as noises, bright lights, a TV, a cell phone, or computer. Having a comfortable mattress and pillow can help promote a good night's sleep. You also sleep better if the temperature in your bedroom is kept on the cool side.

Section 35.2

Alcohol and Its Effects on Sleep

This section includes text excerpted from "Alcohol Effects
and Safer Drinking Habits," U.S. Department of Veterans
Affairs (VA), June 2013.

Alcohol and the Body

Alcohol In

After alcohol enters the stomach, it is absorbed quickly into the
bloodstream through the stomach wall. The rest enters the bloodstream through the small intestine. How fast alcohol is absorbed you're
your bloodstream depends on several things. Higher concentrations of
alcohol like shots are absorbed faster than lower concentrations like
light beer. Absorption is faster for a person who weighs less. If you've
eaten recently, the absorption of alcohol will be slower than if you
drink on an empty stomach.

Alcohol Out

Alcohol leaves your body in several ways. First, 90% is removed
from the blood by the liver. Alcohol is then broken down into several
chemicals, including carbon dioxide and water. The carbon dioxide
and water come out in your urine. The final 10% is not removed by
the liver and is expelled through sweat and breath. The reason why
it is difficult to sober someone up is because the liver can only process
about one drink per hour (this is slow considering the body absorbs
alcohol through the stomach lining in about 10 minutes). There's not
much that can influence how fast your liver processes alcohol. That's
why cold showers, hot coffee or vomiting don't help.

Alcohol Intoxication and Performance

Sleep

Bottom line is alcohol is bad for your sleep. Poor sleep can limit
your ability to think, act quickly and perform well. Alcohol intoxication

shortens the time necessary to fall asleep, but sleep is usually disturbed and fragmented after just a few hours. Restful, restorative sleep decreases during the second half of the night. So, heavy drinking compromises your sleep throughout the night. Poor sleep decreases the body's ability to function optimally. Poor sleep also decreases your physical endurance. If you want peak performance (at work, sports, or other engagements), either plan to abstain from alcohol use altogether or drink in moderation.

Up and down Response to Alcohol in Your Body

The up and down response refers to two different effects that alcohol produces. The up response is feeling stimulated or excited. This is followed by the down response of feeling depressed and tired. The initial up response is associated with low but rising blood alcohol levels (BAL). The BAL is the ratio of alcohol to blood in your bloodstream. The down response is associated more with falling BALs. The up and down response is important because it allows you to test whether "more" alcohol means "better" is really true. It also helps you understand how tolerance affects you physiologically when it comes to drinking alcohol.

Over time, as blood alcohol levels begin to fall, people experience the down effects of alcohol. This is the time when people begin to drink more in an attempt to get back their initial stimulated or excited state. However, the more alcohol that is consumed, the greater both the arousal and the depressant effects will be. At some point, the stimulating effects of a rising BAL will not amount to euphoria. The point at which an increase in BAL will not result in elevated mood or energy is known as the point of diminishing returns. For most people, that point is a BAL of 0.05%.

Table 35.1. Effects of Alcohol on the Body

BAL	Effects of Alcohol on the Body
0.02%	Light to moderate drinkers begin to feel some effect
0.04%	Most people begin to feel relaxed
0.06%	Judgement is somewhat impaired; people are less able to make rational decisions about their capabilities (e.g., driving)
0.08%	Definite impairment of muscle coordination and driving skills. Increased risk of nausea and slurred speech. Legal intoxication.
0.10%	Clear deterioration of reaction time and control.
0.15%	Balance and movement are impaired. Risk of blackouts and accidents.
0.30%	Many people lose consciousness. Risk of death.
0.45%	Breathing stops, death occurs.

Moderating Your Drinking

Decide what you want from drinking alcohol: Think about the pros and cons (short and long-term) for moderating your use versus maintaining your usual drinking behavior. Also consider what you absolutely want to avoid when you drink.

Set Drinking Limits

- What's your upper limit on the number of drinks you consume per week?

- At what point do you decide you've had enough (consider a BAL limit)?

- What's the maximum number of days for drinking you will choose to give yourself?

- Use standard guidelines to determine what constitutes one drink:

(1.25 oz of 80-proof liquor; 4 oz of wine; 10 oz of beer with 5% alcohol (microbrews and "ice" beer); 12 oz of beer with 4% alcohol (standard beer)

Count Your Drinks and Monitor Your Drinking Behavior

Try it! Most people are surprised by what they learn when they actually count how much they drink. Simply observe your behavior–this is like standing outside yourself and watching how you are acting when you are drinking. Some people put the bottle caps in their pockets while drinking to monitor how many beers they have had. You can also make tick marks with a pen on a napkin to monitor the number of drinks.

Alter How and What You Drink

- Switch to drinks that contain less alcohol (e.g., light beers)
- Slow down your pace of drinking
- Space drinks further apart
- Alternate drinking nonalcoholic beverages with alcoholic drinks

Manage Your Drinking in the Moment

- Stay awake and on top of how you drink and what you're drinking when you're at a party

- Choose what's right for you and ask a close friend to help you monitor (preferably the friend that doesn't think being drunk is cool and cooler with company)

Safe Drinking Guideline

- For women, no more than 3 drinks/day; no more than 9 drinks/week.

- For men, no more than 4 drinks/day; no more than 14 drinks/week

Section 35.3

Caffeine and Nicotine and Their Impact upon Sleep

"Caffeine and Nicotine and Their Impact upon Sleep,"
© 2016 Omnigraphics. Reviewed July 2016.

Caffeine has been called the most popular drug in the world. Millions of people consume it on a daily basis in the form of coffee, tea, soft drinks, energy drinks, chocolate, or certain medications. Many people depend on it to help them feel alert and energized throughout the day at work or at school. Some people become addicted to it and experience withdrawal symptoms such as headaches, fatigue, anxiety, and irritability if they do not get their daily dose. Yet most people do not think of caffeine as a drug or realize that it can interfere with sleep.

Caffeine is typically absorbed into the bloodstream within 15 minutes after it is consumed, although it takes about an hour to reach peak levels. It acts as a stimulant to increase the heart rate and blood pressure and promote the production of adrenaline. As a result, caffeine temporarily increases alertness and reduces fatigue by suppressing sleep-inducing chemicals. These effects can last for 4 to 6 hours, although it takes a full 24 hours for the body to completely eliminate caffeine.

By stimulating the body to remain awake, caffeine can also weaken the body's ability to sleep. Consuming too much caffeine may cause insomnia. Most people can safely consume up to 250 milligrams per day, which is equivalent to 2 to 3 cups of coffee, without affecting their sleep. Consumption of 500 milligrams or more per day is considered excessive and can impair sleep.

Caffeine affects sleep in three ways: by making it harder to fall asleep, by reducing the quality of sleep, and by causing nocturia (frequent nighttime urination). These effects are particularly severe if the caffeine is consumed within 4 to 6 hours of bedtime. People with caffeine in their bloodstream are likely to feel jittery, anxious, or wired when they try to go to sleep. If they do manage to fall asleep, the stimulant effects of caffeine will make it difficult for their body to enter a deep, restorative phase of sleep. Finally, they are likely to wake up multiple times during the night to use the bathroom due to the diuretic effects of caffeine.

Although some people have a higher tolerance for caffeine than others, anyone who experiences difficulty sleeping may benefit from limiting caffeine consumption to less than 200 milligrams per day or eliminating it entirely. In addition, any caffeine consumption should take place early in the day—and at least 6 hours before bedtime. Ironically, cutting down on caffeine intake can cause withdrawal symptoms that can temporarily interfere with sleep. Although these symptoms subside over time as the body adjusts, people who are addicted to caffeine may want to reduce their consumption gradually rather than suddenly. Most people who eliminate caffeine find that they experience improvements in sleep afterward.

Nicotine and Sleep

Like caffeine, nicotine is absorbed into the bloodstream quickly and acts as a stimulant, increasing the heart rate and breathing rate and releasing stress hormones in the body. The stimulant effects of nicotine persist for several hours, affecting brain waves, body temperature, and other systems. These effects make it more difficult to fall asleep and stay asleep. As a result, smokers tend to sleep lightly and spend less time in deep, restorative sleep than nonsmokers.

In addition to sleep disruptions from the stimulant effects of nicotine, which tend to occur in the early part of the night, smokers may also experience withdrawal symptoms closer to morning that interfere with sleep. These symptoms may include headaches, nausea, diarrhea or constipation, irritability, anxiety, fatigue, and depression. Although quitting smoking is the best way to avoid the negative effects of nicotine on sleep, the effects can be reduced by avoiding nicotine for at least 2 hours before bedtime.

References

1. "Caffeine, Food, Alcohol, Smoking, and Sleep," Sleep Health Foundation, May 21, 2013.

2. Stewart, Kristin. "The Chemistry of Caffeine, Nicotine, and Sleep," Everyday Health, January 7, 2013.

Chapter 36

Stress and Sleep

Stress is a complex biological response that is designed to help people focus their attention, energy, and physical resources to deal with a problem or threat. Everyone faces sources of stress in their daily lives, such as traffic jams, work deadlines, relationship issues, or hectic schedules. In fact, surveys show that 70% of American adults experience stress, anxiety, or worry on a daily basis. Most people report that stress interferes with their lives, particularly by reducing the quantity and quality of their sleep.

People under stress often have trouble falling asleep because their minds race with thoughts rather than shutting down. Sleep usually gives the brain a chance to rest by switching functions over from the active sympathetic nervous system to the calmer parasympathetic nervous system. Excessive worry prevents this switch from happening, so the brain remains on high alert. Stress also reduces the quantity of sleep by causing people to awaken frequently or toss and turn restlessly during the night. Among American adults, 43% report lying awake at night due to stress, with over half experiencing this problem more than once per week.

Stress also impacts the quality of sleep. Around 42% of American adults report feeling less satisfied with the quality of their sleep when they are under stress. In addition, people who experience ongoing stress have an increased risk of developing sleep disorders and insomnia. In fact, each additional source of stress in a person's life has been

---

shown to increase their risk of insomnia by 19%. As a result, people with high levels of stress report sleeping only 6.2 hours per night on average, with only 33% feeling that they get enough sleep. People with lower levels of stress, on the other hand, sleep an average of 7.1 hours per night, and 79% feel that they get enough sleep.

Compounding the problem, research indicates that sleep deprivation leads to even higher levels of stress. Among people whose sleep is affected by stress or anxiety, 75% report that the lack of sleep increases their levels of stress and anxiety. People with high stress are also more likely to feel the physical and emotional effects of getting too little sleep, such as fatigue, sluggishness, daytime drowsiness, trouble concentrating, irritability, lack of patience, and depression. When stress causes sleep problems, and then sleep problems increase stress levels, people become locked in a vicious cycle that can be hard to break.

Managing Stress and Improving Sleep

There are a number of stress-management tools and techniques available to help people cope with anxiety and thus improve the quantity and quality of their sleep. Some helpful approaches for dealing with stress-related sleep issues include the following:

- Identify sources of stress. The first step in managing stress involves figuring out its main causes, which will vary by individual. Common sources of stress include job, health, finances, trauma, and divorce.

- Reduce exposure to stressors. Once the main sources of stress have been identified, the next step is to find ways to handle them better. With job-related stress, for instance, it may be possible to delegate some responsibilities in order to reduce workload.

- Adjust thought processes and expectations. Often the way of looking at a problem or situation can determine whether or not it is stressful. It is possible to change negative thought patterns and lower expectations in order to reduce stress. It is particularly important to avoid generalizing concerns and blowing small things out of proportion. Many self-help books and websites offer tips and exercises for managing negative thoughts. For instance, one approach might be to write down worries and concerns and then throw away the paper in order to symbolically clear the mind.

- Build a social support system. Spending time relaxing with family and friends is a valuable way to reduce stress. Talking with supportive loved ones can also make problems seem more manageable or lead to positive new approaches and solutions.

- Exercise. Getting regular exercise is a proven way to relieve stress and improve mood. It can also lead to improvements in sleep, although vigorous exercise should be undertaken at least two hours before bedtime to allow body temperature to return to normal.

- Eat a healthy diet. A healthy diet with plenty of fruits, vegetables, whole grains, and lean proteins promotes overall health, increases energy, and helps reduce stress. On the other hand, consuming refined sugars, caffeine, and alcohol can negatively impact sleep and leave people feeling sluggish.

- Try relaxation techniques. Deep-breathing exercises can activate the parasympathetic nervous system and help calm nerves. Yoga, meditation, progressive muscle relaxation, and other techniques can also help quiet the mind and promote sleep.

- Practice good sleep hygiene. Since sleep problems increase stress levels, getting a good night's sleep is vital to effective stress management. Sleep hygiene methods that can improve the quality of sleep include making sleep a priority, blocking out 8 full hours for sleep, establishing a regular sleep schedule and a relaxing bedtime routine, avoiding naps during the day, and creating a comfortable and inviting sleep environment.

If these steps are ineffective in reducing stress and improving sleep, it may be helpful to consult with a doctor. Therapists can help patients identify sources of stress and find productive ways of dealing with them. Sleep specialists can assess patients for sleep disorders and recommend approaches or medications to address the problem. Since stress and sleep often go hand in hand, both kinds of professional help may be needed to enable people to manage stress successfully and sleep soundly through the night.

References

1. Holmes, Lindsay. "Five Ways Stress Wrecks Your Sleep (and What to Do about It)," *Huffington Post,* September 17, 2014.

2. "Stress and Anxiety Interfere with Sleep," Anxiety and Depression Association of America, 2016.

3. "Tips to Reduce Stress and Sleep Better," WebMD, 2016.

Chapter 37

Shift Work and Sleep

The Rewards and Challenges of Shift Work

The rewards and challenges of shift work. As a member of a shift work family, you're already aware of some of the pluses—for example, the extra pay to provide for the family, the freedom of working nontraditional hours and the ability to spend more time with the kids during the day.

- The minuses?

  They include everything from difficulty planning events and family activities to sleep and schedule disruptions.

- It not only affects the shift worker, but everyone in the household.

Living with Shift Work

When you live with a shift worker, you're a shift worker too. Their schedule interrupts your schedule. When they're up, you're up. When

This chapter contains text excerpted from the following sources: Text under the heading "The Rewards and Challenges of Shift Work" is excerpted from "The Rewards and Challenges of Shift Work," National Highway Traffic Safety Administration (NHTSA), February 1, 2001. Reviewed July 2016; Text under the heading "Wake up and Get Some Sleep" is excerpted from "Wake up and Get Some Sleep," National Highway Traffic Safety Administration (NHTSA), February 2, 2002. Reviewed July 2016; Text under the heading "Sleep Disorders, Work Shifts, and Officer Wellness" is excerpted from "Sleep Disorders, Work Shifts, and Officer Wellness," National Institute of Justice (NIJ), June 2012. Reviewed July 2016.

they're driving home late at night, you're up worried in bed. Or on the sofa. Chances are, you could use better quality sleep as much as your shift worker.

So What's Wrong with Losing Sleep?

If you and your shift worker don't get enough sleep, it can result in everything from grumpiness to lowered immune systems, and even depression. It can also lead to something very dangerous—drowsy driving.

Make Sure You and Your Loved One Crash in the Right Spot

Research shows that when you're driving under the strain of sleep deprivation, you're not going to react to situations as quickly as when you're rested and alert. The effect is almost like driving while impaired by alcohol or drugs. And there isn't a big warning sign that flashes every time you're about to fall asleep. Drowsiness creeps up on you. It's almost impossible to predict when you might doze off.

The National Highway Traffic Safety Administration (NHTSA) estimates that more than 100,000 crashes each year are the result of drowsy driving. Some studies reveal that roughly one-quarter of shift workers reported having at least one crash or close call within the last year. So you can see why it's so critical for everyone to get quality sleep. People's lives are at stake

When the Shift Worker Loses Sleep, It's a Family Affair

It's not easy getting quality sleep when the shift worker in the family is coming home from work in the middle of the night or unwinding from a hard shift at three in the morning. Everybody's day (and night) is disturbed. And the whole household must work its schedule around the shift worker's waking and sleeping hours.

Some Tips for the Whole Family to Sleep On

It's important that everybody gets the best quality sleep possible. It's also vital to talk on a regular basis about the challenges, frustrations and issues that come with being a shift work family. Here are a few steps that everybody can take to improve their sleep environment.

Keep the Room Dark. Really Dark

The body has its own natural waking/sleeping clock called the "circadian rhythm." This means a person wants to be active when it's light, and rest when it's dark. Here's what to do to keep everyone, including your shift worker, in the right sleep rhythm.

- **Use black-out or room-darkening shades.**

  They're made to completely eliminate outside light, whether it's the natural light of the sun, or the glow of a street lamp. Also try putting lined curtains over the shades. You'll find them at most home supply centers or department stores.

- **Fix those light leaks.**

  The smallest amount of outside light can disturb sleep. Cover glow-in-the dark alarm clocks with a hand towel, and switch off your nightlights. It may help to block out the shaft of light that leaks under the bedroom door by covering the opening with a rolled-up towel.

- **Wear a sleep mask.**

  It's not just for movie stars anymore. It's ideal for anyone who has trouble

Block out the "Bad" Sounds

Honking cars. Screaming ambulances. Roaring airplanes. Noisy neighbors. Barking dogs. Trying to sleep soundly in the midst of life's daily and nightly sounds isn't easy. Fortunately, there are steps you can take to help the situation.

- **Use earplugs to block outside noise.** Few things are as simple to use or as effective at keeping out sleep-depriving distractions.

- **Purchase a "white noise" machine.** Studies show that shift workers and non-shift workers alike are often lulled to sleep by a steady stream of peaceful sounds, such as ocean waves. White noise machines block out extraneous, not-so-peaceful.

- **Put them to sleep with a noisy old fan**. An old-fashioned oscillating fan is perfect. The new "whisper-quiet" fans don't do a very good job of blocking outside noise.

- **Tune in and fall out. Tune your radio or TV to** just be sure to turn down the brightness or cover the screen so the light doesn't keep you awake.

Set the Temperature

Be sure to keep the sleeping room at a comfortable temperature—not too hot or too cold. Research shows that setting your thermostat to 60-65 degrees Fahrenheit is ideal.

Set Your Schedule

Try to keep a regular sleep schedule—going to sleep and waking up at the same time every day, including weekends. It may not always be possible, but it's important—for the shift worker and everyone in the house.

Follow These Healthy Life Habits and Everybody Will Sleep Better.

The task of getting better sleep is in our control. All it takes is the commitment and desire to live as healthy a life as possible, and the willingness to take a few simple steps.

- **Get everybody involved in a healthy diet and exercise program**. Good health has a positive effect on our ability to sleep. So eat healthy and exercise. Choose nutritious foods that are low in sodium and saturated fat. Pick an activity the whole family likes—such as walking, jogging, swimming or bicycling. And do it together—you're more likely to stick to it that way.

- **Avoid caffeine and alcohol close to bedtime.**

  Caffeine's stimulating effects will peak in two to four hours and may last for several hours afterward. The result is diminished deep sleep and increased awakenings. Alcohol may initially make you fall asleep faster, but when the immediate effects wear off, it deprives your body of deep rest and you end up sleeping in fragments and waking often.

- **Understand the side effects of medication.**

  Read the label. Some medications can make you sleepy and make it dangerous to drive. Other medications can make it harder to fall asleep.

- **Develop a relaxing sleep ritual.**

  Everyone has their own way to unwind. Here are a few suggestions the entire household can use:

246

- Take a warm bath, not a shower. The point is to relax, not just to get clean.

  - Read until you feel sleepy.

  - Listen to quiet, soothing music.

  - Make a list of things you need to do or worry about the next day (or night), so you can clear your mind for sleep.

- **The Better the Communication, the Happier the Household.**

  The goal is to make the most of the time you spend together as a shift work family. So here are some tips everyone in the house can follow:

- **Hold regular family meetings, once or twice a week.**

  - Discuss problems or concerns about the shift worker's schedule, or anything else that comes up. Open up the lines of communication.

  - Try to deal with minor problems early on, before they become major problems.

  - Determine solutions together as a family. Listen, and think about all ideas.

- **Keep household members in touch with the shift worker, and each other.**

  - Set up a bulletin board in your house where everybody can leave notes, school work, drawings, photographs, cartoons, reminders, or anything else to help keep the family connected

  - Rent or purchase a camcorder to capture special moments the shift worker may miss, such as birthday parties, Little League games and school recitals.

  - Select a time each week to relax and talk with your partner.

  - Plan a "family day" once a month.

  - Schedule family events and get-together on the shift worker's days off when he/she is normally awake, such as breakfast or early lunch.

- **Ensure your family feels safe at night.**

  Some research suggests that the safer people feel in their home environment, the better they sleep.

Here are some ideas:

- Install a home security system.

- Get a dog.

- Keep emergency phone numbers (i.e., 911, fire, police) handy by your bedside telephone.

Here's to Better Sleep.

The benefits to getting better sleep include more patience with loved ones, better performance on the job and at school—and most critical of all—safer driving on the road. So get together regularly, talk about what works, and commit to making as many changes as possible.

The key is to be persistent, and to try as many tips as you can, for at least several weeks.

Changing habits doesn't work overnight. It takes time. Everything you've read about here will lead to one common goal: achieving a better quality of life for the whole family

Wake up and Get Some Sleep

Shift work definitely has its rewards — like the extra income, the lack of interruptions, the sense of freedom you get working nontraditional hours, and the ability to be home with the kids during the day. But working night or rotating shifts also has its drawbacks — and one of the biggest is not getting enough restful sleep. That can make you feel tired and grumpy. It can make it hard to get through work. And worst of all, it can cause you to fall asleep behind the wheel while driving home.

Your Body Clock Was Set by Nature

The human body is governed by an internal clock known as the circadian rhythm. In each 24-hour cycle, it makes you want to sleep when it's dark and be awake when it's light. It causes periods of sleepiness between midnight and 6 a.m. — the natural time for humans to sleep — then again in the midafternoon.

But as a shift worker, you have to try to sleep when your body is telling you to be awake, and be awake during those dips in your alertness level when your body is telling you to sleep. And as you get sleepier, you begin to miss things you would normally respond to, resulting in careless and even dangerous errors. Additionally, sleeping during the day can make it difficult to get the amount of sleep your body needs. Some research shows shift workers average five hours of sleep per day, at least one to one-and-a-half hours less than non-shift workers.

Regularly getting less than seven or eight hours of sleep in a 24-hour period really can lead to chronic problem sleepiness and cause irritability, crankiness and depression. It also makes it more likely that you might fall asleep while driving. And the only way to correct the problem is to get more or better sleep.

Dont Learn about Drowsy Driving by Accident

Perhaps one of the most dangerous consequences associated with shift work is sleepiness behind the wheel. The late night and early morning drive times are the most hazardous, with the majority of crashes occurring between the hours of midnight and 6 a.m. when the body naturally experiences sleepiness. This contributes to the high rate of serious injuries and fatalities for several reasons:

- Crashes involving drivers who fall asleep occur more often on highways and roadways where speed limits are higher.

- The driver's eyes are closed so there is no attempt to avoid the crash.

- The driver is usually alone in the vehicle so there's no one to alert the driver to danger.

The National Highway Traffic Safety Administration (NHTSA) estimates that more than 100,000 crashes each year are the result of drowsy driving. Some studies have proven that roughly one-quarter of shift workers report having at least one crash or close call within the last year. In fact, research shows that drivers are just as impaired when they're sleepy as when they've consumed alcohol.

Drowsiness and Drinking Don't Mix

Drinking alcohol when you're sleepy only serves to increase your drowsiness and further impair your judgement, perception, and ability to react to road conditions and other drivers. It's a hazardous combination. How dangerous? NHTSA has found that nearly 20 percent of all sleepiness-related, single-vehicle crashes involve alcohol. Even if you've had just a small amount to drink and are feeling just a little sleepy, the effects of one are intensified by the other.

The Other Driving Forces

The use of certain medications and drugs can also compound sleepiness. And the risk increases for people taking higher doses or more than one sedating medication simultaneously. Another factor to consider is your driving pattern—longer trips in terms of miles or minutes put you at a higher risk.

The Best Thing to Do Is "Sleep on It"

The single most important key to eliminating most problems caused by shift work is to make sleep a number one priority. Set a specific bedtime for yourself. Get good, uninterrupted sleep at the same time every day, even on your days off. And even if you can't sleep more, there are things you can do to make sure you sleep better.

Steps You Can Take to Improve Sleep

- Make your room dark—the darker, the better. As a shift worker, you're waking and sleeping against the natural rhythms of lightness and darkness—the most powerful regulators of our internal clocks. Your body wants to be active when it's light, and craves rest when it's dark. Try using special room-darkening shades, lined drapes or a sleep mask to simulate nighttime. Sleep without a night light, block the light that comes from your doorway, and if your alarm clock is illuminated, cover it up.

- Block outside sounds. Sleep can be easily interrupted by sudden, unexpected sounds—the screech of a passing siren, a plane flying overhead, construction work or a barking dog, to name a few. Use ear plugs, a fan, or turn the FM radio or TV to in between stations so the shhhh blocks out other noises and lulls you to sleep. (Just be sure to turn off the brightness on your TV or cover the screen.) You might even want to consider a white noise machine, which plays a steady stream of lulling sounds such as ocean waves.

- Adjust your thermostat before going to bed. A room that is too hot or too cold can disturb your sleep. Some research shows that 60 to 65 degrees Fahrenheit or 16 to 18 degrees Celsius is ideal.

- Keep a regular schedule. Go to bed and get up at the same time every day. The best way to ensure a good night's sleep is to stick to a regular schedule, even on your days off, holidays or when traveling.

- Maintain or improve your overall health. Eat well and establish a regular exercise routine. It can be as simple as a 20- to 30-minute walk, jog, swim or bicycle ride three times a week. Exercising too close to bedtime may actually keep you awake because your body has not had a chance to unwind. Allow at least three hours between working out and going to bed.

- Avoid caffeine several hours before bedtime. Its stimulating effects will peak two to four hours later and may linger for several hours more. The result is diminished deep sleep and increased awakenings.

- Avoid alcohol before going to sleep. It may initially make you fall asleep faster, but it can make it much harder to stay asleep. As the immediate effects of the alcohol wear off, it deprives your body of deep rest and you end up sleeping in fragments and waking often.

- Know the side effects of medications. Some medications can increase sleepiness and make it dangerous to drive. Other medications can cause sleeping difficulties as a side effect.

- Change the time you go to sleep. After driving home from work, don't go right to bed. Take a few hours to unwind and relax.

- Develop a relaxing sleep ritual. Before going to sleep, try taking a warm bath, listening to soothing music or reading until you feel sleepy — but don't read anything exciting or stimulating.

- Don't make bedtime the time to solve the day's problems. Try to clear your mind. Make a list of things you are concerned about or need to do the next day so you don't worry about them when you're trying to sleep.

- Set house rules. Speak with your family about your sleep schedule and why your sleep time is so important. Establish guidelines for everyone in your household to help maintain a peaceful sleeping environment — such as wearing headphones to listen to music or watch TV, and avoiding vacuuming, dishwashing and noisy games.

- Keep a sleep schedule. Let family and friends know your sleep schedule and ask them to call or visit at times that are convenient for you. Plan ahead for activities together.

- Unplug the phone. Be sure unimportant calls don't wake you up. Unplug the phone in your bedroom and, if necessary, get a beeper so your family can reach you in an emergency.

- Hang a do not disturb sign on your door. Make sure your family understands the conditions under which they should wake you. Make a deal with them. If they let you sleep, you will be less grumpy! And make sure delivery people and solicitors understand your sleeping rules by hanging a do not disturb sign on your front door, too.

When You Sleep Better, You Feel Better

By following as many tips as possible, you should start to experience improvements in the quality of your sleep. It won't happen right away, but if you stick with it for a week or two, you'll begin to notice positive changes. Staying alert on the job will be much easier. Drowsy driving will no longer be a problem. And you'll be able to enjoy more quality time with your family — and they'll enjoy you!

Let's Set the Record Straight

Even getting one hour less sleep per day than your body needs can impair your ability to function. And contrary to popular belief, you usually can't tell when you're about to fall asleep. What's more, when it comes to staying awake behind the wheel, many common remedies just don't work.

These Won't Keep You Awake While Driving

- Turning up the volume of your radio.

- Singing loudly.

- Chewing gum or eating food.

- Getting out of the car and running around.

- Slapping yourself.

- Sticking your head out the window.

The key is to learn to recognize the warning signs of drowsiness and to take corrective action.

Warning Signs of Drowsy Driving

- You can't stop yawning.

- You have trouble keeping your eyes open and focused, especially at stop lights.

- Your mind wanders or you have disconnected thoughts.

- You can't remember driving the last few miles.

- Your driving becomes sloppy – you weave between lanes, tail-gate or miss traffic signals.

- You find yourself hitting the grooves or rumble strips on the side of the road.

Tips to Getting Home Safely

- Avoid driving home from work if you're drowsy. Some experts recommend drinking two cups of coffee, then taking a short 15- to 20-minute nap. You'll get some sleep before the caffeine takes effect, and when it does, you'll wake up and be alert for your drive home.

- Avoid alcohol or any medications that could make you drowsy.

- Carpool if possible, so that you're driving with someone else awake in the car or get a ride from a family member.

- Take a taxi or public transportation.

- If you hit a rumble strip, it's a sure sign that you need to pull off to a safe place, take a nap or get some coffee.

But If You're Still Having Problems

Sometimes making changes in your lifestyle isn't enough. If you continue to have trouble falling asleep, staying asleep or waking too early, or if you or your significant other is a chronic snorer, see your doctor. Nonprescription sleep aids won't help you get better sleep. But rest assured, your doctor or a sleep specialist can prescribe treatment that can make quality sleep more than just a dream.

Sleep Disorders, Work Shifts, and Officer Wellness

Police work is inherently risky. Law enforcement officers face the constant threat of being attacked, wounded or even killed when confronting suspects or handling other dangerous situations in the line of duty. And the risk of being injured during routine traffic stops or roadside emergencies is all too real. In fact, law enforcement officers have one of the highest rates of on-the-job injury and illness.

But one of the greatest dangers to officers and their overall performance on the job is often overlooked—fatigue.

Law enforcement officers work demanding schedules characterized by long hours, frequent night shifts and substantial overtime. Insufficient rest or irregular sleep patterns—coupled with the stress of the job—can lead to sleep deprivation and possibly sleep disorders. The result can be severe fatigue that degrades officers' cognition, reaction time and alertness and impairs their ability to protect themselves and the communities they serve.

So how common are sleep deprivation and sleep disorders among law enforcement? And what role do demanding work schedules play?

There is a small but growing body of research examining the effects of sleep disorders and shift schedules on police officer health, safety and performance. Two recently released studies funded by National Institute of Justice (NIJ) make important additions to this research effort. The first study examines sleep disorders among law enforcement officers, and the second explores the impact of shift length on officer wellness. The findings from both have critical implications for law enforcement officers and agencies across the nation.

Sleep Disorders Common among Officers

Sleep disorders, which are typically associated with poor health, performance and safety outcomes, are twice as prevalent among law enforcement officers compared to the general public—and a new study suggests that they remain largely undiagnosed and untreated.

Researchers at Brigham and Women's Hospital examined sleep disorders and how they affected the health and safety of 4,957 state and local law enforcement officers in the United States and Canada. Using online and onsite screenings and monthly follow-up surveys, the researchers found that just over 40 percent of participating officers had at least one sleep disorder, most of which had not been previously diagnosed.

The most common sleep disorder was obstructive sleep apnea, affecting more than one-third of the officers (33.6 percent or 1,666 of 4,597 respondents). Moderate to severe insomnia came in second (6.5 percent or 281 of 4,298 respondents), followed by shift work disorder (defined as "excessive wake time sleepiness and insomnia associated with night work," affecting 5.4 percent or 269 of 4,597 respondents).

"These findings illustrate the necessity of having proper screening instruments available to detect sleep-related problems among police officers," said Brett Chapman, a social science analyst in NIJ's Office of Research and Evaluation. "Not only is this a health and wellness issue, it is also an issue that can lead to performance problems over the course of their careers."

Having any type of sleep disorder was linked to an increased risk of physical and mental health conditions, including diabetes, depression and cardiovascular disease. The researchers also found that officers with sleep disorders were more likely than their peers to make serious administrative errors or safety violations, fall asleep while driving, and experience "uncontrolled anger" toward suspects.

But the potential risks to officers—and the general public—due to fatigue are even more common than these findings suggest. According to the researchers, excessive sleepiness is common among police officers, whether they have sleep disorders or not. In fact, almost half of all participants (45.9 percent) reported having fallen asleep while driving. Approximately one-quarter (26.1 percent) reported that this occurs one to two times per month.

"This [finding] is despite police officers apparently recognizing the dangers associated with drowsy driving," the researchers wrote. "In a survey of North American police officers, almost 90 percent regarded drowsy driving to be as dangerous as drunk driving."

What Role Does Shift Length Play?

Long hours and demanding work schedules have often been cited as major contributors to officer fatigue and health problems. Traditionally, most police departments placed officers on a 40-hour workweek; officers worked 8-hour shifts for five consecutive days, followed by two days off. In recent years, however, an increasing number of agencies have moved to a compressed work schedule in which officers work, for example, four 10-hour shifts or three 12-hour shifts.

But despite the popularity of this trend, few—if any—rigorous scientific studies have examined the advantages and disadvantages of compressed work schedules for officers and agencies.

"It's clear that agencies of all sizes are increasingly departing from the traditional 40-hour workweek and implementing some type of com- pressed work schedule," said Karen Amendola, Chief Operating

Officer at the Police Foundation. "But what's not clear is the scientific basis for these changes."

"Most of the evidence concerning the benefits—and drawbacks—of a compressed work schedule has been anecdotal up to this point," Amendola added. "The few studies that have been conducted either have methodological flaws or were designed in a way that precludes conclusions about cause and effect. Consequently, agencies are scrambling for information."

To help bring some scientific evidence into the scheduling discussion, Amendola and her colleagues at the Police Foundation conducted a randomized controlled experiment that examined how shift work affects officer performance, safety, health, quality of life, fatigue and extra-duty employment. The researchers randomly assigned 275 officers in Detroit, Mich., and Arlington, Texas, to work three types of shifts for six months: five consecutive 8-hour days, four consecutive 10-hour days and three consecutive 12-hour days. The work included day, evening and midnight shifts.

Officers working the 12-hour shifts reported greater levels of sleepiness and lower levels of alertness at work than those assigned to 8-hour shifts. The researchers noted that because people often underestimate their level of fatigue and because previous research has shown that risk for accidents increases with number of hours worked, caution should be used when considering adopting 12-hour shifts.

Although there were significant differences in the amount of sleep officers got across the three shifts, the researchers found no significant differences in the quality of sleep or in reported sleep disorders.

Quality of Work Life. The data revealed no significant differences in the quality of officers' personal lives among the three shifts. However, officers working 10-hour shifts reported significantly higher quality of work life than those on 8-hour shifts. No quality of work life benefits resulted from the 12-hour shifts.

Overtime. According to the researchers, officers on 8-hour shifts worked more than five times as much overtime as those on

The researchers found that 10-hour shifts offered numerous benefits over the traditionally used 8-hour shifts: Officers get more sleep, report a significantly higher quality of work life and work less overtime.

Sleep and Fatigue. Officers working 10-hour shifts got significantly more sleep per night (more than a half hour) than those working 8-hour shifts, according to the researchers.

"This unique advantage to the 10-hour shift was surprising," admitted Amendola. "Getting a half hour more of sleep a night translates into gaining over 150 hours of sleep a year. This has tremendous implications for police officers' health and on-the-job safety." 10-hour shifts, and more than three times as much as those on 12-hour shifts. Reduced levels of overtime for officers working compressed schedules could lead to possible cost savings for agencies.

Additional Outcomes. The results revealed no significant differences among the three shift lengths on work performance, health or work- family conflict.

More Research Needed

Law enforcement officers will continue to face dangerous and stressful situations in the line of duty. Many risks are obvious—for example, gun violence and vehicle accidents. But other dangers—like fatigue—remain hidden. These all-too-common dangers can greatly hinder performance and threaten the safety of both officers and the public.

"We are all trying to keep officers and our communities safe," said Amendola. "These studies mark a good step in that direction. The findings have broad implications for law enforcement officers and agencies across the country."

"But at the same time, a lot more research is needed," she continued. "There are still questions concerning schedules and officer safety that need to be examined."

Chapter 38

Day Light Savings: Helping Workers to Adapt to the Time Change

Daylight Savings and Its Effect on Sleep

We all know the saying to help us remember to adjust our clocks for the daylight saving time changes (this Sunday in case you are wondering). But, what can we do to help workers adjust to the effects of the time change? A few studies have examined these issues but many questions remain on this topic including the best strategies to cope with the time changes.

By moving the clocks ahead one hour in the Spring, we lose one hour which shifts work times and other scheduled events one hour earlier. This pushes most people to have a one hour earlier bedtime and wake up time. In the Fall, time moves back one hour. We gain one hour which shifts work times and other scheduled events one hour later thereby pushing most people to have a one hour later bedtime and wake up time.

It can take about one week for the body to adjust the new times for sleeping, eating, and activity. Until they have adjusted, people

This chapter includes text excerpted from "Daylight Saving: Suggestions to Help Workers Adapt to the Time Change," Centers for Disease Control and Prevention (CDC), April 22, 2016.

can have trouble falling asleep, staying asleep, and waking up at the right time. This can lead to sleep deprivation and reduction in performance, increasing the risk for mistakes including vehicle crashes. Workers can experience somewhat higher risks to both their health and safety after the time changes. A study by Kirchberger and colleagues reported men and persons with heart disease may be at higher risk for a heart attack during the week after the time changes in the Spring and Fall.

The reason for these problems is thought to be disruption to circadian rhythms and sleep. Circadian rhythms are daily cycles of numerous hormones and other body functions that prepare us for the expected times for sleeping, eating, and activity. Circadian rhythms have difficulty adjusting to an abrupt one hour time change.

Other hazards for workers related to the time change in the Fall include a sudden change in the driving conditions in the late afternoon rush hour–from driving home from work during daylight hours to driving home in darkness. People may not have changed their driving habits to nighttime driving and might be at somewhat higher risk for a vehicle crash. Additionally, the Spring time change leads to more daylight in the evening which may disturb some people's sleep.

To help reduce risks about one and a half weeks before the time changes in the Fall and Spring, employers can relay these points to help their workers.

- Remind workers that several days after the time changes are associated with somewhat higher health and safety risks due to disturbances to circadian rhythms and sleep.

- It can take one week for the body to adjust sleep times and circadian rhythms to the time change so consider reducing demanding physical and mental tasks as much as possible that week to allow oneself time to adjust.

- Remind workers to be especially vigilant while driving, at work, and at home to protect themselves since others around them may be sleepier and at risk for making an error that can cause a vehicle crash or other accident.

- Research found men and people with existing heart disease may be at risk for a heart attack after the time change.

- Workers can improve their adaptation to the time change by using these suggestions. Circadian rhythms and sleep are strongly influenced by several factors including timing of exposure to light and darkness, times of eating and exercise, and time of work. One way to help the body adjust is to gradually change the times for sleep, eating, and activity.

- For the Spring time change, starting about three days before, one can gradually move up the timing of wakening and bedtime, meals, exercise, and exposure to light earlier by 15–20 minutes each day until these are in line with the new time. About one hour before bedtime, keep the lights dim and avoid electronic lit screens on computers, tablets, etc. to help the body move earlier the time it is ready to wake up in the morning and go to sleep at night.

- For the Fall time change, starting about three days before, one can gradually move the timing of wakening and bedtime, meals, exercise, and exposure to light later by 15–20 minutes each day until these are in line with the new time. About 1 hour after awakening in the morning, you can keep the lights dim and avoid electronic lit screens on computers, tablets, and so forth can help the body move to a later time that it is ready to wake up in the morning and go to sleep at night.

- Being sleep deprived before the time change will increase the health and safety risks so make it a priority to get enough sleep and be well rested several days before the time change.

Does the Time Change Effect Everyone Equally?

In short, no. People who sleep seven or less hours per day tend to have more problems with the time changes. Additionally, a person's natural tendency to get up early and go to bed early or get up late and go to bed late may also influence their ability to adjust to the one hour time changes in the Spring and Fall. Those prone to naturally follow an "early to bed and early to rise" pattern (morningness) will tend to have more difficulties adjusting to the Fall time change because this goes against their natural tenancies. Conversely, those who naturally follow a "late to bed and late to rise" routine (eveningness) will tend to have more trouble with the Spring time change.

Morningness/eveningness tends to change as people age. Teenagers and young adults tend to be "evening" types, and researchers theorize this may be due to brain and body development at those ages. Younger workers therefore may have more difficulty adjusting to the Spring time change. Morningness increases as people age, so older adults tend to be "morning" types.

As a result, older workers may have more trouble adjusting to the Fall time change. Finally, people who are on the extreme end of the eveningness or the morningness trait may tend to have more trouble adjusting their sleep to the time changes.

Chapter 39

Bedding and
Sleep Environment

Although sleep is vital to emotional and physical health, millions of people do not get the recommended 8 hours of sleep per night. Some have chronic, long-term sleep disorders, while others experience occasional trouble sleeping. Sleep deprivation can lead to daytime drowsiness, poor concentration, stress, irritability, and a weakened immune system. Among the many factors that can impact the amount and quality of sleep, bedding and the sleep environment are perhaps the easiest to control or change. Choosing a high-quality mattress, selecting the right pillow, and creating a comfortable, inviting sleep sanctuary can help people improve their sleep as well as their overall quality of life.

Environmental factors—such as light, noise, temperature, color, accessories, and bedding—play an important role in the sleep experience. Choosing comfortable bedding, making sure the bedroom temperature is neither too hot nor too cold, and eliminating sources of distracting noise or light can make a big difference in helping people get a good night's sleep. The goal is to turn the bedroom into a soothing, relaxing, indulgent escape from the everyday pressures and hassles of life. Inviting colors and attractive accessories are available from many sources to fit any space or budget.

"Bedding and Sleep Environment," © 2016 Omnigraphics. Reviewed July 2016.

Choosing a Mattress

The centerpiece of any bedroom, and the most important aspect of ensuring a comfortable, high-quality night's sleep, is the mattress. Mattresses generally have a lifespan of five to seven years, depending on usage, before the comfort and support they offer begins to decline. At this point, experts recommend evaluating the mattress and comparing it to newer models. A mattress is likely to need replacing if it shows signs of wear, such as sagging, lumps, or exposed springs. A new mattress may also be warranted if users tend to sleep better elsewhere or frequently wake up with numbness, stiffness, or pain. Research has shown that 70% of people report significant improvements in sleep comfort, 62% report improvements in sleep quality, and more than 50% report reductions in back pain and spine stiffness when sleeping on a new mattress rather than one that is five years old.

The search for a new mattress begins at a reputable mattress store with educated salespeople who can explain the various options and guide customers through the purchasing process. Since quality mattresses are major expenditures, it is important for customers to test different types and models to find the one that best meets their personal needs. Testing a mattress involves lying down for several minutes in various sleep positions while concentrating on the feel of each surface.

The main qualities to look for in a new mattress include comfort, support, durability, and size. Many types of cushioning materials are available to create a soft, plush feel. Beneath the surface, the mattress and foundation should provide gentle support that keeps the spine in alignment. The quality of materials and construction determine the durability of the mattress. The main mattress sizes, from smallest to largest, are:

- twin (38" × 75")
- full or double (53" × 75")
- queen (60" × 80")
- California king (72" × 84")
- king (76" × 80")

Since twin- and full-sized mattresses are only 75" long, they may be too short to accommodate taller adults. If two people will be sharing a bed, experts recommend buying a queen-sized or larger mattress. King-sized mattresses provide maximum sleeping space. Since an average person shifts position between 40 and 60 times per night, many people feel that a larger mattress provides them with greater freedom to move around comfortably.

There are many different types of mattresses to choose from, including:

- Innerspring, which features tempered steel coils for support beneath layers of insulation and cushioning for comfort;

- Foam, which can be made of solid foam or layers of different kinds of foam, including visco-elastic "memory" foam that molds to individual sleepers;

- Airbeds, which feature an air-filled core rather than springs for support and are usually adjustable to fit sleepers' preferences;

- Waterbeds, which feature a water-filled core for support beneath layers of upholstery for comfort and insulation;

- Adjustable beds, which feature an electric motor to allow sleepers to change the position of the head and foot of the bed to increase comfort; and

- Futons, which offer a space-saving alternative by converting into a sofa during the day.

Caring for a Mattress

After purchasing a new mattress, proper care is key to getting the most out of the investment. The first step is to ensure that the mattress and foundation are properly installed. If they have a slight "new product" odor, proper ventilation should solve the problem within a few hours. Although it is not illegal to remove the tag, it is best to leave it attached to the mattress in case it is required for a warranty claim.

Sleep sets retain their comfort and support longer if they are placed on a sturdy, high-quality bed frame. Boards should never be placed beneath the mattress to increase support. Instead, the mattress should be replaced when it reaches that stage. To keep the mattress fresh and prevent stains, it is important to use a washable mattress pad. If the mattress should require cleaning, the recommended methods are vacuuming or spot cleaning with mild soap and cold water. Mattresses should never be dry cleaned, which can damage the material, or soaked with water.

Basic mattress care involves not allowing children to jump on the bed, which can damage its interior construction. In addition, periodically rotating the mattress from top to bottom and end to end will

265

help extend its useful life. For other issues, it is best to follow the manufacturer's guidelines.

Choosing a Pillow

Pillows, like mattresses, need to be replaced periodically to ensure that they provide adequate support and comfort. The useful life of a pillow depends on its quality and the amount of use it receives. Most pillows should be replaced on an annual basis. A pillow generally must be replaced when it becomes lumpy or shows signs of dirt, stains, or wear and tear. An easy test to see whether a pillow has lost its capacity to support the head involves folding it in half and squeezing the air out. If it springs back to its original shape quickly, it still retains its support. If not, it may be time to buy a new pillow.

Ideally, a pillow should support the head in the same position as if the person were standing with an upright posture. Different amounts of cushioning are available for different sleeping positions. People who sleep on their side may want a firm pillow, while people who sleep on their back may want a somewhat softer pillow. A wide variety of pillows are available to fit any budget. Some of the different types of pillows include feather, down, memory foam, microbead, neck, lumbar, body, and wedge. Special pillows are also available for people who are pregnant or have sleep apnea.

References

1. "The Better Sleep Guide," Better Sleep Council, n.d.

2. "Pillows," Better Sleep Council, n.d.

Chapter 40

Exercise and Sleep

Overview

Exercise is an essential aspect of a healthy lifestyle. It not only promotes physical fitness, cardiovascular health, and weight management, but it can also help people sleep better. Regular exercise has been shown to reduce stress and anxiety, which often contribute to sleep problems. It can also improve physical health conditions that contribute to sleep disorders. For instance, exercise can help people lose weight, which can reduce the symptoms of sleep apnea. Improvements in sleep duration and quality, in turn, lead to greater energy, vitality, and mood—all of which can increase people's motivation to exercise, as well as improve their athletic performance.

The link between exercise and sleep is particularly important for people who are middle-aged or older. Around half of adults in this age group experience symptoms of chronic insomnia. Regular aerobic exercise can help this population combat insomnia without medication and improve their sleep and overall health. A 2010 study followed a group of sedentary women aged 60 or older who had been diagnosed with chronic insomnia. Half of the group remained inactive, while the other half engaged in a moderate exercise program over a four-month period. By the end of the study, the women who exercised 30 minutes per day were sleeping 45 to 60 minutes longer each night than the women who did not exercise. They also reported sleeping more soundly,

"Exercise and Sleep," © 2016 Omnigraphics. Reviewed July 2016.

waking up fewer times during the night, and feeling more refreshed in the morning.

Enhancing the Effects of Exercise on Sleep

Although exercise has the potential to positively impact sleep, getting the full effect depends on the timing and intensity of the workout, as well as the length of time that an exercise program is sustained. The following tips can help people with sleep difficulties maximize the benefits of exercise:

- Time workouts at least 5 to 6 hours before bedtime, if possible. Body temperature tends to rise during exercise and slowly drop back to normal afterward. This process can take several hours. Since cooler body temperatures coincide with feelings of drowsiness, exercising too close to bedtime can interfere with sleep. On the other hand, exercising in the late afternoon or early evening can help people fall asleep faster at night.

- Exercise at a moderate intensity. It is not necessary to exercise at peak intensity or to the point of exhaustion to see improvements in sleep. In fact, moderate aerobic activities such as brisk walking or bicycling seem to provide the maximum benefits. Although any increase in physical activity can lead to improvements in insomnia, studies have shown that the more people exercise, the better they tend to sleep.

- Stick with the program for at least three months. For people with insomnia or other sleep issues, research has shown that it takes time for an exercise regimen to show results. At first, they may not sleep any better than they did before starting to exercise. Researchers theorize that people with existing sleep problems have highly aroused stress systems, and that it may take several months for the effects of regular exercise to overcome this stress response. Eventually, however, people with insomnia can see improvements in sleep duration and quality that are better than those offered by other treatments or medications.

Finally, it is important to note that the connection between exercise and sleep works both ways. Just as exercise can help people sleep better, getting a good night's sleep can help people feel motivated to exercise and remain active. Studies have shown that people with insomnia often shorten or skip their workouts following nights when they have trouble sleeping. Sleep deprivation makes exercise feel harder and more tiring, and it can also detract from athletic performance. On the flip side, getting a good night's sleep can help athletes reach their potential. One study showed that college basketball players ran faster and made a higher percentage of shots when they got extra sleep the night before.

References

1. Andrews, Linda Wasmer. "How Exercise Helps You Get a Good Night's Sleep," Health Grades, November 10, 2014.

2. Hendrick, Bill. "Exercise Helps You Sleep," WebMD, September 17, 2010

3. Reynolds, Gretchen. "How Exercise Can Help Us Sleep Better," *New York Times,* August 21, 2013.

Chapter 41

Recognizing Sleep Disorders

Chapter Contents

Section 41.1

What Are the Common Symptoms of Sleep Disorder?

This section includes text excerpted from "Your Guide
to Healthy Sleep," National Heart, Lung, and Blood
Institute (NHLBI), August 2011. Reviewed July 2016.

Common Sleep Disorders

A number of sleep disorders can disrupt your sleep quality and make you overly sleepy during the day, even if you spent enough time in bed to be well rested.

More than 70 sleep disorders affect at least 40 million Americans and account for an estimated $16 billion in medical costs each year, not counting costs due to lost work time, car accidents, and other factors.

The four most common sleep disorders are insomnia, sleep apnea, restless legs syndrome, and narcolepsy. Additional sleep problems include chronic insufficient sleep, circadian rhythm abnormalities, and "parasomnias" such as sleep walking, sleep paralysis, and night terrors.

Common Signs of a Sleep Disorder

Look over this list of common signs of a sleep disorder, and talk to your doctor if you have any of them on three or more nights a week:

- It takes you more than 30 minutes to fall asleep at night.

- You awaken frequently in the night and then have trouble falling back to sleep again.

- You awaken too early in the morning.

- You often don't feel well rested despite spending 7–8 hours or more asleep at night.

- You feel sleepy during the day and fall asleep within 5 minutes if you have an opportunity to nap, or you fall asleep unexpectedly or at inappropriate times during the day.

- Your bed partner claims you snore loudly, snort, gasp, or make choking sounds while you sleep, or your partner notices that your breathing stops for short periods.

- You have creeping, tingling, or crawling feelings in your legs that are relieved by moving or massaging them, especially in the evening and when you try to fall asleep.

- You have vivid, dreamlike experiences while falling asleep or dozing.

- You have episodes of sudden muscle weakness when you are angry or fearful, or when you laugh.

- You feel as though you cannot move when you first wake up.

- Your bed partner notes that your legs or arms jerk often during sleep.

- You regularly need to use stimulants to stay awake during the day.

Also keep in mind that, although children can show some of these signs of a sleep disorder, they often do not show signs of excessive daytime sleepiness. Instead, they may seem overactive and have difficulty focusing and concentrating. They also may not do their best in school.

Section 41.2

Diagnosing Sleep Disorders

This section includes text excerpted from "Diagnosing Sleep Disorders," National Institutes of Health (NIH), December 2012. Reviewed July 2016.

If You Don't Sleep Well

If you are often tired during the day and don't feel that you sleep well, you should discuss this with your doctor or healthcare provider. Many primary care providers can diagnose sleep disorders and offer suggestions and treatments that can improve your sleep.

Keep a Sleep Diary

Before you visit the doctor, it may be very helpful for you to ask for and keep a sleep diary for a week or more. A sleep diary will give you and your doctor a picture of your sleep habits and schedules and help determine whether they may be affecting your sleep.

What to Share with Your Doctor

During your appointment your doctor will ask you about your symptoms and may have you fill out questionnaires that measure the severity of your sleep problem. It is also helpful to have your bed partner come with you to your appointment since he or she may be able to report symptoms unknown to you like loud snoring, breathing pauses, or movements during sleep.

Since older people are more likely to take medications and to have medical problems that may affect sleep, it is important for your doctor to be aware of any health condition or medication you are taking. Don't forget to mention over-the-counter medications, coffee or caffeine use, and alcohol since these also may have an impact on your sleep.

What Your Doctor Will Look For

The doctor will then perform a physical examination. During the exam the doctor will look for signs of other diseases that may affect sleep, such as Parkinson disease, stroke, heart disease, or obesity. If your doctor feels more information is needed, he or she may refer you to a sleep center for more testing.

Sleep Tests

Sleep centers employ physicians and others who are experts in problems that affect sleep. If the sleep specialist needs more information, he or she may ask you to undergo an overnight sleep study, also called a polysomnogram, and/or a daytime sleepiness, or a nap test. A polysomnogram is a test that measures brain waves, heart rate, breathing patterns and body movements.

A common sleepiness test is the multiple sleep latency test. During this test, the person has an opportunity to nap every two hours during the daytime. If the person falls asleep too quickly it may mean that he or she has too much daytime sleepiness.

Table 41.1. Daily Sleep Diary

Daily Sleep Diary					
Today's Date					
1. Last night, I took sleep medication. (yes or no)					
2. What time did you go to bed last night?					
3. After turning the lights off, how long did it take you to fall asleep?					
4. How long were you awake during the night?					
5. What time did you wake up this morning? (your last awakening in the morning)					
6. Overall, my sleep last night was_____: 1 = very restless 2 = restless 3 = average quality 4 = sound 5 = very sound					
Comments:					

Chapter 42

What You Need to Know about Sleep Studies

What Are Sleep Studies?

Sleep studies are tests that measure how well you sleep and how your body responds to sleep problems. These tests can help your doctor find out whether you have a sleep disorder and how severe it is.

Sleep studies are important because untreated sleep disorders can raise your risk for heart disease, high blood pressure, stroke, and other medical conditions. Sleep disorders also have been linked to an increased risk of injury, such as falling (in the elderly) and car accidents.

People usually aren't aware of their breathing and movements while sleeping. They may never think to talk to their doctors about issues that might be related to sleep problems.

However, sleep disorders can be treated. Talk with your doctor if you snore regularly or feel very tired while at work or school most days of the week.

You also may want to talk with your doctor if you often have trouble falling or staying asleep, or if you wake up too early and aren't able to go back to sleep. These are common signs of a sleep disorder.

This chapter includes text excerpted from "Sleep Studies," National Heart, Lung, and Blood Institute (NHLBI), March 29, 2012. Reviewed July 2016.

Your doctor might be able to diagnose a sleep disorder based on your sleep schedule and habits. However, he or she also might need the results from sleep studies and other medical tests to diagnose a sleep disorder.

Sleep studies can help diagnose:

- Sleep-related breathing disorders, such as sleep apnea

- Sleep-related seizure disorders

- Sleep-related movement disorders, such as periodic limb movement disorder

- Sleep disorders that cause extreme daytime tiredness, such as narcolepsy

Doctors might use sleep studies to help diagnose or rule out restless legs syndrome (RLS). However, RLS usually is diagnosed based on signs and symptoms, medical history, and a physical exam.

Types of Sleep Studies

To diagnose sleep-related problems, doctors may use one or more of the following sleep studies:

- Polysomnogram, or PSG

- Multiple sleep latency test, or MSLT

- Maintenance of wakefulness test, or MWT

- Home-based portable monitor

Your doctor may use actigraphy if he or she thinks you have a circadian rhythm disorder. This is a disorder that disrupts your body's natural sleep–wake cycle.

Polysomnogram

For a PSG, you usually will stay overnight at a sleep center. This study records brain activity, eye movements, heart rate, and blood pressure.

A PSG also records the amount of oxygen in your blood, air movement through your nose while you breathe, snoring, and chest movements. The chest movements show whether you're making an effort to breathe.

PSG results are used to help diagnose:

- Sleep-related breathing disorders, such as sleep apnea

- Sleep-related seizure disorders

- Sleep-related movement disorders, such as periodic limb movement disorder

- Sleep disorders that cause extreme daytime tiredness, such as narcolepsy (PSG and MSLT results will be reviewed together)

Your doctor also may use a PSG to find the right setting for you on a CPAP (continuous positive airway pressure) machine. CPAP is a treatment for sleep apnea.

Sleep apnea is a common disorder in which you have one or more pauses in breathing or shallow breaths while you sleep. In obstructive sleep apnea, the airway collapses or becomes blocked during sleep. A CPAP machine uses mild air pressure to keep your airway open while you sleep.

If your doctor thinks that you have sleep apnea, he or she might schedule a split-night sleep study. During the first half of the night, your sleep is checked without a CPAP machine. This will show whether you have sleep apnea and how severe it is.

If the PSG shows that you have sleep apnea, you'll use a CPAP machine during the second half of the split-night study. A technician will help you select a CPAP mask that fits and is comfortable.

While you sleep, the technician will check the amount of oxygen in your blood and whether your airway stays open. He or she will adjust the flow of air through the mask to find the setting that's right for you. This process is called CPAP titration.

Sometimes the entire study isn't done during the same night. Some people need to go back to the sleep center for the CPAP titration study.

Also, some people might need more than one PSG. For example, your doctor may recommend a follow up PSG to:

- Adjust your CPAP settings after weight loss or weight gain

- Recheck your sleep if symptoms return despite treatment with CPAP

- Find out how well surgery has worked to correct a sleep-related breathing disorder

Multiple Sleep Latency Test

This daytime sleep study measures how sleepy you are. It typically is done the day after a PSG. You relax in a dark, quiet room for about 30 minutes while a technician checks your brain activity.

279

The MSLT records whether you fall asleep during the test and what types and stages of sleep you're having. Sleep has two basic types: rapid eye movement (REM) and non-REM. Non-REM sleep has three distinct stages. REM sleep and the three stages of non-REM sleep occur in regular cycles throughout the night.

The types and stages of sleep you have can help your doctor diagnose sleep disorders such as narcolepsy, idiopathic hypersomnia, and other sleep disorders that cause daytime tiredness.

An MSLT takes place over the course of a full day. This is because your ability to fall asleep changes throughout the day.

Maintenance of Wakefulness Test

This daytime sleep study measures your ability to stay awake and alert. It's usually done the day after a PSG and takes most of the day.

Results can show whether your inability to stay awake is a public or personal safety concern. Results also can show how you're responding to treatment.

Home-Based Portable Monitor

Your doctor may recommend a home-based sleep test with a portable monitor. The portable monitor will record some of the same information as a PSG. For example, it may record:

- The amount of oxygen in your blood
- Air movement through your nose while you breathe
- Your heart rate
- Chest movements that show whether you're making an effort to breathe

A sleep specialist might use the results from a home-based sleep test to help diagnose sleep apnea. He or she also might use the results to see how well some treatments for sleep apnea are working.

Home-based testing is appropriate only for some people. Talk with your doctor to find out whether a portable monitor is an option for you. If your doctor recommends this test, you'll need to visit a sleep center or your doctor's office to pick up the equipment and learn how to use it.

If you're diagnosed with sleep apnea, your doctor may prescribe treatment with CPAP. If so, he or she will need to find the correct airflow setting for your CPAP machine. To do this, you may need to go to a sleep center to have a PSG. Or, you may be able to find the correct setting at home with an autotitrating CPAP machine.

An autotitrating CPAP machine automatically finds the right air-flow setting for you. These machines work well for some people who have sleep apnea. A technician or a doctor will teach you how to use the machine.

Actigraphy

Actigraphy is a test that's done while you do your normal daily routine. This test is useful for all age groups and doesn't require an overnight stay at a sleep center.

An actigraph is a simple device that's usually worn like a wrist-watch. Your doctor may ask you to wear the device for several days and nights, except when bathing or swimming.

Actigraphy gives your doctor a better idea about your sleep schedule, such as when you sleep or nap and whether the lights are on while you sleep.

Doctors can use actigraphy to help diagnose many sleep disorders, including circadian rhythm disorders (such as jet lag and shift work disorder). Doctors also may use the test to check how well sleep treatments are working.

Actigraphy might be used with a PSG or alone.

Who Needs a Sleep Study?

Your doctor might not detect a sleep problem during a routine office visit because you're awake. Thus, you should let your doctor know if you or a family member/sleep partner thinks you might have a sleep problem.

For example, talk with your doctor if you:

- Have chronic (ongoing) snoring
- Often feel sleepy during the day, even though you've spent enough time in bed to be well rested
- Don't wake up feeling refreshed and alert
- Have trouble adapting to shift work

Your doctor might be able to diagnose a sleep disorder based on your sleep schedule and habits. However, he or she also might need the results from sleep studies and other medical tests to diagnose a sleep disorder.

Sleep studies often are used to diagnose sleep-related breathing disorders, such as sleep apnea. Signs of these disorders include loud snoring, gasping, or choking sounds while you sleep or pauses in breathing during sleep.

Other common signs and symptoms of sleep disorders include the following:

- It takes you more than 30 minutes to fall asleep at night.

- You often wake up during the night and then have trouble falling asleep again, or you wake up too early and aren't able to go back to sleep.

- You feel sleepy during the day and fall asleep within 5 minutes if you have a chance to nap, or you fall asleep at inappropriate times during the day.

- You have creeping, tingling, or crawling feelings in your legs that you can relieve by moving or massaging them, especially in the evening and when you try to fall asleep.

- You have vivid, dreamlike experiences while falling asleep or dozing.

- You have episodes of sudden muscle weakness when you're angry, fearful, or when you laugh.

- You feel as though you can't move when you first wake up.

- Your bed partner notes that your legs or arms jerk often during sleep.

- You regularly feel the need to use stimulants, such as caffeine, to stay awake during the day.

Many of the same signs and symptoms of sleep disorders can occur in infants and children. If your child snores or has other signs or symptoms of sleep problems, talk with his or her doctor.

If you've had a sleep disorder for a long time, you may not notice how it affects your daily routine.

Your doctor will work with you to decide whether you need a sleep study. A sleep study allows your doctor to observe sleep patterns and diagnose a sleep disorder, which can then be treated.

Certain medical conditions have been linked to sleep disorders, such as heart failure, kidney disease, high blood pressure, diabetes, stroke, obesity, and depression.

If you have or have had one of these conditions, ask your doctor whether it would be helpful to have a sleep study.

What to Expect before a Sleep Study

Before a sleep study, your doctor may ask you about your sleep habits and whether you feel well rested and alert during the day.

Your doctor also may ask you to keep a sleep diary. You'll record information such as when you went to bed, when you woke up, how many times you woke up during the night, and more.

What to Bring with You

Depending on what type of sleep study you're having, you may need to bring:

- Notes from your sleep diary. These notes may help your doctor.

- Pajamas and a toothbrush for overnight sleep studies.

- A book or something to do between testing periods if you're having a maintenance of wakefulness test (MWT) or multiple sleep latency test (MSLT).

How to Prepare

Your doctor may advise you to stop or limit the use of tobacco, caffeine, and other stimulants before having a sleep study.

Your doctor also may ask whether you're taking any medicines. Make sure you tell your doctor about all of the medicines you're taking, including over-the-counter products. Some medicines can affect the sleep study results.

Your doctor also may ask about any allergies you have.

You should try to sleep well for 2 nights before having a sleep study. If you're being tested as a requirement for a transportation- or safety-related job, you might be asked to take a drug-screening test.

If you're going to have a home-based sleep test with a portable monitor, you'll need to visit a sleep center or your doctor's office to pick up the equipment. Your doctor or a technician will show you how to use the equipment.

What to Expect during a Sleep Study

Sleep studies are painless. The polysomnogram (PSG), multiple sleep latency test (MSLT), and maintenance of wakefulness test (MWT) usually are done at a sleep center.

The room the sleep study is done in may look like a hotel room. A technician makes the room comfortable for you and sets the temperature to your liking.

Most of your contact at the sleep center will be with nurses or technicians. They can answer questions about the test itself, but they usually can't give you the test results.

During a Polysomnogram

Sticky patches with sensors called electrodes are placed on your scalp, face, chest, limbs, and a finger. While you sleep, these sensors record your brain activity, eye movements, heart rate and rhythm, blood pressure, and the amount of oxygen in your blood.

Elastic belts are placed around your chest and belly. They measure chest movements and the strength and duration of inhaled and exhaled breaths.

Wires attached to the sensors transmit the data to a computer in the next room. The wires are very thin and flexible. They are bundled together so they don't restrict movement, disrupt your sleep, or cause other discomfort.

If you have signs of sleep apnea, you may have a split-night sleep study. During the first half of the night, the technician records your sleep patterns. At the start of the second half of the night, he or she wakes you to fit a CPAP (continuous positive airway pressure) mask over your nose and/or mouth.

A small machine gently blows air through the mask. This creates mild pressure that keeps your airway open while you sleep.

The technician checks how you sleep with the CPAP machine. He or she adjusts the flow of air through the mask to find the setting that's right for you.

At the end of the PSG, the technician removes the sensors. If you're having a daytime sleep study, such as an MSLT, some of the sensors might be left on for that test.

Parents usually are required to spend the night with their child during the child's PSG.

During a Multiple Sleep Latency Test

The MSLT is a daytime sleep study that's usually done after a PSG. This test often involves sensors placed on your scalp, face, and chin. These sensors record brain activity and eye movements. They show various stages of sleep and how long it takes you to fall asleep. Sometimes your breathing is checked during an MSLT.

A technician in another room watches these recordings as you sleep. He or she fixes any problems that occur with the recordings.

About 2 hours after you wake from the PSG, you're asked to relax and try to fall asleep in a dark, quiet room. The test is repeated four or five times throughout the day. This is because your ability to fall asleep changes throughout the day.

You get 2-hour breaks between tests. You need to stay awake during the breaks.

The MSLT records whether you fall asleep during the test and what types and stages of sleep you have. Sleep has two basic types: rapid eye movement (REM) and non-REM. Non-REM sleep has three distinct stages. REM sleep and the three stages of non-REM sleep occur in regular cycles throughout the night.

The types and stages of sleep you have during the day can help your doctor diagnose sleep disorders such as narcolepsy, idiopathic hypersomnia, and other sleep disorders that cause daytime tiredness.

During a Maintenance of Wakefulness Test

This sleep study usually is done the day after a PSG, and it takes most of the day. Sensors on your scalp, face, and chin are used to measure when you're awake and asleep.

You sit quietly on a chair in a comfortable position and look straight ahead. Then you simply try to stay awake for a period of time.

An MWT typically includes four trials lasting about 40 minutes each. If you fall asleep, the technician will wake you after about 90 seconds. There usually are 2-hour breaks between trials. During these breaks, you can read, watch television, etc.

If you're being tested as a requirement for a transportation- or safety-related job, you may need a drug-screening test before an MWT.

During a Home-Based Portable Monitor Test

If you're having a home-based portable monitor test, you'll need to set up the equipment at home before you go to sleep.

When you pick up the equipment at the sleep center or your doctor's office, someone will show you how to use it. In some cases, a technician will come to your home to help you prepare for the study.

During Actigraphy

You don't have to go to a sleep center for this test. An actigraph is a small device that's usually worn like a wristwatch. You can do your normal daily routine while you wear it. You remove it while bathing or swimming.

The actigraph measures your sleep–wake behavior over 3 to 14 days and nights. Results give your doctor a better idea about your sleep habits, such as when you sleep or nap and whether the lights are on while you sleep.

Your doctor may ask you to keep a sleep diary while you wear an actigraph.

About 1.5 to 3 hours after you wake from the PSG, you're asked to relax in a quiet room for about 30 minutes. The test is repeated four or five times throughout the day. This is because your ability to fall asleep changes throughout the day.

You get 2-hour breaks between tests. You need to stay awake during the breaks.

The MSLT records whether you fall asleep during the test and what types and stages of sleep you have. Sleep has two basic types: rapid eye movement (REM) and non-REM. Non-REM sleep has three distinct stages. REM sleep and the three stages of non-REM sleep occur in patterns throughout the night.

The types and stages of sleep you have during the day can help your doctor diagnose sleep disorders such as narcolepsy and idiopathic hypersomnia.

What to Expect after a Sleep Study

Once the sensors are removed after a polysomnogram (PSG), multiple sleep latency test, or maintenance of wakefulness test, you can go home. If you used an actigraph or a home-based portable monitor, you'll return the equipment to a sleep center or your doctor's office.

You won't receive a diagnosis right away. A sleep specialist and your primary care doctor will review the results of your sleep study. They will use your medical history, your sleep history, and the test results to make a diagnosis.

You may not get the sleep study results for a couple of weeks. Usually, your doctor, nurse, or sleep specialist will explain the test results and work with you to develop a treatment plan.

What Do Sleep Studies Show?

Sleep studies allow doctors to look at sleep patterns and note sleep-related problems that patients don't know about or can't describe during routine office visits. Sleep studies are needed to diagnose certain sleep disorders, such as sleep apnea and narcolepsy.

Your sleep study results might include information about sleep and wake times, sleep stages, abnormal breathing, the amount of oxygen in your blood, and any movement during sleep.

Your doctor will use your sleep study results and your medical history to make a diagnosis and create a treatment plan.

Results from a Polysomnogram

Polysomnogram (PSG) results are used to help diagnose:

- Sleep-related breathing disorders, such as sleep apnea

- Sleep-related seizure disorders

- Sleep-related movement disorders, such as periodic limb movement disorder

- Sleep disorders that cause extreme daytime tiredness, such as narcolepsy (PSG and MSLT results will be reviewed together)

If you have sleep apnea, your doctor also may use a PSG to find the correct setting for you on a CPAP(continuous positive airway pressure) machine.

A CPAP machine supplies air to your nose and/or mouth through a special mask. Finding the right setting involves adding just enough extra air to create mild pressure that keeps your airway open while you sleep.

Your doctor may recommend a follow up PSG to:

- Adjust your CPAP settings after weight loss or weight gain

- Recheck your sleep if symptoms return despite treatment with CPAP

- Find out how well surgery has worked to correct a sleep-related breathing disorder

Technicians also use PSGs to record the number of abnormal breathing events that occur with sleep-related breathing disorders, such as sleep apnea. These events include pauses in breathing or dips in the level of oxygen in your blood.

Results from a Multiple Sleep Latency Test

MSLT results are used to help diagnose narcolepsy, idiopathic hypersomnia, and other sleep disorders that cause daytime sleepiness.

For narcolepsy, technicians study how quickly you fall asleep. The MSLT also shows how long it takes you to reach different types and stages of sleep.

Sleep has two basic types: rapid eye movement (REM) and non-REM. Non-REM sleep has three distinct stages. REM sleep and the three stages of non-REM sleep occur in regular cycles throughout the night.

People who fall asleep in less than 5 minutes or quickly reach REM sleep may need treatment for a sleep disorder.

Results from a Maintenance of Wakefulness Test

Maintenance of wakefulness test (MWT) results can show whether your inability to stay awake is a public or personal safety concern. This test also is used to show how well treatment for a sleep disorder is working.

Results from a Home-Based Portable Monitor Test

Home-based portable monitors might be used to help diagnose sleep apnea. Portable monitors also can show how well some treatments for sleep apnea are working.

Sometimes, home-based monitors don't record enough information. If this happens, you might have to take the monitor home again and repeat the test, or your sleep specialist may ask you to have a PSG.

Results from Actigraphy

Actigraphy results give your doctor a better idea about your sleep habits, such as when you sleep or nap and whether the lights are on while you sleep. This test also is used to help diagnose circadian rhythm disorders.

What Are the Risks of Sleep Studies?

Sleep studies are painless. There's a small risk of skin irritation from the sensors. The irritation will go away once the sensors are removed.

Although the risks of sleep studies are minimal, these studies take time (at least several hours). If you're having a daytime sleep study, bring a book or something to do during the test.

Chapter 43

Sleep Medication

Chapter Contents

Section 43.1

Prescription Sleep Aid Use among Adults

This section includes text excerpted from "Prescription Sleep Aid
Use among Adults: United States, 2005–2010," Centers for Disease
Control and Prevention (CDC), August 2013.

Key Findings

Data from the National Health and Nutrition Examination Survey, 2005–2010

- About 4% of U.S. adults aged 20 and over used prescription
  sleep aids in the past month.

- The percentage of adults using a prescription sleep aid increased
  with age and education. More adult women (5.0%) used prescription sleep aids than adult men (3.1%).

- Non-Hispanic white adults were more likely to use sleep aids
  (4.7%) than non-Hispanic black (2.5%) and Mexican-American
  (2.0%) adults.

- Prescription sleep aid use varied by sleep duration and was
  highest among adults who sleep less than 5 hours (6.0%) or sleep
  9 or more hours (5.3%).

- One in six adults with a diagnosed sleep disorder and one in
  eight adults with trouble sleeping reported using sleep aids.

Sedative and hypnotic medications, often referred to as sleep aids,
are used to induce or maintain sleep by suppressing activities in the
central nervous system. In the past two decades, both popular media
and pharmaceutical companies have reported an increased number
of prescriptions filled for sleep aids in the United States. In fact, a
market research firm has reported a tripling in sleep aid prescriptions
from 1998 to 2006 for young adults aged 18–24. This report presents
person-based nationally representative estimates on prescription sleep
aid use in the past 30 days, describes sociodemographic differences in
use, and examines sleep aid use by self-reported sleep duration and
insomnia.

Prescription Sleep Aid Use in the past 30 Days Increased with Age

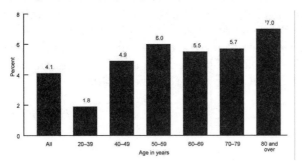

Figure 43.1. *Percentage of adults aged 20 and over who used prescription sleep aids in the past 30 days, by age: United States, 2005–2010*

Sleep aids include all hypnotic drugs and four antidepressant or sedative medications commonly prescribed for insomnia or depression.
SOURCE: CDC/NCHS, National Health and Nutrition Examination Survey.

During 2005–2010, about 4% of U.S. adults aged 20 and over reported that they took prescription sleep aids in the past 30 days. Prevalence of use was lowest among the youngest age group (those aged 20–39) at about 2%, increased to 6% among those aged 50–59, and reached 7% among those aged 80 and over.

Prescription Sleep Aid Use in the past 30 Days Varied by Sex and Race and Ethnicity

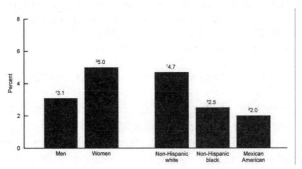

Figure 43.2. *Prescription sleep aid use in the past 30 days varied by sex and race and ethnicity.*

Data are age-adjusted to the 2000 projected U.S. standard population using the age groups 20–39, 40–59, and 60 and over. Sleep aids include all hypnotic drugs and four antidepressant or sedative medications commonly prescribed for insomnia or depression.
SOURCE: CDC/NCHS, National Health and Nutrition Examination Survey.

Reported prescription sleep aid use in the past 30 days was higher among women (5.0%) than men (3.1%). Non-Hispanic white adults reported higher use of sleep aids (4.7%) than non-Hispanic black (2.5%) and Mexican-American (2.0%) adults. No difference was shown between non-Hispanic black adults and Mexican-American adults in use of prescription sleep aids (Figure 43.2.).

Prescription Sleep Aid Use in the past 30 Days Increased with Higher Education

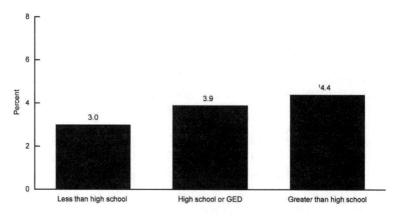

Figure 43.3. *Age-adjusted percentage of adults aged 20 and over who used prescription sleep aids in the past 30 days, by education: United States, 2005–2010*

GED is General Educational Development high school equivalency diploma. Data are age-adjusted to the 2000 projected U.S. standard population using the age groups 20–39, 40–59, and 60 and over. Sleep aids include all hypnotic drugs and four antidepressant or sedative medications commonly prescribed for insomnia or depression.
SOURCE: CDC/NCHS, National Health and Nutrition Examination Survey.

Three percent of adults with less than a high school education reported using sleep aids in the past 30 days, compared with 3.9% with a high school diploma and 4.4% of adults with greater than a high school education (Figure 43.3.).

Prescription Sleep Aid Use in the past 30 Days Varied by Sleep Duration

The National Sleep Foundation suggests that 7 hours of sleep is the minimum amount of sleep that adults need on a regular basis for optimal performance, thus 7 hours is used as the reference point for sleep duration. Compared with those who reported 7 hours of sleep (3.2%), adults with 5 or fewer hours of sleep per night had the highest use of sleep aids in the past 30 days (6.0%). Those with 6 hours of sleep (3.8%) did not significantly differ from the reference group, whereas those with 8 hours (4.1%) or 9 or more hours (5.3%) of sleep showed higher usage of sleep aids. In other words, when sleep duration was greater or less than 7 hours, the use of sleep aids increased (Figure 43.4.).

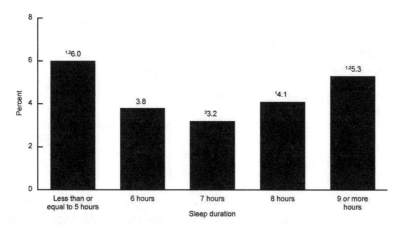

Figure 43.4. *Age-adjusted percentage of adults aged 20 and over who used prescription sleep aids in the past 30 days, by sleep duration: United States, 2005–2010*

Data are age-adjusted to the 2000 projected U.S. standard population using the age groups 20–39, 40–59, and 60 and over. Sleep aids include all hypnotic drugs and four antidepressant or sedative medications commonly prescribed for insomnia or depression. SOURCE: CDC/NCHS, National Health and Nutrition Examination Survey.

Prescription Sleep Aid Use in the past 30 Days Was Higher among Adults with Diagnosed Sleep Disorders and among Adults with Trouble Sleeping

Over 16% of adults who reported a physician's diagnosis of a sleep disorder reported using sleep aids in the past 30 days, which was more than five times higher than those who did not report such a diagnosis. About 13% of adults who told their doctor that they had trouble sleeping reported sleep aid use, which was nearly 12 times higher than those who did not report any trouble sleeping (Figure 43.5.).

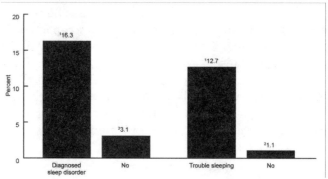

Figure 43.5. **Age-adjusted percentage of adults aged 20 and over who** *used prescription sleep aids in the past 30 days, by physician-diagnosed sleep disorder and self-reported trouble going to sleep: United States, 2005–2010*
Data are age-adjusted to the 2000 projected U.S. standard population using the age groups 20–39, 40–59, and 60 and over. Sleep aids include all hypnotic drugs and four antidepressant or sedative medications commonly prescribed for insomnia or depression.
SOURCE: CDC/NCHS, National Health and Nutrition Examination Survey.

Summary

According to estimates, 50–70 million Americans suffer from sleep disorders or deprivation, which can not only hinder daily functioning, but can also adversely affect their health. Prescription sleep aids are one of the treatment options for trouble going into or maintaining sleep. However, long-term use of sleep aids has been linked to adverse outcomes in health.

So far, studies on sleep aid use are mostly based on administrative claims data, which describe the number of times sleep aid prescriptions are filled rather than how many people have actually used prescription sleep aids. This report provides the first person-based national data on prescription sleep aid use among the noninstitutionalized U.S. adult population. Approximately 4% of adults aged 20 and over reported using a prescription sleep aid in the past month. Use increased with age and was more common among women, non-Hispanic white adults, and those with greater than a high school education. Use also varied by sleep duration and was significantly higher among adults who reported sleep disorders or trouble sleeping.

Section 43.2

Medicines to Help You Sleep

This section contains text excerpted from the following sources: Text in this section begins with excerpts from "Sleep Problems," U.S. Food and Drug Administration (FDA), September 28, 2015; Text under the heading "Prescription Insomnia Drugs" is excerpted from "Sleep Disorder (Sedative-Hypnotic) Drug Information," U.S. Food and Drug Administration (FDA), July 8, 2015.

There are medicines that may help you fall asleep or stay asleep. You need a doctor's prescription for some sleep drugs. You can get other over-the-counter (OTC) medicines without a prescription.

Prescription

Prescription sleep medicines work well for many people but they can cause serious side effects.

- Talk to your doctor about all of the risks and benefits of using prescription sleep medicines.

- Sleep drugs taken for insomnia can affect your driving the morning after use.

- Sleep drugs can cause rare side effects like:

  - Severe allergic reactions

  - Severe face swelling

  - Behaviors like making phone calls, eating, having sex or driving while you are not fully awake

Over-the-Counter (OTC)

OTC sleep drugs have side effects too. Read the 'Drug Facts Label' to learn more about the side effects of your OTC sleep medicine.

Tips for Better Sleep

Making some changes to your night time habits may help you get the sleep you need.

- Go to bed and get up at the same times each day
- Sleep in a dark, quiet room.
- Avoid caffeine and nicotine.
- Don't drink alcohol before bedtime.
- Do something to help you relax before bedtime.
- Don't exercise before bedtime.
- Don't take a nap after 3 p.m.
- Don't eat a large meal before you go to sleep.

Talk to your healthcare provider if you have trouble sleeping almost every night for more than 2 weeks.

Prescription Insomnia Drugs

- Ambien, Ambien CR (zolpidem tartrate)
- Butisol sodium (butabarbital sodium)
- Carbtrital (pentobarbital and carbromal)
- Dalmane (flurazepam hydrochloride)
- Doral (quazepam)
- Edluar (zolpidem tartrate)
- Halcion (triazolam)
- Intermezzo (zolpidem)
- Lunesta (eszopiclone)
- Placidyl (ethchlorvynol)
- Prosom (estazolam)
- Restoril (temazepam)
- Rozerem (ramelteon)
- Seconal (secobarbital sodium)
- Silenor (doxepin hydrochloride)

- Sonata (zaleplon)

- Zolpimist (zolpidem tartrate)

Over-the-Counter (OTC) Insomnia Drugs

- Benadryl (diphenhydramine)

- Unisom (doxylamine)

Section 43.3

Side Effects of Sleep Drugs

This section contains text excerpted from the following sources:
Text in this section begins with excerpts from "Side Effects of Sleep
Drugs," U.S. Food and Drug Administration (FDA), April 11, 2016;
Text beginning with the heading "Some Sleep Drugs Can Impair
Driving" is excerpted from "Some Sleep Drugs Can Impair Driving,"
U.S. Food and Drug Administration (FDA), April 11, 2016.

Eating a little bit of chocolate was a treat that Teresa Wood looked forward to after work. The Fairfax Station, Va., resident allowed herself two small pieces of chocolate candy a day.

But after taking a drug to help her sleep at night, Wood awoke in the morning to find an empty box on the table in place of a pound of chocolates that had been there the night before.

"I couldn't believe it," says Wood. "I started looking all around the house—I even looked under the bed. I thought for sure someone came into the house during the night and ate them." But she was alone.

A few weeks later, Wood awoke to find a near-full box of chocolates gone again. "I just don't remember eating all that candy," she says.

Complex Sleep-Related Behaviors

Wood and her doctor determined that she had been getting up during the night and "sleep eating," an occurrence known as a complex sleep-related behavior. Other behaviors include making phone calls, having sex, and getting into the car and driving while not fully awake. Most people do not remember these events later.

Complex behaviors are a potential side effect of sedative-hypnotic products—a class of drugs used to help a person fall asleep and stay asleep.

"Complex behaviors, such as sleep-driving, could be potentially dangerous to both the patients and to others," says Russell Katz, M.D., Director of the U.S. Food and Drug Administration's (FDA) Division of Neurology Products.

Allergic Reactions

Other rare but potential side effects of sedative-hypnotic drugs are a severe allergic reaction (anaphylaxis) and severe facial swelling (angioedema), which can occur as early as the first time the product is taken.

"Severe allergic reactions can affect a patient's ability to breathe and can affect other body systems as well, and can even be fatal at times," says Katz. "Although these allergic reactions are probably very rare, people should be aware that they can occur, because these reactions may be difficult to notice as people are falling asleep."

Stronger Warnings

To make known the risks of these products, FDA requested in early 2007 that all manufacturers of sedative-hypnotic drug products strengthen their product labeling to include warnings about complex sleep-related behaviors and anaphylaxis and angioedema.

"There are a number of prescription sleep aids available that are well-tolerated and effective for many people," says Steven Galson, M.D., M.P.H., Director of FDA's Center for Drug Evaluation and Research. However, after reviewing the available information on adverse events that occurred after the sedative-hypnotic drugs were on the market, FDA concluded that labeling changes were necessary to inform healthcare providers and consumers about risks, says Galson.

In addition to the labeling changes, FDA has requested that manufacturers of sedative-hypnotic products

- send letters to healthcare providers to notify them about the new warnings.

- develop Patient Medication Guides for the products to inform consumers about risks and advise them of precautions that can be taken. (Patient Medication Guides are handouts given to patients, families, and caregivers when a medicine is dispensed. The guides will contain FDA-approved information, such as proper use and the recommendation to avoid ingesting alcohol or other central nervous system depressants.)

- conduct clinical studies to investigate the frequency with which sleep-driving and other complex behaviors occur in association with individual drug products.

The revised labeling and other actions to make risks known affect these sedative-hypnotic products:

- Ambien, Ambien CR (zolpidem tartrate)
- Butisol sodium
- Carbrital (pentobarbital and carbromal)
- Dalmane (flurazepam hydrochloride)
- Doral (quazepam)
- Halcion (triazolam)
- Lunesta (eszopiclone)
- Placidyl (ethchlorvynol)
- Prosom (estazolam)
- Restoril (temazepam)
- Rozerem (ramelteon)
- Seconal (secobarbital sodium)
- Sonata (zaleplon)

Precautions

FDA advises people who are treated with any of these products to take the following precautions:

- Talk to your healthcare provider before you start these medications and if you have any questions or concerns.

- Read the Medication Guide, when available, before taking the product.

- Do not increase the dose prescribed by your healthcare provider. Complex sleep-related behaviors are more likely to occur with higher than appropriate doses.

- Do not drink alcohol or take other drugs that depress the nervous system.

- Do not discontinue the use of these medications without first talking to your healthcare provider.

Over-the-Counter Sleep Aids

Not all sleep medications are prescription. FDA has approved over-the-counter (OTC) medications for use up to two weeks to help relieve occasional sleepiness in people ages 12 and older. "If you continue to have sleeping problems beyond two weeks, you should see a doctor," says Marina Chang, R.Ph., pharmacist and team leader in FDA's Division of Nonprescription Regulation Development.

OTC sleep aids are non-habit-forming and do not present the risk of allergic reactions and complex sleep-related behaviors that are known to occur with sedative-hypnotic drugs.

But just because they're available over-the-counter doesn't mean they don't have side effects, says Chang. "They don't have the same level of precision as the prescription drugs. They don't completely stop working after 8 hours—many people feel drowsy for longer than 8 hours after taking them."

Chang advises reading the product label and exercising caution when taking OTC sleep aids until you learn how they will affect you. "They affect people differently," she says. "They are not for everybody."

Some Sleep Drugs Can Impair Driving

Many people take sedatives to help them sleep. The U.S. Food and Drug Administration (FDA) is reminding consumers that some drugs to treat insomnia could make them less able the next morning to perform activities for which they must be fully alert, including driving a car.

FDA has informed manufacturers that the recommended dose should be lowered for sleep drugs approved for bedtime use that contain a medicine called zolpidem. FDA is also evaluating the risk of next-morning impairment in other insomnia medications.

People with insomnia have trouble falling or staying asleep. Zolpidem, which belongs to a class of medications called sedative-hypnotics, is a common ingredient in widely prescribed sleep medications. Some sleep drugs contain an extended-release form of zolpidem that stays in the body longer than the regular form.

FDA is particularly concerned about extended-release forms of zolpidem. They are sold as generic drugs and under the brand name Ambien CR. New data show that the morning after use, many people who take products containing extended-release zolpidem have drug levels that are high enough to impair driving and other activities. FDA says that women are especially vulnerable because zolpidem is cleared from the body more slowly in women than in men.

FDA also found that some medicines containing the immediate-release form of zolpidem can impair driving and other activities the next morning. They are marketed as generic drugs and under the following brand names:

- Ambien (oral tablet)
- Edluar (tablet placed under the tongue)
- Zolpimist (oral spray)

FDA has informed the manufacturers of products containing zolpidem that the recommended dose for women for both immediate- and extended-release products should be lowered. FDA is also suggesting a lower dose range for men.

Drowsiness is already listed as a side effect in the drug labels of insomnia drugs, along with warnings that patients may still feel drowsy the day after taking these products. However, people with high levels of zolpidem in their blood can be impaired even if they feel wide awake. "All insomnia drugs are potent medications, and they must be used carefully," says Russell Katz, M.D., director of FDA's Division of Neurology Products.

Recommended Doses

FDA has informed manufacturers that changes to the dosage recommendations for the use of zolpidem products should be made:

For women, dosing should be cut in half, from 10mg to 5mg for products containing the regular form of zolpidem (Ambien, Edluar, Zolpimist) and from 12.5 mg to 6.25 mg for zolpidem extended-release products (Ambien CR).

For men, the lower dose of 5mg for immediate-release zolpidem and 6.25 mg for extended-release should be considered.

Intermezzo, a more recently approved drug containing zolpidem, is used when middle-of-the-night wakening is followed by difficulty returning to sleep and at least 4 hours remain available for sleep. The recommended dose for Intermezzo remains at 1.75 mg for women and 3.5 mg for men.

FDA is evaluating the risk of next-day impairment with other insomnia drugs, both prescription and over-the-counter (OTC) drugs.

Most Widely Used Sleep Drug

Zolpidem—which has been on the market for nearly 20 years—is by far the most widely used active ingredient in prescription sleep medications, says Ronald Farkas, M.D., Ph.D., a medical team leader in FDA's neurology products division. About 9 million patients received products containing zolpidem from retail pharmacies in 2011.

FDA's Adverse Event Reporting System has logged approximately 700 reports of zolpidem use and impaired driving ability and/or traffic accidents. However, FDA cannot be certain that those incidents are conclusively linked to zolpidem. Many of those reports lacked important information, such as the dose of zolpidem and the time at which it was taken, the time of the accident, and whether alcohol or other drugs had also been used.

"We have had longstanding concern about sleep medications and driving. However, only recently have data from clinical trials and specialized driving simulation studies become available that enabled FDA to better establish the risk of driving impairment and to make new recommendations about dosing," Farkas says.

An Individual Decision

FDA is urging healthcare professionals to caution patients who use these products about the risks of next-morning impairment and its effect on activities, such as driving, that require alertness.

The agency recommends that people who take sleep medications talk to their healthcare professional about ways to take the lowest effective dose. It should not be assumed that OTC sleep medicines are necessarily safer alternatives.

With zolpidem, Farkas notes that people must be aware of how this drug affects them personally. "Even with the new dosing recommendations, it's important to work with your healthcare professional to find the sleep medicine and dose that work best for you," he says.

Patients are asked to contact FDA's MedWatch program if they suffer side effects from the use of zolpidem or another insomnia medication.

Section 43.4

Risk of Next-Morning Impairment after Use of Zolpidem and Other Insomnia Drugs

This section includes text excerpted from "Drug Safety and Availability," U.S. Food and Drug Administration (FDA), December 23, 2014.

FAQs on Zolpidem and Other Insomnia Drugs

What Is Zolpidem?

Zolpidem is a sedative-hypnotic (sleep) medicine that is used in adults for the treatment of insomnia. Zolpidem is available as an oral tablet (Ambien and generics), an extended-release tablet (Ambien CR and generics), a sublingual (under-the-tongue) tablet (Edluar), and an oral spray (Zolpimist).

Zolpidem is also available under the brand name Intermezzo, a lower dose sublingual tablet that is approved for use as needed for the treatment of insomnia when a middle-of-the-night awakening is followed by difficulty returning to sleep.

Why Is FDA Requiring the Manufacturers of Certain Zolpidem-Containing Products to Revise the Labeling to Lower the Recommended Dose of Zolpidem for Women and to Recommend Consideration of the Lower Dose in Men?

FDA is requiring the manufacturers of certain zolpidem-containing products to revise the labeling to lower the recommended dose of zolpidem-containing medicines for women and to recommend that healthcare professionals consider prescribing the lower dose for men because next-morning blood levels of zolpidem may be high enough to impair activities that require alertness, including driving. Patients with high levels of zolpidem can be impaired even if they feel fully awake. Zolpidem is eliminated from the body more slowly in women, so the drug can stay in their systems longer than it does in men.

What Should Patients Currently Taking the 10 Mg or 12.5 Mg Dose of Zolpidem-Containing Insomnia Medicines Do Now?

If you are currently taking the 10 mg or 12.5 mg dose of zolpidem-containing insomnia medicine, continue taking your prescribed dose as directed until you have contacted your healthcare professional to ask for instructions on how to safely continue to take your medicine. Each patient and situation is unique, and the appropriate dose should be discussed with your healthcare professional.

Will a Lower Dose of Zolpidem Be Effective in Treating Insomnia?

FDA has informed the manufacturers that the recommended dose of zolpidem for women should be lowered from 10 mg to 5 mg for immediate-release products (Ambien, Edluar, and Zolpimist) and from 12.5 mg to 6.25 mg for extended-release products (Ambien CR). For men, FDA has informed the manufacturers that the labeling should recommend that healthcare professionals consider prescribing these lower doses. These lower doses of zolpidem (5 mg for immediate-release products and 6.25 mg for extended-release products) will be effective in most women and many men.

Is FDA Requiring the Manufacturer of Intermezzo (Zolpidem Tartrate) Sublingual Tablets to Also Change the Dosing Recommendations?

No. When Intermezzo was FDA-approved in November 2011, the label already recommended a lower dosage in women compared to men. The recommended and maximum dose of Intermezzo is 1.75 mg for women and 3.5 mg for men, taken only once per night as needed if a middle-of-the-night awakening is followed by difficulty returning to sleep.

Do Any Other Factors, Such as a Patient's Age, Weight or Ethnicity, Have an Effect on Zolpidem Levels?

Based on data from pharmacokinetic trials, no relationship was evident between the zolpidem blood level and patients' body weight or ethnicity. In elderly patients, zolpidem blood levels can be higher, and the lower doses are already recommended. In contrast to younger patients, zolpidem blood levels in elderly patients are not affected by gender.

Why Is FDA Informing the Public about This Safety Risk Now, after Zolpidem Has Been on the Market for Nearly 20 Years?

Since the approval of zolpidem, FDA has been continually monitoring the drug's safety profile. As more data became available, FDA continued to assess the benefits and risks of zolpidem treatment. Over the years, FDA has received reports of possible driving impairment and motor vehicle accidents associated with zolpidem; however, in most cases it was difficult to determine if the driving impairment was related to zolpidem or to specific zolpidem blood levels because information about time of dosing and time of the impairment was often not reported. Recently, data from clinical trials and driving simulation studies have become available that allowed FDA to better characterize the risk of driving impairment caused by specific blood levels of zolpidem and to recognize the increased risk of driving-impairing blood levels of zolpidem in women. This led FDA to require the manufacturers of certain zolpidem-containing products to revise the dosing recommendations.

Is Next-Morning Impairment the Same as Complex Sleep-Related Behaviors?

No, they are different. Next-morning impairment occurs when patients are awake the next morning, but levels of the insomnia medicine in their blood remain high enough to impair activities that require alertness, including driving.

Complex sleep-related behaviors occur when patients get out of bed while not fully awake, and sleep walk or do an activity such as drive a car, prepare and eat food, make phone calls, or have sex.

Both problems are made worse by high levels of zolpidem. The changes that FDA is requiring to the dosing recommendations in the drug labeling are expected to decrease the risk of both next-morning impairment and complex sleep-related behaviors.

Is FDA Requiring the Manufacturers of Other Insomnia Medicines to Revise Their Dosing Recommendations?

No. At this time, FDA is only requiring the manufacturers of certain zolpidem-containing products to revise their dosing recommendations.

FDA is continuing to evaluate ways to lower the risk of next-morning impairment with other insomnia medicines.

Do Other Insomnia Medicines Have the Same Gender Effect as Zolpidem?

FDA is currently evaluating other insomnia medicines to determine if they affect men and women differently.

Do Over-the-Counter (OTC) Insomnia Medicines That Are Available without a Prescription Have a Risk of Next-Morning Impairment?

Yes. OTC insomnia medicines also have a risk for next-morning impairment. FDA is not recommending that patients who are currently taking prescription insomnia medicines switch to OTC insomnia medicines.

Patients who drive or perform activities that require full alertness the next morning should discuss with their healthcare professional if the insomnia medicine they are using is right for them.

What Can Patients Do to Decrease Their Risk of Next-Morning Impairment with Insomnia Medicines?

Patients can decrease their risk of next-morning impairment by taking the lowest dose of their insomnia medicine that treats their symptoms. It is important for patients to take their insomnia medicine exactly as prescribed. Taking a higher dose than prescribed or using more than one insomnia medicine is dangerous if patients drive or perform activities that require full alertness the next morning, even if the drugs are taken at the beginning of the night. In addition, patients should not take insomnia medicine intended for bedtime use if less than a full night's sleep (7–8 hours) remains. Likewise, patients should not take Intermezzo, a zolpidem product that is approved for use in the middle of the night, if less than 4 hours of sleep remain.

FDA on Zolpidem

The U.S. Food and Drug Administration (FDA) is notified the public of information about zolpidem, a widely prescribed insomnia drug. FDA recommends that the bedtime dose be lowered because the data show that blood levels in some patients may be high enough the morning after use to impair activities that require alertness, including driving. The announcement focused on zolpidem products approved for bedtime use, which are marketed as generics and under the brand names Ambien, Ambien CR, Edluar, and Zolpimist.

FDA is also reminded the public that all drugs taken for insomnia can impair driving and activities that require alertness the morning after use. Drowsiness is already listed as a common side effect in the drug labels of all insomnia drugs, along with warnings that patients may still feel drowsy the day after taking these products. Patients who take insomnia drugs can experience impairment of mental alertness the morning after use, even if they feel fully awake.

FDA urged healthcare professionals to caution all patients (men and women) who use these zolpidem products about the risks of next-morning impairment for activities that require complete mental alertness, including driving. For zolpidem products, data show the risk for next-morning impairment is highest for patients taking the extended-release forms of these drugs (Ambien CR and generics). Women appear to be more susceptible to this risk because they eliminate zolpidem from their bodies more slowly than men.

Because use of lower doses of zolpidem will result in lower blood levels in the morning, the manufacturers of Ambien, Ambien CR, Edluar, and Zolpimist are required by the FDA to lower the recommended dose. FDA has informed the manufacturers that the recommended dose of zolpidem for women should be lowered from 10 mg to 5 mg for immediate-release products (Ambien, Edluar, and Zolpimist) and from 12.5 mg to 6.25 mg for extended-release products (Ambien CR). FDA also informed the manufacturers that, for men, the labeling should recommend that healthcare professionals consider prescribing the lower doses 5 mg for immediate-release products and 6.25 mg for extended-release products.

Section 43.5

Harmful Effects of CNS Depressants

This section includes text excerpted from "CNS Depressants,"
National Institute on Drug Abuse (NIDA), November 2014.

What Are CNS Depressants?

CNS depressants, sometimes referred to as sedatives and tranquilizers, are substances that can slow brain activity. This property makes them useful for treating anxiety and sleep disorders. Among the medications commonly prescribed for these purposes are the following:

- **Benzodiazepines**, such as diazepam (Valium) and alprazolam (Xanax), are sometimes prescribed to treat anxiety, acute stress reactions, and panic attacks. The more sedating benzodiazepines, such as triazolam (Halcion) and estazolam (ProSom) are prescribed for short-term treatment of sleep disorders. Usually, benzodiazepines are not prescribed for long term use because of the risk for developing tolerance, dependence, or addiction.

- **Non-benzodiazepine sleep medications**, such as zolpidem (Ambien), eszopiclone (Lunesta), and zalepon (Sonata), have a different chemical structure, but act on some of the same brain receptors as benzodiazepines. They are thought to have fewer side effects and less risk of dependence than benzodiazepines.

- **Barbiturates**, such as mephobarbital (Mebaral), phenobarbital (Luminal Sodium), and pentobarbital sodium (Nembutal), are used less frequently to reduce anxiety or to help with sleep problems because of their higher risk of overdose compared to benzodiazepines. However, they are still used in surgical procedures and for seizure disorders.

How Do CNS Depressants Affect the Brain and Body?

Most CNS depressants act on the brain by affecting the neurotransmitter gamma aminobutyric acid (GABA). Neurotransmitters are brain chemicals that facilitate communication between brain cells. Although the different classes of CNS depressants work in unique ways, it is through their ability to increase GABA—and thereby inhibit brain activity—that they produce a drowsy or calming effect beneficial to those suffering from anxiety or sleep disorders.

What Are the Possible Consequences of CNS Depressant Use and Abuse?

Despite their many beneficial effects, benzodiazepines and barbiturates have the potential for abuse and should be used only as prescribed. The use of non-benzodiazepine sleep aids is less well studied, but certain indicators have raised concern about their abuse liability as well. During the first few days of taking a prescribed CNS depressant, a person usually feels sleepy and uncoordinated, but as the body becomes accustomed to the effects of the drug and tolerance develops, these side effects begin to disappear. If one uses these drugs long term, larger doses may be needed to achieve the therapeutic effects. Continued use can also lead to physical dependence and withdrawal when use is abruptly reduced or stopped. Because all CNS depressants work by slowing the brain's activity, when an individual stops taking them, there can be a rebound effect, resulting in seizures or other harmful consequences.

Although withdrawal from benzodiazepines can be problematic, it is rarely life threatening, whereas withdrawal from prolonged use of barbiturates can have life-threatening complications. Therefore, someone who is thinking about discontinuing CNS depressant therapy or who is suffering withdrawal from a CNS depressant should speak with a physician or seek immediate medical treatment.

Is It Safe to Use CNS Depressants with Other Medications?

Only under a physician's supervision is it safe to use CNS depressants with other medications. Typically, they should not be combined with any other medication or substance that causes CNS depression, including prescription pain medicines, some OTC cold and allergy medications, and alcohol. Using CNS depressants with these other substances—particularly alcohol—can affect heart rhythm, slow respiration, and even lead to death.

Over-the-Counter Medicines

Over-the-counter (OTC) medications, such as certain cough suppressants, sleep aids, and antihistamines, can be abused for their psychoactive effects. This typically means taking doses higher than recommended or combining OTC medications with alcohol, or with illicit or prescription drugs. Either practice can have dangerous results, depending on the medications involved. Some contain aspirin or acetaminophen (e.g., Tylenol), which can be toxic to the liver at high doses. Others, when taken for their "hallucinogenic" properties, can cause confusion, psychosis, coma, and even death.

Cough syrups and cold medications are the most commonly abused OTC medications. In 2010, for example, 6.6 percent of high school seniors took cough syrup "to get high." At high doses, dextromethorphan—a key ingredient found in cough syrup—can act like PCP or ketamine, producing dissociative or out-of-body experiences.

311

Chapter 44

Dietary Supplements and Complementary and Alternative Medicine (CAM) for Sleep Disorders

Chapter Contents

Section 44.1

Melatonin

This section includes text excerpted from "Melatonin: In Depth," National Center for Complementary and Integrative Health (NCCIH), April 4, 2016.

What Is Melatonin?

Melatonin is a natural hormone that plays a role in sleep. Melatonin production and release in the brain is related to time of day, rising in the evening and falling in the morning. Light at night blocks its production. Melatonin dietary supplements have been studied for sleep disorders, such as jet lag, disruptions of the body's internal "clock," insomnia, and problems with sleep among people who work night shifts. It has also been studied for dementia symptoms.

What the Science Says about the Effectiveness of Melatonin

For Sleep Disorders

Studies suggest that melatonin may help with certain sleep disorders, such as jet lag, delayed sleep phase disorder (a disruption of the body's biological clock in which a person's sleep-wake timing cycle is delayed by 3 to 6 hours), sleep problems related to shift work, and some sleep disorders in children. It's also been shown to be helpful for a sleep disorder that causes changes in blind peoples' sleep and wake times. Study results are mixed on whether melatonin is effective for insomnia in adults, but some studies suggest it may slightly reduce the time it takes to fall asleep.

Jet lag. Jet lag is caused by rapid travel across several time zones; its symptoms include disturbed sleep, daytime fatigue, indigestion, and a general feeling of discomfort.

- In a 2009 research review, results from six small studies and two large studies suggested that melatonin may ease jet lag.

- In a 2007 clinical practice guideline, the American Academy of Sleep Medicine supported using melatonin to reduce jet lag symptoms and improve sleep after traveling across more than one time zone.

Delayed Sleep Phase Disorder. Adults and teens with this sleep disorder have trouble falling asleep before 2 a.m. and have trouble waking up in the morning.

- In a 2007 review of the literature, researchers suggested that a combination of melatonin supplements, a behavioral approach to delay sleep and wake times until the desired sleep time is achieved, and reduced evening light may even out sleep cycles in people with this sleep disorder.

- In a 2007 clinical practice guideline, the American Academy of Sleep Medicine recommended timed melatonin supplementation for this sleep disorder.

Shift Work Disorder. Shift work refers to job-related duties conducted outside of morning to evening working hours. About 2 million Americans who work afternoon to nighttime or nighttime to early morning hours are affected by shift work disorder.

- A 2007 clinical practice guideline and 2010 review of the evidence concluded that melatonin may improve daytime sleep quality and duration, but not nighttime alertness, in people with shift work disorder.

- The American Academy of Sleep Medicine recommended taking melatonin prior to daytime sleep for night shift workers with shift work disorder to enhance daytime sleep.

Insomnia. Insomnia is a general term for a group of problems characterized by an inability to fall asleep and stay asleep.

- **In adults.** A 2013 analysis of 19 studies of people with primary sleep disorders found that melatonin slightly improved time to fall asleep, total sleep time, and overall sleep quality. In a 2007 study of people with insomnia, aged 55 years or older, researchers found that prolonged-release melatonin significantly improved quality of sleep and morning alertness.

- **In children.** There's limited evidence from rigorous studies of melatonin for sleep disorders among young people. A 2011 literature review suggested a benefit with minimal side effects in healthy children as well as youth with attention-deficit hyper-activity disorder, autism, and several other populations. There's insufficient information to make conclusions about the safety and effectiveness of long-term melatonin use.

For Other Conditions

While there hasn't been enough research to support melatonin's use for other conditions:

- Researchers are investigating whether adding melatonin to standard **cancer care** can improve response rates, survival time, and quality of life.

- Results from a few small studies in people (clinical trials) have led investigators to propose additional research on whether melatonin may help to improve mild cognitive impairment in patients with **Alzheimer disease (AD)** and prevent cell damage associated with **amyotrophic lateral sclerosis (ALS**, also known as **Lou Gehrig's disease**). An analysis of the research suggested that adding sustained-release melatonin (but not fast-release melatonin) to high blood pressure management reduced **elevated nighttime blood pressure.**

What the Science Says about Safety and Side Effects of Melatonin

Melatonin appears to be safe when used short-term, but the lack of long-term studies means we don't know if it's safe for extended use.

- In one study, researchers noted that melatonin supplements may worsen mood in people with dementia.

- In 2011, the U.S. Food and Drug Administration (FDA) issued a warning to a company that makes and sells "relaxation brownies," stating that the melatonin in them hasn't been deemed a safe food additive.

- Side effects of melatonin are uncommon but can include drowsiness, headache, dizziness, or nausea. There have been no reports of significant side effects of melatonin in children.

More to Consider

- If you or a family member has trouble sleeping, see your healthcare provider.

- When you take a melatonin supplement is important because it may affect your biological clock.

- FDA regulates dietary supplements such as melatonin, but the regulations for dietary supplements are different and less strict than those for prescription or over-the-counter drugs.

- Some dietary supplements may interact with medications or pose risks if you have medical problems or are going to have surgery.

- Most dietary supplements haven't been tested in pregnant women, nursing mothers, or children. If you're pregnant or nursing a child, it's especially important to see your healthcare provider before taking any medication or supplement, including melatonin.

- To use dietary supplements, such as melatonin safely, read and follow label instructions, and recognize that "natural" does not always mean "safe."

- Tell all your healthcare providers about any complementary or integrative health approaches you use. Give them a full picture of what you do to manage your health. This will help ensure safe and coordinated care.

Section 44.2

Valerian

This section includes text excerpted from "Valerian," Office of Dietary Supplements (ODS), National Institutes of Health (NIH), March 15, 2013.

What Is Valerian?

Valerian *(Valeriana officinalis)*, a member of the Valerianaceae family, is a perennial plant native to Europe and Asia and natu-ralized in North America. It has a distinctive odor that many find unpleasant. Other names include setwall (English), Valerianae radix

(Latin), Baldrianwurzel (German), and phu(Greek). The genus Valerian includes over 250 species, but *V. officinalis* is the species most often used in the United States and Europe and is the only species discussed in this section.

What Are Common Valerian Preparations?

Preparations of valerian marketed as dietary supplements are made from its roots, rhizomes (underground stems), and stolons (horizontal stems). Dried roots are prepared as teas or tinctures, and dried plant materials and extracts are put into capsules or incorporated into tablets.

There is no scientific agreement as to the active constituents of valerian, and its activity may result from interactions among multiple constituents rather than any one compound or class of compounds. The content of volatile oils, including valerenic acids; the less volatile sesquiterpenes; or the valepotriates (esters of short-chain fatty acids) is sometimes used to standardize valerian extracts. As with most herbal preparations, many other compounds are also present.

Valerian is sometimes combined with other botanicals. Because this section focuses on valerian as a single ingredient, only clinical studies evaluating valerian as a single agent are included.

What Clinical Studies Have Been Done on Valerian and Sleep Disorders?

In a systematic review of the scientific literature, nine randomized, placebo-controlled, double-blind clinical trials of valerian and sleep disorders were identified and evaluated for evidence of efficacy of valerian as a treatment for insomnia. Reviewers rated the studies with a standard scoring system to quantify the likelihood of bias inherent in the study design. Although all nine trials had flaws, three earned the highest rating (5 on a scale of 1 to 5) and are described below. Unlike the six lower-rated studies, these three studies described the randomization procedure and blinding method that were used and reported rates of participant withdrawal.

The first study used a repeated-measures design; 128 volunteers were given 400 mg of an aqueous extract of valerian, a commercial preparation containing 60 mg valerian and 30 mg hops, and a placebo. Participants took each one of the three preparations three times in random order on nine nonconsecutive nights and filled out a questionnaire the morning after each treatment. Compared with the placebo, the valerian extract resulted in a statistically significant subjective improvement in time required to fall asleep (more or less difficult than usual), sleep quality (better or worse than usual), and number of nighttime awakenings (more or less than usual).This result was more pronounced in a subgroup of 61 participants who identified themselves as poor sleepers on a questionnaire administered at the beginning of the study. The commercial preparation did not produce a statistically significant improvement in these three measures. The clinical significance of the use of valerian for insomnia cannot be determined from the results of this study because having insomnia was not a requirement for participation. In addition, the study had a participant withdrawal rate of 22.9%, which may have influenced the results.

In the second study, eight volunteers with mild insomnia (usually had problems falling asleep) were evaluated for the effect of valerian on sleep latency (defined as the first 5-minute period without movement). Results were based on nighttime motion measured by activity meters worn on the wrist and on responses to questionnaires about sleep quality, latency, depth, and morning sleepiness filled out the morning after each treatment. The test samples were 450 or 900 mg of an aqueous valerian extract and a placebo. Each volunteer was randomly assigned to receive one test sample each night, Monday through Thursday, for 3 weeks for a total of 12 nights of evaluation. The 450-mg test sample of valerian extract reduced average sleep latency from about 16 to 9 minutes, which is similar to the activity of prescription benzodiazepine medication (used as a sedative or tranquilizer). No statistically significant shortening of sleep latency was seen with the 900-mg test sample. Evaluation of the questionnaires showed a statistically significant improvement in subjectively measured sleep. On a 9-point scale, participants rated sleep latency as 4.3 after the 450-mg test sample and 4.9 after the placebo. The 900-mg test sample increased the sleep improvement but participants noted an increase in sleepiness the next morning. Although statistically significant, this 7-minute reduction in sleep latency and the improvement in subjective sleep rating are probably not clinically significant. The small sample size makes it difficult to generalize the results to a broader population.

The third study examined longer-term effects in 121 participants with documented nonorganic insomnia. Participants received either 600 mg of a standardized commercial preparation of dried valerian root or placebo for 28 days. Several assessment tools were used to evaluate the effectiveness and tolerance of the interventions, including questionnaires on therapeutic effect (given on days 14 and 28), change in sleep patterns (given on day 28), and changes in sleep quality and well-being (given on days 0, 14, and 28). After 28 days, the group receiving the valerian extract showed a decrease in insomnia symptoms on all the assessment tools compared with the placebo group. The differences in improvement between valerian and placebo increased between the assessments done on days 14 and 28.

The reviewers concluded that these nine studies are not sufficient for determining the effectiveness of valerian to treat sleep disorders. For example, none of the studies checked the success of the blinding, none calculated the sample size necessary for seeing a statistical effect, only one partially controlled pre bedtime variables, and only one validated outcome measures.

Two other randomized, controlled trials published after the systematic review described above are presented below:

- In a randomized, double-blind study, 75 participants with documented nonorganic insomnia were randomly assigned to receive 600 mg of a standardized commercial valerian extract (LI 156) or 10 mg oxazepam (a benzodiazepine medication) for 28 days. Assessment tools used to evaluate the effectiveness and tolerance of the interventions included validated sleep, mood scale, and anxiety questionnaires as well as sleep rating by a physician (on days 0, 14, and 28). Treatment result was determined via a 4-step rating scale at the end of the study (day 28). Both groups had the same improvement in sleep quality but the valerian group reported fewer side effects than did the oxazepam group. However, this study was designed to show superiority, if any, of valerian over oxazepam and its results cannot be used to show equivalence.

- In a randomized, double-blind, placebo-controlled crossover study, researchers evaluated sleep parameters with polysomnographic techniques that monitored sleep stages, sleep latency, and total sleep time to objectively measure sleep quality and stages. Questionnaires were used for subjective measurement of sleep parameters. Sixteen participants with medically documented nonorganic insomnia were randomly assigned to receive either a single dose and a 14-day administration of 600 mg of a standardized commercial preparation of valerian (LI 156) or placebo. Valerian had no effect on any of the 15 objective or subjective measurements except for a decrease in slow-wave sleep onset (13.5 minutes) compared with placebo (21.3 minutes). During slow-wave sleep, arousability, skeletal muscle tone, heart rate, blood pressure, and respiratory frequency decreased.

Increased time spent in slow-wave sleep may decrease insomnia symptoms. However, because all but 1 of the 15 endpoints showed no difference between placebo and valerian, the possibility that the single endpoint showing a difference was the result of chance must be considered. The valerian group reported fewer adverse events than did the placebo group.

Although the results of some studies suggest that valerian may be useful for insomnia and other sleep disorders, results of other studies do not. Interpretation of these studies is complicated by the fact the studies had small sample sizes, used different amounts and sources of valerian, measured different outcomes, or did not consider potential bias resulting from high participant withdrawal rates. Overall, the evidence from these trials for the sleep-promoting effects of valerian is inconclusive.

How Does Valerian Work?

Many chemical constituents of valerian have been identified, but it is not known which may be responsible for its sleep-promoting effects in animals and in in vitro studies. It is likely that there is no single active compound and that valerian's effects result from multiple constituents acting independently or synergistically.

Two categories of constituents have been proposed as the major source of valerian's sedative effects. The first category comprises the major constituents of its volatile oil including valerenic acid and its derivatives, which have demonstrated sedative properties in animal studies. However, valerian extracts with very little of these components also have sedative properties, making it probable that other components are responsible for these effects or that multiple constituents contribute to them. The second category comprises the iridoids, which include the valepotriates. Valepotriates and their derivatives are active as sedatives in vivo but are unstable and break down during storage or in an aqueous environment, making their activity difficult to assess.

A possible mechanism by which a valerian extract may cause sedation is by increasing the amount of gamma aminobutyric acid (GABA, an inhibitory neurotransmitter) available in the synaptic cleft. Results from an in vitro study using synaptosomes suggest that a valerian extract may cause GABA to be released from brain nerve endings and then block GABA from being taken back into nerve cells. In addition, valerenic acid inhibits an enzyme that destroys GABA.

Valerian extracts contain GABA in quantities sufficient to cause a sedative effect, but whether GABA can cross the blood-brain barrier to contribute to valerian's sedative effects is not known. Glutamine is present in aqueous but not in alcohol extracts and may cross the blood-brain barrier and be converted to GABA. Levels of these constituents vary significantly among plants depending on when the plants are harvested, resulting in marked variability in the amounts found in valerian preparations.

What Is the Regulatory Status of Valerian in the United States?

In the United States, valerian is sold as a dietary supplement, and dietary supplements are regulated as foods, not drugs. Therefore, premarket evaluation and approval by the U.S. Food and Drug Administration (FDA) are not required unless claims are made for specific disease prevention or treatment. Because dietary supplements are not always tested for manufacturing consistency, the composition may vary considerably between manufacturing lots.

Can Valerian Be Harmful?

Few adverse events attributable to valerian have been reported for clinical study participants. Headaches, dizziness, pruritus, and gastrointestinal disturbances are the most common effects reported in clinical trials but similar effects were also reported for the placebo. In one study an increase in sleepiness was noted the morning after 900 mg of valerian was taken. Investigators from another study concluded that 600 mg of valerian (LI 156) did not have a clinically significant effect on reaction time, alertness, and concentration the morning after ingestion. Several case reports described adverse effects, but in one case where suicide was attempted with a massive overdose it is not possible to clearly attribute the symptoms to valerian.

Valepotriates, which are a component of valerian but are not necessarily present in commercial preparations, had cytotoxic activity in vitro but were not carcinogenic in animal studies.

Who Should Not Take Valerian?

- Women who are pregnant or nursing should not take valerian without medical advice because the possible risks to the fetus or infant have not been evaluated.

- Children younger than 3 years old should not take valerian because the possible risks to children of this age have not been evaluated.

- Individuals taking valerian should be aware of the theoretical possibility of additive sedative effects from alcohol or sedative drugs, such as barbiturates and benzodiazepines

Does Valerian Interact with Any Drugs or Supplements or Affect Laboratory Tests?

Valerian might have additive therapeutic and adverse effects if taken with sedatives, other medications, or certain herbs and dietary supplements with sedative properties. These include the following:

- Benzodiazepines such as Xanax®, Valium®, Ativan®, and Halcion®.

- Barbiturates or central nervous system (CNS) depressants such as phenobarbital (Luminal®), morphine, and propofol (Diprivan®).

- Dietary supplements such as St. John's wort, kava, and melatonin.

Individuals taking these medications or supplements should discuss the use of valerian with their healthcare providers.

Although valerian has not been reported to influence laboratory tests, this has not been rigorously studied.

Section 44.3

Complementary and Alternative Medicine

This section includes text excerpted from "5 Things to Know about Sleep Disorders and Complementary Health Approaches," *Eunice Kennedy Shriver* National Institute of Child Health and Human Development (NICHD), September 24, 2015.

Things to Know about Sleep Disorders and Complementary Health Approaches

Chronic, long-term sleep disorders affect millions of Americans each year. These disorders and the sleep deprivation they cause can interfere with work, driving, social activities, and overall quality of life, and can have serious health implications. Sleep disorders account for an estimated $16 billion in medical costs each year, plus indirect costs due to missed days of work, decreased productivity, and other factors.

People who have trouble sleeping often try various dietary supplements, relaxation therapies, or other complementary health approaches in an effort to fall asleep faster, stay asleep longer, and improve the overall quality of their sleep. Here are 5 things to know about what the science says about sleep disorders and complementary health approaches.

Relaxation Techniques May Be Helpful for Insomnia

Evidence indicates that using relaxation techniques before bedtime can be helpful components of a successful strategy to improve sleep habits. Other components include maintaining a consistent sleep schedule; avoiding caffeine, alcohol, heavy meals, and strenuous exercise too close to bedtime; and sleeping in a quiet, cool, dark room.

Melatonin Supplements May Be Helpful for Some People with Insomnia or Sleep Problems Caused by Shift Work or Jet Lag

Research on the use of melatonin for children is more limited; available research suggests some benefit in children, but those studies were small and only addressed short-term use of melatonin. The long-term safety of melatonin has not been investigated.

Current Evidence regarding Other Mind and Body Approaches Such as Mindfulness-Based Stress Reduction (a Type of Meditation), Yoga, Massage Therapy, and Acupuncture Is Either Too Preliminary or Inconsistent to Draw Conclusions about Whether They Are Helpful for Sleep Disorders

These mind and body practices are generally considered safe for healthy people and when performed by an experienced practitioner.

Various Herbs and Dietary Supplements Sometimes Used as Sleep Aids, including Valerian, Kava, Chamomile, and L-Tryptophan and 5-Hydroxytryptophan (5-HTP) Have Not Been Shown to Be Effective for Insomnia, and Important Safety Concerns Have Been Raised about a Few

For example, the use of L-tryptophan supplements has been linked to eosinophilia-myalgia syndrome (EMS), a complex, potentially fatal disorder with multiple symptoms including severe muscle pain. Kava supplements have been linked to a risk of severe liver damage.

If You Are Considering a Complementary Health Approach for Sleep Problems, Talk to Your healthcare Providers

Trouble sleeping can be an indication of a more serious condition, and some prescription and over-the-counter drugs can contribute to sleep problems. So, it's important to discuss your sleep-related symptoms with your healthcare providers before trying any complementary health product or practice.

Chapter 45

How Is Insomnia Treated?

How Is Insomnia Diagnosed?

Your doctor will likely diagnose insomnia based on your medical and sleep histories and a physical exam. He or she also may recommend a sleep study. For example, you may have a sleep study if the cause of your insomnia is unclear.

Medical History

To find out what's causing your insomnia, your doctor may ask whether you:

- Have any new or ongoing health problems

- Have painful injuries or health conditions, such as arthritis

- Take any medicines, either over-the-counter or prescription

- Have symptoms or a history of depression, anxiety, or psychosis

- Are coping with highly stressful life events, such as divorce or death

---

This chapter contains text excerpted from the following sources: Text under the heading "How Is Insomnia Diagnosed?" is excerpted from "Insomnia," National, Heart, Lung, and Blood Institute (NHLBI), December 13, 2011, Reviewed July 2016; Text under the heading "Examples of Treatments for Insomnia in Adults Studied in the Literature" is excerpted from "Treatment of Insomnia Disorder," Agency for Healthcare Research and Quality (AHRQ), April 3, 2014.

Your doctor also may ask questions about your work and leisure habits. For example, he or she may ask about your work and exercise routines; your use of caffeine, tobacco, and alcohol; and your long-distance travel history. Your answers can give clues about what's causing your insomnia.

Your doctor also may ask whether you have any new or ongoing work or personal problems or other stresses in your life. Also, he or she may ask whether you have other family members who have sleep problems.

Sleep History

To get a better sense of your sleep problem, your doctor will ask you for details about your sleep habits. Before your visit, think about how to describe your problems, including:

- How often you have trouble sleeping and how long you've had the problem

- When you go to bed and get up on workdays and days off

- How long it takes you to fall asleep, how often you wake up at night, and how long it takes to fall back asleep

- Whether you snore loudly and often or wake up gasping or feeling out of breath

- How refreshed you feel when you wake up, and how tired you feel during the day

- How often you doze off or have trouble staying awake during routine tasks, especially driving

- To find out what's causing or worsening your insomnia, your doctor also may ask you:

- Whether you worry about falling asleep, staying asleep, or getting enough sleep

- What you eat or drink, and whether you take medicines before going to bed

- What routine you follow before going to bed

- What the noise level, lighting, and temperature are like where you sleep

- What distractions, such as a TV or computer, are in your bedroom

To help your doctor, consider keeping a sleep diary for 1 or 2 weeks. Write down when you go to sleep, wake up, and take naps. (For example, you might note: Went to bed at 10 a.m.; woke up at 3 a.m. and couldn't fall back asleep; napped after work for 2 hours.)

Also write down how much you sleep each night, as well as how sleepy you feel throughout the day.

Physical Exam

Your doctor will do a physical exam to rule out other medical problems that might cause insomnia. You also may need blood tests to check for thyroid problems or other conditions that can cause sleep problems.

Sleep Study

Your doctor may recommend a sleep study called a polysomnogram (PSG) if he or she thinks an underlying sleep disorder is causing your insomnia.

You'll likely stay overnight at a sleep center for this study. The PSG records brain activity, eye movements, heart rate, and blood pressure.

A PSG also records the amount of oxygen in your blood, how much air is moving through your nose while you breathe, snoring, and chest movements. The chest movements show whether you're making an effort to breathe.

How is Insomnia Treated?

Lifestyle changes often can help relieve acute (short-term) insomnia. These changes might make it easier to fall asleep and stay asleep.

A type of counseling called cognitive-behavioral therapy (CBT) can help relieve the anxiety linked to chronic (ongoing) insomnia. Anxiety tends to prolong insomnia.

Several medicines also can help relieve insomnia and re-establish a regular sleep schedule. However, if your insomnia is the symptom or side effect of another problem, it's important to treat the underlying cause (if possible).

Lifestyle Changes

If you have insomnia, avoid substances that make it worse, such as:

Caffeine, tobacco, and other stimulants. The effects of these substances can last as long as 8 hours.

Certain over-the-counter and prescription medicines that can disrupt sleep (for example, some cold and allergy medicines). Talk with your doctor about which medicines won't disrupt your sleep.

Alcohol. An alcoholic drink before bedtime might make it easier for you to fall asleep. However, alcohol triggers sleep that tends to be lighter than normal. This makes it more likely that you will wake up during the night.

Try to adopt bedtime habits that make it easier to fall asleep and stay asleep. Follow a routine that helps you wind down and relax before bed. For example, read a book, listen to soothing music, or take a hot bath.

Try to schedule your daily exercise at least 5 to 6 hours before going to bed. Don't eat heavy meals or drink a lot before bedtime.

Make your bedroom sleep-friendly. Avoid bright lighting while winding down. Try to limit possible distractions, such as a TV, computer, or pet. Make sure the temperature of your bedroom is cool and comfortable. Your bedroom also should be dark and quiet.

Go to sleep around the same time each night and wake up around the same time each morning, even on weekends. If you can, avoid night shifts, alternating schedules, or other things that may disrupt your sleep schedule.

Cognitive-Behavioral Therapy

CBT for insomnia targets the thoughts and actions that can disrupt sleep. This therapy encourages good sleep habits and uses several methods to relieve sleep anxiety.

For example, relaxation techniques and biofeedback are used to reduce anxiety. These strategies help you better control your breathing, heart rate, muscles, and mood.

CBT also aims to replace sleep anxiety with more positive thinking that links being in bed with being asleep. This method also teaches you what to do if you're unable to fall asleep within a reasonable time.

CBT also may involve talking with a therapist one-on-one or in group sessions to help you consider your thoughts and feelings about sleep. This method may encourage you to describe thoughts racing through your mind in terms of how they look, feel, and sound. The goal is for your mind to settle down and stop racing.

CBT also focuses on limiting the time you spend in bed while awake. This method involves setting a sleep schedule. At first, you will limit your total time in bed to the typical short length of time you're usually asleep.

This schedule might make you even more tired because some of the allotted time in bed will be taken up by problems falling asleep.

However, the resulting tiredness is intended to help you get to sleep more quickly. Over time, the length of time spent in bed is increased until you get a full night of sleep.

For success with CBT, you may need to see a therapist who is skilled in this approach weekly over 2 to 3 months. CBT works as well as prescription medicine for many people who have chronic insomnia. It also may provide better long-term relief than medicine alone.

For people who have insomnia and major depressive disorder, CBT combined with antidepression medicines has shown promise in relieving both conditions.

Medicines

Prescription Medicines

Many prescription medicines are used to treat insomnia. Some are meant for short-term use, while others are meant for longer use.

Talk to your doctor about the benefits and side effects of insomnia medicines. For example, insomnia medicines can help you fall asleep, but you may feel groggy in the morning after taking them.

Rare side effects of these medicines include sleep eating, sleep walking, or driving while asleep. If you have side effects from an insomnia medicine, or if it doesn't work well, tell your doctor. He or she might prescribe a different medicine.

Some insomnia medicines can be habit forming. Ask your doctor about the benefits and risks of insomnia medicines.

Over-the-Counter Products

Some over-the-counter (OTC) products claim to treat insomnia. These products include melatonin, L-tryptophan supplements, and valerian teas or extracts.

The Food and Drug Administration doesn't regulate "natural" products and some food supplements. Thus, the dose and purity of these substances can vary. How well these products work and how safe they are isn't well understood.

Some OTC products that contain antihistamines are sold as sleep aids. Although these products might make you sleepy, talk to your doctor before taking them.

Antihistamines pose risks for some people. Also, these products may not offer the best treatment for your insomnia. Your doctor can advise you whether these products will benefit you.

Table 45.1. Examples of Treatments for Insomnia in Adults Studied in the Literature

Treatment Category	Treatment
Behavioral/psychological	Aroma therapy
	Bright-light therapy
	Brief behavioral therapy
	Biofeedback
	Cognitive behavioral therapy (CBT)
	Exercise
	Music therapy
	Relaxation training
	Sleep hygiene education
	Sleep restriction
CAM	Acupuncture
	Acupressure
	Cupping
	Homeopathy
	Hypnotherapy
	Reflexology
	Tai Chi
	Yoga
CAM – herbal/dietary supplements	Bach Flower
	Isoflavones
	L-tryptophan
	Magnesium
	Melatonin
	Valerian

Table 45.2. Examples of Treatments for Insomnia in Adults Studied in the Literature

Medications	Drug Name
Antihistamines	Diphenhydramine
	Doxylamine
Prescription antidepressants	Amitriptyline
	Doxepin*

Table 45.2. Continued

Medications	Drug Name
	Trazodone
	Mirtazapine
Prescription antipsychotics	Olanzapine
	Quetiapine
Prescription hypnotics	Benzodiazepines
	Estazolam*
	Flurazepam*
	Lorazepam
	Quazepam*
	Temazepam*
	Triazolam*
	Non-Benzodiazepines
	Eszopiclone*
	Zaleplon*
	Zolpidem*
Melatonin receptor agonist	Ramelteon*
Prescription antipsychotics	Gabapentin
	Pregabalin

Chapter 46

Continuous Positive Airway Pressure (CPAP)

What Is CPAP?

CPAP, or continuous positive airway pressure, is a treatment that uses mild air pressure to keep the airways open. CPAP typically is used by people who have breathing problems, such as sleep apnea.

CPAP also may be used to treat preterm infants whose lungs have not fully developed. For example, doctors may use CPAP to treat infants who have respiratory distress syndrome or bronchopulmonary dysplasia.

The main focus of this chapter is CPAP treatment for sleep apnea, although treatment in preterm infants is discussed briefly.

Overview

CPAP treatment involves a CPAP machine, which has three main parts:

- A mask or other device that fits over your nose or your nose and mouth. Straps keep the mask in place while you're wearing it.

- A tube that connects the mask to the machine's motor.

- A motor that blows air into the tube.

This chapter includes text excerpted from "CPAP," National Heart, Lung, and Blood Institute (NHLBI), December 13, 2011. Reviewed July 2016.

Some CPAP machines have other features as well, such as heated humidifiers. CPAP machines are small, lightweight, and fairly quiet. The noise that they make is soft and rhythmic.

CPAP often is the best treatment for obstructive sleep apnea. Sleep apnea is a common disorder that causes pauses in breathing or shallow breaths while you sleep. As a result, not enough air reaches your lungs.

In obstructive sleep apnea, your airway collapses or is blocked during sleep. When you try to breathe, any air that squeezes past the blockage can cause loud snoring. Your snoring may wake other people in the house.

The mild pressure from CPAP can prevent your airway from collapsing or becoming blocked.

The animation below shows how CPAP works to treat sleep apnea. Click the "start" button to play the animation. Written and spoken explanations are provided with each frame. Use the buttons in the lower right corner to pause, restart, or replay the animation, or use the scroll bar below the buttons to move through the frames.

If your doctor prescribes CPAP, you'll work with someone from a home equipment provider to select a CPAP machine. (Home equipment providers sometimes are called durable medical equipment, or DME.)

Your doctor will work with you to make sure the settings that he or she prescribes for your CPAP machine are correct. He or she may recommend an overnight sleep study to find the correct settings for you. Your doctor will want to make sure the air pressure from the machine is just enough to keep your airway open while you sleep.

Your doctor will work with you to make sure the settings that he or she prescribes for your CPAP machine are correct. He or she may recommend an overnight sleep study to find the correct settings for you. Your doctor will want to make sure the air pressure from the machine is just enough to keep your airway open while you sleep.

Outlook

CPAP has many benefits. It can:

- Keep your airway open while you sleep

- Correct snoring so others in your household can sleep

- Improve your quality of sleep

- Relieve sleep apnea symptoms, such as excessive daytime sleepiness

- Decrease or prevent high blood pressure

Many people who use CPAP report feeling better once they begin treatment. They feel more attentive and better able to work during the day. They also report fewer complaints from bed partners about snoring and sleep disruption.

In some preterm infants whose lungs have not fully developed, CPAP improves survival. It also can reduce the need for steroid treatment for the lungs.

Also, in some infants, CPAP prevents the need to insert a breathing tube through the mouth and into the windpipe to deliver air from a ventilator. (A ventilator is a machine that supports breathing.)

CPAP treatment is less invasive than ventilator therapy. Research suggests that CPAP is an appropriate first treatment for some preterm newborns.

Who Needs CPAP?

Your doctor may recommend CPAP if you have obstructive sleep apnea. CPAP often is the best treatment for adults who have this condition.

Children also can have obstructive sleep apnea. The most common treatment for children is surgery to remove the tonsils and adenoids. If symptoms don't improve after surgery, or if the condition is severe, CPAP may be an option.

If you have sleep apnea symptoms, your doctor may recommend an overnight sleep study. A sleep study measures how much and how well you sleep. It also can show whether you have sleep problems and how severe they are.

Your doctor will likely refer you to a sleep specialist for the sleep study. Sleep specialists are doctors who diagnose and treat people who have sleep problems.

A special type of CPAP device is used to treat breathing disorders that are similar to sleep apnea, such as chronic hypoventilation or central sleep apnea.

In these conditions, the airways aren't blocked. However, the brain may not send the signals needed for proper breathing. This causes breaths that are too shallow or slow to meet your body's needs.

In central sleep apnea, you may stop breathing for brief periods. This disorder can occur alone or with obstructive sleep apnea. Only a sleep study can find out which type of sleep apnea you have and how severe it is.

In addition to CPAP, there are other positive airway pressure devices. If you don't feel that CPAP is working for you, ask your sleep specialist about other possible options.

Besides treating sleep apnea and other similar disorders, CPAP also is used to treat preterm infants whose lungs have not fully developed. For example, doctors may use CPAP to treat infants who have respiratory distress syndrome or bronchopulmonary dysplasia.

Treatment with CPAP can improve a preterm infant's chance of survival and reduce the need for other treatments and therapies.

What to Expect before Using CPAP

Before your sleep specialist prescribes CPAP, you'll likely have a sleep study called a polysomnogram (PSG).

You'll probably stay overnight at a sleep center for a PSG. The study records brain activity, eye movements, heart rate, blood pressure, and other data while you sleep.

What to Expect during a Polysomnogram

Your sleep specialist may suggest a split-night sleep study. During the first half of the night, a technician will check how you sleep without a CPAP machine. This will show whether you have sleep apnea and how severe it is.

If the PSG shows that you have sleep apnea, you might use a CPAP machine during the second half of the split-night study. The technician will help you select a CPAP mask that fits and is comfortable.

While you sleep, the technician will check the amount of oxygen in your blood and whether your airway stays open. He or she will adjust the flow of air through the mask to find the setting that works best for you. This process is called CPAP titration.

Sometimes the CPAP titration study is done on a different night. Your sleep specialist will decide which type of study is best for you and leave instructions with the technician.

What to Expect after a Polysomnogram

Your sleep specialist will review the results from your sleep study. If CPAP will benefit you, he or she will prescribe the type of CPAP machine and the correct settings for you.

Most health insurance companies cover CPAP treatment. You might want to contact your health insurance provider to learn more about your coverage.

Your sleep specialist can refer you to a local home equipment provider. The home equipment provider will use your prescription to set up your CPAP machine. Ask your sleep specialist to recommend a home equipment provider that has a lot of experience with CPAP.

As you adjust to CPAP treatment, continue to work with your sleep specialist. Talk with him or her about how to handle followup questions. Your sleep specialist can answer some questions, but your home equipment provider may need to address others.

Selecting a CPAP Machine and Mask

CPAP units come with many features designed to improve fit and comfort. Your home equipment provider will help you select a machine based on your prescription and the features that meet your needs.

You might be able to use the CPAP unit for a trial period to make sure you're happy with your choice.

There are many types of CPAP masks. The fit of your mask is important, not only for comfort, but also to keep air from leaking out. A mask that fits will help maintain proper air pressure and keep your airway open.

CPAP masks come in many shapes, sizes, and materials. Some fit over your nose and mouth; others cover only your nose. Some masks can be worn with eyeglasses. If you need oxygen, masks are available that have room for an oxygen tube.

You may want to try nasal pillows instead of a mask. Nasal pillows are small, flexible, mushroom-shaped cones that fit into each nostril.

Let your home equipment provider know whether you sleep on your back, side, or stomach. Different types of plastic tubing connect the mask to the CPAP machine. Some types may make it easier for you to sleep on your side or stomach.

What to Expect while Using CPAP

CPAP is a long-term treatment. Many people have questions when they first start using CPAP.

Talk with your sleep specialist about how to handle followup questions. He or she can answer some questions, but your home equipment provider may need to address others. Ask your sleep specialist to recommend a home equipment provider that has a lot of experience with CPAP.

To achieve the full benefits of CPAP, use it every time you sleep—during naps and at night. Most people should use CPAP for at least 7.5 hours each night for the best results.

The CPAP Machine

Adjusting to the CPAP machine can take time. You may feel strange wearing a mask on your face at night or feeling the flow of air. Some people feel confined by the mask. If you feel this way, slowly adjusting to the mask may help.

First, hold the mask up to your face for short periods during the day. Next, try wearing it with the straps for short periods. Then, add the hose.

Breathing with a machine doesn't feel natural. If your machine has a "ramp" feature, you can use it to slowly "ramp up" from a lower air pressure to the pressure that's needed to keep your airways open during sleep. Once you're comfortable using CPAP during the day, try using it at night while you sleep.

Relaxation exercises help some people adjust to using CPAP. Talk with your doctor about whether relaxation exercises might help you.

If you're having trouble adjusting to the mask or the CPAP machine, contact your home equipment provider. Your provider may have staff who can help you adjust to CPAP. Also, you may want to try a different mask that has fewer straps or less contact with your skin.

Follow-Up Care

Your sleep specialist may ask you to schedule a follow-up visit about a month after you begin using CPAP. He or she will want to see how well you are adjusting to treatment. After that, you may have followup care every 6 or 12 months.

Your sleep specialist might need to adjust the air pressure setting of your CPAP machine if:

- You gain or lose a lot of weight

- Your symptoms, such as daytime sleepiness, persist or recur

- You have another treatment for sleep apnea, such as upper airway surgery or a mouthpiece

Benefits of CPAP

CPAP has many benefits. It can:

- Keep your airway open while you sleep

- Correct snoring so others in your household can sleep

- Improve your quality of sleep

- Relieve sleep apnea symptoms, such as excessive daytime sleepiness

- Decrease or prevent high blood pressure

With CPAP, you may fall asleep faster and wake fewer times during the night. The pauses in breathing that are typical with sleep apnea won't disrupt your sleep.

Studies also show that treatment with CPAP is linked to a decrease in reported car accidents and near accidents. Some studies have shown that CPAP improves reaction time, concentration, and memory in people who use the treatment.

Many people who use CPAP report feeling better once they begin treatment. They feel more attentive and better able to work during the day. They also report fewer complaints from bed partners about snoring and sleep disruption.

You may feel better after the first night of using CPAP. You may wake feeling refreshed, alert, and in a better mood. You also may feel less tired during the day.

However, it can take a week to a month to adjust to CPAP. Some people have trouble falling asleep when they first start using CPAP. This problem usually is short term and goes away as you adjust to the treatment.

Even if you don't notice a change right away, stick with the treatment. The benefits are worthwhile. Once you adjust to using CPAP, you'll sleep better.

What Are the Risks of CPAP?

CPAP is a safe, painless treatment. Side effects and other problems usually are minor, and they can be treated or fixed. Talk with your doctor if you're having problems using CPAP. He or she can suggest ways to handle or treat these problems.

Although these problems can be frustrating, stick with the treatment. The benefits of CPAP are worthwhile.

Side Effects

Mask Allergies and Skin Irritation

CPAP masks can cause skin allergies or skin irritation. If this happens, try a different type of mask.

CPAP masks come in many shapes, sizes, and materials. Some have fewer straps and less contact with your face. Some masks may irritate your skin less than others.

If you have trouble finding a mask that works for you, ask your sleep specialist about nasal pillows. These are small, flexible, mushroom-shaped cones that fit into each nostril.

Dry Mouth

Dry mouth can be caused by the CPAP itself or from breathing through your mouth at night. A CPAP machine that has a heated humidifier can help relieve this side effect.

If dry mouth persists, your sleep specialist may suggest a chin strap to keep your mouth closed or a different type of mask.

Talk to your sleep specialist if dry mouth continues. Your mask might be leaking air into your open mouth, causing dry mouth.

Congestion, Runny Nose, Sneezing, Sinusitis, and Nosebleeds

Congestion, runny nose, sneezing, sinusitis, and nosebleeds can occur while using CPAP. A CPAP machine that has a heated humidifier can help relieve these side effects. Also, make sure that your CPAP mask fits well.

Some people find that using a saline nasal spray at bedtime prevents these side effects. If these steps don't work, talk to your sleep specialist. He or she may prescribe a steroid nasal spray.

Stomach Bloating and Discomfort

A problem with the air pressure setting on your CPAP machine might cause stomach bloating and discomfort. If you have these side effects, talk to your sleep specialist. He or she may adjust the settings of your machine to relieve these problems.

Problems with the CPAP Equipment

Mask Leaks

Many factors can cause a CPAP mask to leak. To avoid a leak, follow the instructions that come with the mask. Try washing the mask daily. Also, wash your face and use a moisturizer so your skin is moist before you put on the mask.

You might find it helpful to adjust the mask's straps. When straps are too loose or too tight, a leak can happen. You may need to select a different size or type of mask.

If your CPAP mask leaks air, you won't get the proper amount of air pressure. Also, leaks can lead to skin or eye irritation.

Very small leaks don't stop the machine from producing the correct amount of air pressure. But small leaks can cause a shrill sound that disturbs the sleep of others in the house.

Don't use tape or grease on a mask to prevent leaks, unless advised by your home equipment provider or sleep specialist.

Air Pressure Problems

The air pressure from CPAP makes some people feel like it's hard to exhale (breathe out) or like they're choking or suffocating. Some people swallow air, which may cause burping.

If you have problems with the air pressure from CPAP, it may help to use the "ramp" feature on your CPAP machine. This feature allows the machine to slowly "ramp up" from a lower air pressure to the pressure that's needed to keep your airway open during sleep.

If your machine doesn't have this feature or if it doesn't help, talk to your sleep specialist. He or she may suggest a different CPAP machine. If that doesn't work, your sleep specialist may suggest another type of positive airway pressure.

Mask Removal

To get the full benefit of CPAP, you should use it every time you sleep. Some people remove the CPAP mask while they're asleep. If this happens, you might be able to solve the problem by:

- Finding a mask that fits better.

- Using a CPAP machine that has a humidifier. This might make the treatment more comfortable and stop you from removing the mask.

- Using a chin strap to hold the mask in place.

Some CPAP machines come with an alarm that makes noise if the mask comes off.

Noise

Most new CPAP machines are fairly quiet. The noise that they make is soft and rhythmic. If the noise bothers you, check the air filter to make sure the machine is working properly. Your sleep specialist or home equipment provider also can check the machine for you.

If the CPAP machine is working properly, but the noise still bothers you, try using earplugs or a white-noise sound machine.

Chapter 47

Treating Sleep Problems of People in Recovery from Substance Use Disorders

Sleep Disturbances and Substance Use

Many Americans suffer from unhealthy sleep-related behaviors. The prevalence of insomnia symptoms (difficulty initiating or maintaining sleep) in the general population is estimated at 33 percent, with an estimated 6 percent having a diagnosis of insomnia. According to a 12-state survey conducted by the Centers for Disease Control and Prevention (CDC).

- 35.3 percent of survey respondents obtain less than 7 hours of sleep on average during a 24-hour period.

- 48.0 percent snore.

- 37.9 percent unintentionally fall asleep during the day

This chapter contains text excerpted from the following sources: Text under the heading "Sleep Disturbances and Substance Use" is excerpted from "Treating Sleep Problems of People in Recovery from Substance Use Disorders," Substance Abuse and Mental Health Services Administration (SAMHSA),October 23, 2014; Text under the heading "Chronic Cocaine Abusers Have Occult Insomnia in Early Abstinence" is excerpted from "Chronic Cocaine Abusers Have Occult Insomnia in Early Abstinence," National Institute on Drug Abuse (NIDA), March 2008. Reviewed July 2016.

Substance/medication-induced sleep disorder is recognized in the *Diagnostic and Statistical Manual of Mental Disorders, Fifth Edition*. Substance use can exacerbate sleep difficulties, which in turn present a risk factor for substance use or relapse to use. The types of sleep problems vary by substance used and can include insomnia, sleep latency (the time it takes to fall asleep), disturbances in sleep cycles and sleep continuity, or hypersomnia (excessive daytime sleepiness). Specific findings on the relationship between sleep disturbances and substance use are presented below.

Alcohol Abuse

Insomnia and other sleep disturbances are common symptoms of alcohol dependence. Many people with alcohol use disorder (AUD) have insomnia before entering treatment. Reported rates of sleep problems among people with AUD in treatment range from 25 to 72 percent. Some people in recovery from AUD may continue to have sleep problems, including insomnia or sleep-disordered breathing (such as sleep apnea), for weeks, months, or sometimes years after initiating abstinence.

Illicit Drug Use

Sleep disturbances are common among people abstaining from chronic substance use. People stopping marijuana use can experience sleep problems in the first days of withdrawal, and these problems can last for weeks. People in detoxification from opioids often report symptoms of insomnia. A study that objectively measured sleep in people who chronically use cocaine found that sleep quality deteriorated during a period of abstinence, even though the subjects perceived their sleep to be improving. Another study of people in withdrawal from cocaine found that three-quarters experienced poor sleep quality. In a study of college students, those who reported a history of nonmedical psychostimulant use or current use reported worse subjective and overall sleep quality and more sleep disturbance compared with those who had not used such substances.

The Effects of Sleep Loss during Recovery

Sleep loss can have significant negative effects on the physical, mental, and emotional well-being of people in recovery. It can also interfere with substance abuse treatment. Persistent sleep complaints after withdrawal are associated with relapse to alcohol use. Poor sleep quality before a quit attempt from cannabis use is a risk factor for lapsing back into use within 2 days.

Medication-Assisted Treatment and Sleep Disorders

Disrupted sleep, including central sleep apnea and related daytime sleepiness, is prevalent in people on methadone maintenance therapy for opioid dependence. Methadone dose and duration of opioid use prior to treatment correlate linearly with sleep problems. The prevalence of sleep problems is attributable to the methadone, which is a full μ-opioid agonist, and to concurrent factors that often affect patients in recovery from opioid addiction, such as mental disorders, benzodiazepine abuse, and chronic pain. Buprenorphine, a partial μ-opioid agonist, at routine therapeutic doses has also been found to induce significant alterations of breathing during sleep.

Assessing Sleep Disorders

If a patient initiating withdrawal from a substance or recovering from an substance use disorder (SUD) complains of a sleep disturbance, the healthcare provider should assess for causes by doing the following:

- Determine the duration of recovery and medications used for SUD treatment

- Ask questions about difficulty falling asleep, waking during the night, amount of sleep per night, snoring, sleep apnea, excessive movements during sleep, uncontrollable movements that are relieved by getting up and walking, and excessive daytime sleepiness. If possible, ask significant others the same questions about the patient.

- Rule out other causes of the sleep problem, such as stress, a life crisis, or side effects of medications the patient is taking

- Ask the patient to write in a sleep diary or log immediately on awakening. The patient should record total time in bed, time of sleep onset, number of times awakened, and total time spent awake

- Determine the frequency and duration of symptoms of insomnia. If difficulties occur two or three nights per week and

347

last for 1 month or more, the patient warrants a diagnosis of insomnia

Note that some patients tend to overestimate the quality and duration of their sleep on self-report questionnaires and in sleep logs. If warranted, a referral for an objective sleep study in a sleep laboratory can be made.

Treatments

The association between insomnia and relapse calls for treatment that addresses insomnia during recovery. The first step in treating insomnia should focus on the status of the patient's recovery. Patients should be receiving treatment from an appropriate substance abuse treatment program. It is important to address other psychological, social, and medical problems that may contribute to insomnia, such as co-occurring mental and medical disorders, use of medications that disturb sleep, and nicotine use.

Nonpharmacological Treatments

Nonpharmacological treatments are preferred because many pharmacological treatments for insomnia have the potential for abuse and can interfere with SUD recovery. Research on cognitive–behavioral therapy (CBT) to treat insomnia has shown positive results, generally and also in patients who are alcohol dependent. Exhibit 1 lists several nonpharmacological interventions that have shown some degree of effectiveness. Combining approaches may be more effective than using one approach.

Healthcare providers can educate patients about simple nonpharmacological techniques that can improve sleep (see Exhibit 2). Sleep education includes teaching about sleep, the effects of recovery from substance use on sleep, and health practices and environmental factors that affect sleep. Sleep can be improved by limiting bedroom activities to sleeping (e.g., refraining from activities such as reading the newspaper, paying bills, or working on electronic devices) and going to bed only when sleepy and at about the same time each day. These activities help reassociate the bed and bedroom with going to sleep. Establishing a relaxing pre sleep routine, which can include progressive muscle relaxation, imagery, or a warm bath, also promotes sleep. Some patients may benefit from referral to a sleep medicine specialist.

What Healthcare Providers Can Do

- Screen for insomnia among people in recovery from SUDs.

- Include questions about sleep during the routine patient history.

- Rule out other causes of sleep problems (e.g., stress, medications).

- Educate patients about sleep hygiene, and make referrals to a specialist if necessary.

- Conduct a careful evaluation, and consider risk factors, before prescribing sedative–hypnotic medications to treat insomnia.

- Monitor patients for signs of abuse or diversion of scheduled medications prescribed to treat insomnia and other sleep disorders.

Exhibit 1. Nonpharmacological Treatments

- **Mindfulness meditation**. The patient moves into a state of restful, present-moment alertness, which reduces stress and improves self-control

- **Progressive muscle relaxation**. The patient concentrates on tensing and relaxing groups of muscles

- **Biofeedback**. The patient becomes aware of physiologic stress responses and how to control them

- **CBT for insomnia**. The patient's dysfunctional beliefs and behaviors are modified to improve his or her emotional state

- **Stimulus control**. The patient reassociates the bedroom with the rapid onset of sleep

- **Exercise**. Regular physical activity relieves stress and tires the patient

- **Sleep restriction therapy**. The patient limits sleep to a few hours and progressively increases it until the desired amount of sleep time is achieved

- **Bright-light therapy**. Exposure to a natural bright light while awake helps promote normal sleep patterns

- **Dental devices and continuous positive airway pressure machines**. These devices help the patient with obstructive sleep apnea breathe more easily during sleep.

Pharmacological Treatments

Over-the-Counter Medications and Dietary Supplements

Some people who have trouble sleeping have tried over the-counter sleep medications or dietary supplements to help them sleep. Patients may ask about these, and care should be taken to explain their safety and efficacy. Many over-the-counter sleep medications contain antihistamines that cause sedation. They are not recommended as a long-term treatment for insomnia because they negatively affect the natural sleep cycle and have side effects such as morning grogginess, daytime sleepiness, and impaired alertness and judgement. Furthermore, evidence supporting their long-term effectiveness is insufficient.

Popular dietary supplements taken with the intent to promote sleep include valerian and melatonin. Valerian, an herb, is thought to have sedative effects. However, studies of valerian offer mixed results, and evidence supporting the supplement's efficacy is insufficient to warrant its use. In addition, valerian could damage the liver. Melatonin is a brain hormone that helps regulate sleep patterns. Limited evidence shows that it can treat chronic insomnia in some people and, to date, there is no evidence that it is harmful

Prescription Medications without Known Abuse Potential

Medications without known abuse potential should be the first treatment option when pharmacotherapy is necessary to treat insomnia during recovery. Ramelteon and doxepin are the only unscheduled prescription medications approved by the U.S. Food and Drug Administration (FDA) for the treatment of insomnia. Ramelteon decreases the amount of time it takes to fall asleep. Doxepin, originally FDA approved as an antidepressant, has been approved for treating insomnia typified by problems staying asleep. These medications may be suitable for treating insomnia in patients in recovery, because they do not appear to have potential for abuse.

Exhibit 2. Promoting Sleep Hygiene: Tips for a Good Night's Sleep

- Go to bed and get up at the same times each day.

- Use natural light (that comes through a window) to remind yourself of when it's time to be asleep and awake. This can help you set a healthy sleep–wake cycle.

- Exercise regularly.

- If you take naps, keep them short and before 5 p.m.

- Don't eat or drink too much when it is close to bedtime.

- Avoid caffeine (in coffee, tea, chocolate, cola, and some pain relievers) and nicotine for several hours before bedtime.

- Wind down before going to bed (e.g., take a warm bath, do light reading, practice relaxation exercises).

- Keep the bedroom a relaxing place—avoid working or paying bills in bed.

- Sleep in a dark, quiet room that isn't too hot or too cold.

- Don't lie in bed awake. If you can't fall asleep within 20 minutes, get up and do something relaxing.

Off-Label Medications

Other medications are often prescribed off label (for purposes other than the medication's FDA-approved use) to treat insomnia. According to a survey of addiction medicine physicians, the sedating antidepressant trazodone is the medication most often prescribed for the management of sleep disorders in patients in early recovery from AUD. One study found that its use among people in recovery from AUD improved sleep efficiency. Studies of its effects on abstinence and relapse in persons with AUD are conflicting. A 2008 study comparing trazodone with placebo for people after detoxification from alcohol showed that the trazodone group had improved sleep quality but had less improvement in the proportion of days abstinent while taking the medication. Furthermore, when the medication was discontinued, the trazodone group experienced less improvement in abstinence days and an increase in the number of drinks per drinking day. In contrast, a study published in 2011 of patients discharged from residential treatment did not find an association between trazodone use and relapse or return to heavy drinking. A study of patients on methadone maintenance treatment found that trazodone use provided no improvement in sleep.

Other sedating antidepressants that have been used to treat insomnia include amitriptyline, mirtazapine, nefazodone, and nortriptyline. In a study of the use of mirtazapine on subjects with cocaine dependence and co-occurring depression, the medication decreased sleep latency; however, it had no measurable effect on treatment for cocaine dependence and depressive symptoms.

Gabapentin, an anticonvulsant with sedative properties, also has evidence of efficacy for treating insomnia. It has been found to be more effective in promoting sleep than lorazepam (an anxiolytic commonly prescribed to treat insomnia) among people withdrawing from alcohol. It has also been found to be more effective than trazodone in promoting sleep among those in early recovery.

Acamprosate, a medication used to maintain alcohol abstinence, may also improve sleep during withdrawal from alcohol.

Prescription Medications with Known Abuse Potential

Sedative–hypnotic medications, such as benzodiazepines and non-benzodiazepines, are commonly prescribed to treat sleep problems. However, these medications should be avoided by people with histories of SUDs, who are at increased risk for abusing them. Benzodiazepines, such as alprazolam, diazepam, and triazolam, are especially risky for use with people with SUDs because they are potentially addicting. They can also cause residual daytime sedation, cognitive impairment, motor incoordination, and rebound insomnia. Long-term treatment of insomnia with benzodiazepines may lead to withdrawal symptoms (e.g., anxiety, irritability, seizures) when patients stop taking the medications. A careful clinical evaluation is needed to ensure appropriate prescribing. Measures to prevent abuse include the following:

- Observe closely and perform ongoing evaluations.

- Prescribe a few tablets at a time.

- Schedule frequent office visits.

- Conduct occasional urine screenings.

- Use one source to dispense the medication.

- Occasionally taper the medication.

- Be attentive to risk factors such as antisocial personality disorder and dependence on multiple substances.

Alternatives to benzodiazepines include sedative–hypnotic medications such as zaleplon, eszopiclone, and zolpidem. These medications all have the same mechanism of action as benzodiazepines but lack some of the negative side effects. However, some research indicates that at high doses they may have the same side effects as benzodiazepines. The three medications are Schedule IV controlled substances, indicating abuse potential. For these reasons, these medications should be used only for short-term treatment of insomnia in people with a history of SUDs.

Chronic Cocaine Abusers Have Occult Insomnia in Early Abstinence

Patients in early treatment may not recognize their own sleep impairment or its impact on their performance.

Chronic cocaine abusers may feel they are sleeping better and better during early abstinence, but objective measures show the opposite happens. A team of NIDA-funded addiction and sleep researchers at the Yale and Harvard Schools of Medicine found evidence of insomnia, with learning and attentional deficits, on days of taking the drug and after 2.5 weeks of abstinence. The researchers believe cocaine may impair the brain's ability to gauge its own need for sleep, and patients' ability to benefit from early treatment may suffer as a result.

"Problems in memory and attention are linked with increased treatment dropout and likely affect patients' ability to 'take in' lessons from drug abuse counseling," says Dr. Robert Malison of Yale, a co-investigator on the study. If the results are confirmed, clinicians and patients may want to consider addressing sleep disorders in early therapy, perhaps with the use of medications or behavioral treatments.

The researchers recruited 10 men and two women aged 24 to 49 who, on average, had abused cocaine for 17 years and had used $500 worth of the drug per week. All the participants declined an offer of drug abuse treatment. Urine tests indicated that cocaine was the only drug any of them had abused during the week before the study.

At the outset of the study, participants self-administered cocaine from a pump under physician oversight, building up to a dose of 32 mg/kg of body weight over 1.5 hours, then repeating this dose essentially at will, but no less than 5 minutes apart, for another 1.5 hours. Subsequently, they self-administered the higher dose with the same minimal restriction for 2 hours on each of three consecutive days, either on days 4-6 or 18-20. This schedule simulated chronic cocaine abusers' typical bingeing pattern of drug abuse and allowed researchers to monitor each participant's sleep and cognitive performance for 17 days after a binge.

Research staff made sure the participants stayed awake from 7:45 AM to 9:30 PM, and let them sleep through the night. At night, the participants wore Nightcap sleep monitors, a bandana-like device that records eye and body movements that indicate whether someone is awake, asleep and dreaming, or sleeping dreamlessly. On most nights participants also wore polysomnographic (PSG) devices that continuously assessed brain activity with electroencephalography (EEG) and measured eye and muscle movements associated with different sleep stages. Combining the information gathered by these measures with participants' responses to daily questionnaires on their sleep experience and with cognitive testing, the researchers demonstrated that the participants had:

- Sleep deficits—After 14 to 17 days of abstinence, the study group exhibited sleep deficits on several measures, relative to healthy, age-matched peers who participated in prior studies. For example, they had less total sleep time (336 versus 421-464 minutes) and took longer to fall asleep (19 versus 6-16 minutes).

- Declines in sleep quantity and quality—The time participants took to fall asleep and their total time asleep transiently improved during the first week of abstinence, but then reverted to the patterns recorded on days of cocaine taking. On abstinence days 14-17, participants took an average of 20 minutes to fall asleep (from a low of 11) and slept for 40 minutes less than their minimum. Slow-wave sleep—a deep sleep that often increases following sleep deprivation—rose during the binge and on abstinence days 10-17.

- Lack of awareness of their sleep problems—In contrast to the evidence of objective measures, the study participants reported steadily improving sleep from the beginning to the end of their days of abstinence.

- Impairments in learning and attention—As with sleep quality, participants' performance on tests of alertness and motor-skills learning initially improved and then deteriorated. On abstinence day 17, they registered their lowest scores on alertness and ability to learn a new motor skill.

Increased Risk of Relapse

"Unlike most people with chronic insomnia, including alcoholics, cocaine abusers do not perceive sleep problems and may not ask clinicians for treatment to improve sleep," says Dr. Malison. The problem often goes unaddressed and persists as a result, and the accompanying impairments in attention and learning may affect how well they respond to drug abuse treatment. Clinical studies have shown that poor objective sleep during the first 2 weeks of abstinence predicts relapse to alcohol 5 months after treatment.

In fact, the insidious nature of cocaine-related insomnia may directly trigger relapse, suggests Dr. Peter Morgan, lead investigator of the study. "Addicted people may take cocaine to improve sleep-related cognitive functioning deficits—unaware that they are abusing, in part, to 'solve' these problems."

Dr. Morgan adds, "Cocaine abusers who recognize their cognitive problems often report that it takes them 6 months to a year to turn the corner—a clinical observation that points to the need for longer term studies of sleep and treatment outcomes among this population." In addition to studies with larger numbers of participants, the investigators say there is a need to investigate possible gender differences in cocaine-related sleep problems. Dr. Morgan and his team are currently testing two medications, tiagabine and modafinil, to see if they can improve cocaine abusers' sleep and restore cognitive performance.

"Experts believe that not getting enough sleep is an unmet public health problem in the general population. These findings highlight this important problem in cocaine abusers," says Dr. Harold Gordon of NIDA's Division of Clinical Neuroscience and Behavioral Research.

Part Six

A Special Look at Pediatric Sleep Issues

Chapter 48

Infants and Sleep-Related Concerns

Chapter Contents

Section 48.1

Safe Sleeping and Bed-Sharing

Text in this section under the heading "Safe Sleeping Environment
for Infants" is excerpted from "What Is a Safe Sleep Environment?"
National Institutes of Health (NIH), September 11, 2015;
Remaining text in this section is from "Bed-Sharing," © 1995–2016.
The Nemours Foundation/KidsHealth®. Reprinted with permission.

Safe Sleeping Environment for Infants

There are ways parents and caregivers can reduce the risk of sudden infant death syndrome (SIDS) and other sleep-related causes of infant death. Learn how to create a safe sleep environment for your baby. To start, select the crib.

Always Place Your Baby on His or Her Back to Sleep, for Naps and at Night, to Reduce the Risk of SIDS.

The back position is the safest: Babies who sleep on their backs are much less likely to die of SIDS than are babies who sleep on their stomachs or sides.

Babies who are used to sleeping on their backs but who are then placed on their stomachs, such as for a nap, are at very high risk for SIDS. So remember, every sleep time counts.

Use a Firm Sleep Surface, Such as a Mattress in a Safety-Approved Crib, Covered by a Fitted Sheet, to Reduce the Risk of SIDS and Other Sleep-Related Causes of Infant Death.

Firm sleep surfaces can include safety-approved* cribs, bassinets, and portable play areas. Do not use a car seat, carrier, swing, or similar product as baby's everyday sleep area.

Babies who sleep on a soft surface, such as an adult mattress, or under a soft surface, such as a soft blanket or quilt, are more likely to die of SIDS and other sleep-related causes of infant death. Never place baby to sleep on soft surfaces, such as couches or sofas, pillows, quilts, sheepskins, or blankets.

Give Your Baby a Dry Pacifier—Not Attached to a String—for Naps and at Night to Reduce the Risk of SIDS.

But don't force the baby to take the pacifier.

If the pacifier falls out of the baby's mouth during sleep, you do not need to replace it.

Wait until your baby is used to breastfeeding before trying a pacifier.

Do Not Let Your Baby Get Too Hot during Sleep.

Because blankets can make a baby too warm during sleep, use them as decoration in the room instead of in the crib with the baby.

Dress your baby in no more than one layer of clothing more than an adult would wear to be comfortable, and leave the blanket out of the crib. A one-piece sleeper or sleep sack can be used for sleep clothing. If you notice baby sweating or breathing rapidly, he or she may be too warm.

Have the Baby Share Your Room, Not Your Bed.

Room sharing—keeping baby's sleep area separate from your sleep area in the same room where you sleep—reduces the risk of SIDS and other sleep-related causes of infant death, such as accidental suffocation.

Your baby should not sleep in an adult bed, on a couch, or on a chair alone, with you, or with anyone else.

Keeping the baby's sleep area next to you makes it easier to feed and check on your baby. If you bring baby into your bed to feed, make sure to put him or her back in a separate sleep area, such as a safety-approved* crib, bassinet, or portable play area, in your room next to where you sleep when you are finished.

Keep Soft Objects, Toys, Crib Bumpers, and Loose Bedding out of Your Baby's Sleep Area to Reduce the Risk of SIDS and Other Sleep-Related Causes of Infant Death.

Stuffed animals and toys are great for when baby is awake, but keep them and other objects out of the sleep area.

Don't use pillows, blankets, quilts, sheepskins, or crib bumpers anywhere in your baby's sleep area.

Why no crib bumpers? Evidence does not support using crib bumpers to prevent injuries. In fact, crib bumpers can cause serious injuries and even death. Keeping them out of baby's sleep area is the best way to avoid these dangers.

Do Not Let Your Baby Get Too Hot during Sleep.

Keep the room at a temperature that is comfortable for an adult. Dress your baby in no more than one layer of clothing more than an adult would wear to be comfortable, and do not use a blanket. A one-piece sleeper or sleep sack can be used for sleep clothing.

Put Your Baby on His or Her Back to Sleep for All Sleep Times, including Daytime Naps and Overnight, to Reduce the Risk of SIDS. The back position is the safest: Babies who sleep on their backs are much less likely to die of SIDS than are babies who sleep on their stomachs or sides.

Every sleep time counts: Babies who are used to sleeping on their backs but who are then placed on their stomachs, such as for a nap, are at very high risk for SIDS.

Great Job! You've helped to create a safe sleep environment for your baby and learned some ways to reduce the risk of SIDS and other sleep-related causes of infant death.

Consider these other ways to reduce your baby's risk of SIDS and other sleep-related causes of infant death:
Women should:
Get regular healthcare during pregnancy, and
Not drink alcohol or use illegal drugs during pregnancy or after the baby is born.

Do not allow smoking around your baby to reduce the risk of SIDS. Don't smoke during pregnancy, and don't smoke or allow smoking around your baby.

Breastfeed your baby to reduce the risk of SIDS. Breastfeeding also has many health benefits for mother and baby.

Follow healthcare provider guidance on your baby's vaccines and regular health checkups.

Avoid products that claim to reduce the risk of SIDS and other sleep-related causes of death. These wedges, positioners, and other products have not been tested for safety or effectiveness.

Do not use home heart or breathing monitors to reduce the risk of SIDS. If you have questions about using these types of monitors for other health conditions, talk with your baby's healthcare provider.

Give your baby plenty of Tummy Time when he or she is awake and when someone is watching. Supervised Tummy Time helps baby's neck, shoulder, and arm muscles get stronger. It also helps to prevent flat spots on the back of your baby's head. Holding baby upright and limiting time in carriers and bouncers can also help prevent flat spots on the back of baby's head.

Co-Sleeping, Room-Sharing, and Bed-Sharing

Many people use the terms "bed-sharing" and "co-sleeping" to describe the same thing, but there are differences:

- **Co-sleeping**: This is when a parent and child sleep within a "sensory" distance of each other, meaning that each can tell that the other is nearby their touch, sight, or even smell. (Co-sleeping is sometimes also called sleep-sharing.)

Room-sharing and bed-sharing are types of co-sleeping:

- **Room-sharing**: This is when parents have a crib in the room with them, a bassinet or portable crib near the bed, a separate crib attached to the bed, or a similar arrangement.

- **Bed-sharing**: This is when parents share their bed with their children (sometimes called the "family bed"). This is what has raised concerns with pediatricians and others.

Why Some People Bed-Share

Bed-sharing supporters believe—and some studies support their beliefs—that bed-sharing:

- encourages breastfeeding by making nighttime breastfeeding more convenient

- makes it easier for a nursing mother to get her sleep cycle in sync with her baby's

- helps babies fall asleep more easily, especially during their first few months and when they wake up in the middle of the night

- helps babies get more nighttime sleep (because they awaken more often with shorter feeding time, which can add up to a greater amount of sleep throughout the night)

- helps parents regain closeness with their infant after being separated from their babies during the workday

Is Bed-Sharing Safe?

In some non-Western cultures, bed-sharing is common and the number of infant deaths related to it is lower than in the West. Differences in mattresses, bedding, and other cultural practices may account for the lower risk in these countries.

Despite the possible pros, various U.S. medical groups warn parents not to place their infants to sleep in adult beds due to serious safety risks. Bed-sharing puts babies at risk of suffocation, strangulation, and sudden infant death syndrome (SIDS). Studies have found that bed-sharing is the most common cause of deaths in babies, especially those 3 months and younger.

An adult bed has many safety risks for a baby, including:

- suffocation from lying face-down on a waterbed, a regular mattress, or soft bedding such as pillows, blankets, or a quilt, or due to an infant's head being covered by such items

- suffocation, when an infant gets trapped or wedged between a mattress and headboard, wall, or other object

- strangulation in a bed frame that allows part of an infant's body to pass through an area while trapping the baby's head

Among older infants (4 to12 months old) who died due to bed-sharing, having an additional item (like a pillow or a blanket) on the bed increased the risk of death. Babies should always be placed to sleep on their backs on a firm mattress without any pillows, blankets, toys, stuffed animals, or other items.

Because of the risks involved, both the American Academy of Pediatrics (AAP) and the U.S. Product Safety Commission (CPSC) advice against bed-sharing. The AAP does recommend the practice of room-sharing without bed-sharing. Room-sharing is thought to help lower the risk of SIDS.

Besides the potential safety risks, sharing a bed with a baby sometimes prevent parents from getting a good night's sleep. And infants who co-sleep might learn to associate sleep with being close to a parent in the parent's bed, which can become a problem at naptime or when the baby needs to go to sleep before the parent is ready.

Bed-Sharing and SIDS

Some studies suggest that bed-sharing increases the risk of SIDS, especially in infants younger than 12 weeks old.

Factors that can increase this risk include:

- a baby sleeping on a couch alone or with a parent

- a baby sleeping between two parents

- a mother who smokes

- parents who are extremely tired

- a parent who has recently used alcohol or drugs

- bed-sharing with pillows or bed covers

It's safer to use room-sharing without bed-sharing. Experts note that parents and babies sleeping in the same room can reduce the risk of SIDS because they tend to wake up more often throughout the night.

How to Room-Share Safely

To avoid the risks of bed sharing while enjoying the benefits of room-sharing, parents have lots of options. To keep your little one close by, but not in your bed, you could:

- Put a bassinet, play yard, or crib next to your bed. This lets you keep that desired closeness, which can be especially important if you're breastfeeding. The AAP says that having an infant sleep in a separate crib, bassinet, or play yard in the same room as the mother reduces the risk of SIDS.

- Buy a device that looks like a bassinet or play yard with one side that is lower, which attaches to your bed to allow you and baby to be next to each other while eliminating the possibility of rolling over onto your infant.

How to Bed-Share as Safely as Possible

Despite the risks of bed-sharing, some parents decide this sleeping arrangement is best for their family. If you do choose to share your bed with your baby, follow these precautions:

- Don't share a bed with an infant under 4 months of age—a bassinet or crib next to the bed is a better choice.

- Always place your baby on his or her back to sleep to reduce the risk of SIDS.

- Dress your baby in minimal clothing to avoid overheating.

- Don't place a baby to sleep alone in an adult bed.

- Don't place a baby on a soft surface to sleep, such as a soft mattress, sofa, or waterbed.

- Make sure your bed's headboard and footboard don't have openings or cutouts that could trap your baby's head.

- Make sure your mattress fits snugly in the bed frame so that your baby won't become trapped between the frame and the mattress.

- Don't cover your child's head while sleeping.

- Don't use pillows, comforters, quilts, and other soft or plush items on the bed. You can dress your baby in a sleeper instead of using blankets.

- Don't drink alcohol or use medicines or drugs that could keep you from waking or might cause you to roll over onto, and therefore suffocate, your baby.

- Don't place your bed near draperies or blinds where your child could be get caught in and strangled by cords.

- Don't fall asleep with a baby on your chest.

- Don't sleep on couches, recliners, or rockers with a baby.

Who Shouldn't Share a Bed with a Baby?

If an infant and a parent are bed-sharing, keep the following people out of the sleep environment:

- other children—particularly toddlers—because they might not be aware of the baby's presence

- parents who are under the influence of alcohol or any drug because that could lower their awareness of the baby

And nobody should smoke in the room, as this increases the risk of SIDS.

Moving Out of the Parent's Bed

Eventually, the bed-sharing routine will be end at some point, either because the child wants to or by the parents' choice.

If you've been bed-sharing with your little one and would like to stop, talk to your doctor about making a plan for when your baby will sleep in a crib. Moving to a crib by 6 months of age is usually easier—for both parents and baby—before the bed-sharing habit is ingrained and other developmental issues (such as separation anxiety) come into play.

Section 48.2

Flat Head Syndrome (Positional Plagiocephaly)

This section includes text excerpted from "Flat Head Syndrome (Positional Plagiocephaly)," © 1995–2016. The Nemours Foundation/ KidsHealth®. Reprinted with permission.

What Is Flat Head Syndrome?

Babies are born with soft heads to allow for the amazing brain growth that occurs in the first year of life. As a result, their heads are easily "molded."

Passage through the birth canal during childbirth can cause a newborn's head to look pointy or too long. So it's normal for a baby's skull, which is made up of several bones that eventually fuse together, to be a bit oddly shaped during the few days or weeks after birth.

But if a baby develops a lasting flat spot, either on one side or the back of the head, it could be **flat head syndrome**, also called positional plagiocephaly. Flat head syndrome usually happens when a baby sleeps in the same position most of the time or because of problems with the neck muscles.

This problem does not harm brain development or cause any lasting appearance problems. And, fortunately, it does not require surgery. Simple practices like changing a baby's sleep position, holding your baby, and providing lots of "tummy time" can help.

Causes

The most common cause of a flattened head is a baby's sleep position. Because infants sleep for so many hours on their backs, the head sometimes flattens in one spot. Placing babies in devices where they lie down often during the day (infant car seats, carriers, strollers, swings, and bouncy seats) also adds to this problem.

Premature babies are more likely to have a flattened head. Their skulls are softer than those of full-term babies. They also spend a lot of time on their backs without being moved or picked up because of their medical needs and extreme fragility after birth, which usually requires a stay in the neonatal intensive care unit (NICU).

A baby might even start to develop flat head syndrome before birth, if pressure is placed on the baby's skull by the mother's pelvis or a twin. In fact, many babies from multiple births are born with heads that have some flat spots.

Being cramped in the womb can also cause torticollis, which can lead to a flattened head. Babies with torticollis have a hard time turning their heads because of tight neck muscles on one side of the neck. Since it's hard to turn the head, they tend to keep their heads in the same position when lying down. This can cause flattening.

Likewise, many babies who started out with flat head syndrome develop torticollis. Because it takes a lot of energy for them to turn their heads, babies with severe flattening on one side tend to stay on that side, so their necks become stiff from lack of use.

Signs and Symptoms

Flattened head syndrome is usually easy for parents to notice. Typically, the back of the child's head, called the occiput, is flattened on one side. There is usually less hair on that part of the baby's head. If a person is looking down at the baby's head, the ear on the flattened side may be pushed forward.

In severe cases, the head might bulge on the side opposite from the flattening, and the forehead may be uneven. If torticollis is the cause, the neck, jaw, and face may be uneven as well.

Diagnosis

Doctors usually diagnose flat head syndrome simply by looking a child's head. To check for torticollis, the doctor may watch how a baby moves the head and neck. Lab tests, X-rays, and computed tomography (CT scans) usually are not needed.

The doctor may monitor a child over a few visits to see how the shape of the head changes. If repositioning the child's head during sleep helps to improve the skull over time, the problem is likely due to flat head syndrome. If it doesn't, the cause could be due to another condition, such as craniosynostosis.

Craniosynostosis happens when a child's skull bones fuse together before they're supposed to (normally, around age 4). This fusion restricts brain growth and causes skull deformities. Children with craniosynostosis need treatment to correct the problem.

If the doctor suspects craniosynostosis or another condition, the child will be referred to a pediatric neurosurgeon or a craniofacial plastic surgeon who may order other tests, like X-rays or a CT scan.

Treatment

If your child has flat head syndrome that's caused by a sleeping or lying position, there is a lot you can do at home to help treat it:

- **Change the head position while your baby sleeps**. Reposition your baby's head (from left to right, right to left) when your baby is sleeping on the back. Even though your baby will probably move around throughout the night, it's still a good idea to place your child with the rounded side of the head touching the mattress and the flattened side facing up. The American Academy of Pediatrics (AAP) does not recommend using any wedge pillows or other devices to keep your baby in one position.

- **Alternate positions in the crib**. Consider how you lay your baby down in the crib. Most right-handed parents carry small infants cradled in their left arms and lay them down with the heads to their left. In this position, the infant must turn to the right to look out into the room—and, indeed, torticollis to the right with flattening of the right side of the head is far more common than the left. Whichever side of your infant's head is flattened, you will want to position your baby in the crib to encourage active turning of the head to the other side.

- **Hold your baby more often**. Reduce the amount of time your child spends lying on the back or often being in a position where the head is resting against a flat surface (such as in car seats, strollers, swings, bouncy seats, and play yards). For instance, if your baby has fallen asleep in a car seat during travel, take your baby out of the seat when you get home rather than leaving your little one snoozing in the seat. Pick up and hold your baby often, which will take pressure off the head overall.

- **Practice tummy time**. Provide plenty of supervised time for your baby to lie on the stomach while awake during the day. Not only does "tummy time" promote normal shaping of the back the head, it also helps in other ways. Looking around from a new perspective encourages your baby's learning and discovery of the world. Plus, it helps babies strengthen their neck muscles and learn to push up on their arms, which helps develop the muscles needed for crawling and sitting up.

As most infants with plagiocephaly have some degree of torticollis, physical therapy and a home exercise program will usually be part of the recommended treatment. A physical therapist can teach you exercises to do with your baby involving stretching techniques that are gradual and progressive. Most moves will involve stretching your child's neck to the side opposite the tilt. In time, the neck muscles will get longer and the neck will straighten itself out. Although they're very simple, the exercises must be done correctly.

For kids with severe flat head syndrome in which repositioning for 2-3 months doesn't help, doctors may prescribe a custom-molded helmet or head band. While helmets might not work for all children, some kids with severe torticollis can benefit from them.

The helmets work best if used between the ages of 4 and 12 months, when a child grows the fastest and the bones are most moldable. They work by applying gentle but constant pressure on a baby's growing skull in an effort to redirect the growth.

Never purchase or use any devices like these without first having your child seen by a doctor. Only a small percentage of babies wear helmets. The decision to use helmet therapy is made on a case-by-case basis (for example, if the condition is so severe that a baby's face is becoming misshapen).

Outlook

The outlook for babies with flat head syndrome is excellent. As babies grow, they begin to reposition themselves naturally during sleep much more often than they did as newborns, which allows their heads to be in different positions throughout the night.

After babies are able to roll over, the AAP still recommends that parents put them to sleep on their backs, but then allow them to move into the position that most suits them without repositioning them onto their backs.

As a general rule, once an infant can sit independently, a flat spot will not get any worse. Then, over months and years, as the skull grows, even in severe cases the flattening will improve. The head may never be perfectly symmetrical, but for a variety of reasons the asymmetry becomes less apparent as well. For example, in later childhood the face becomes more prominent in relation to the skull, hair thickens, and children are always on the go. Experience and clinical research have shown that by school age, a flattened head is no longer a social or cosmetic problem.

It's important to remember that having a flattened head does not affect a child's brain growth or cause developmental delays or brain damage.

Prevention

Babies should be put down to sleep on their backs to help prevent sudden infant death syndrome (SIDS), despite the possibility of developing an area of flattening on the back of the head.

However, alternating their head position every night when you put them down to sleep and providing lots of tummy time and stimulation during the day while they're awake can reduce the risk of flat head syndrome.

Section 48.3

Sudden Infant Death Syndrome and Sleep

This section contains text excerpted from the following sources:
Text under the heading "What Is SIDS?" is excerpted from "About
SIDS and Safe Infant Sleep," National Institute of Child Health and
Human Development (NICHD), October 29, 2015; Text under the
heading "Ways to Reduce the Risk of SIDS and Other Sleep-Related
Causes of Infant Death" is excerpted from "Ways to Reduce the Risk
of SIDS and Other Sleep-Related Causes of Infant Death," National
Institute of Child Health and Human Development (NICHD),
January 20, 2016.

What Is SIDS?

Sudden infant death syndrome (SIDS) is the sudden, unexplained
death of a baby younger than 1 year of age that doesn't have a known
cause even after a complete investigation. This investigation includes
performing a complete autopsy, examining the death scene, and
reviewing the clinical history.

When a baby dies, healthcare providers, law enforcement personnel,
and communities try to find out why. They ask questions, examine the
baby, gather information, and run tests. If they can't find a cause for
the death, and if the baby was younger than 1 year old, the medical
examiner or coroner will call the death SIDS.

If there is still some uncertainty as to the cause after it is determined to be fully unexplained, then the medical examiner or coroner
might leave the cause of death as "unknown."

Fast Facts about SIDS

- SIDS is the leading cause of death among babies between 1
  month and 1 year of age.

- More than 2,000 babies died of SIDS in 2010, the last year for
  which such statistics are available.

- Most SIDS deaths occur when in babies between 1 month and
  4 months of age, and the majority (90%) of SIDS deaths occur

before a baby reaches 6 months of age. However SIDS deaths can occur anytime during a baby's first year.

- SIDS is a sudden and silent medical disorder that can happen to an infant who seems healthy.

- SIDS is sometimes called "crib death" or "cot death" because it is associated with the timeframe when the baby is sleeping. Cribs themselves don't cause SIDS, but the baby's sleep environment can influence sleep-related causes of death.

- Slightly more boys die of SIDS than do girls.

- In the past, the number of SIDS deaths seemed to increase during the colder months of the year. But today, the numbers are more evenly spread throughout the calendar year.

- SIDS rates for the United States have dropped steadily since 1994 in all racial and ethnic groups. Thousands of infant lives have been saved, but some ethnic groups are still at higher risk for SIDS.

SIDS Is Not...

Sudden infant death syndrome is **not** the cause of every sudden infant death.

Each year in the United States, thousands of babies die suddenly and unexpectedly. These deaths are called SUID, which stands for "Sudden Unexpected Infant Death."

SUID includes all unexpected deaths: those without a clear cause, such as SIDS, and those from a known cause, such as suffocation. One-half of all SUID cases are SIDS. Many unexpected infant deaths are accidents, but a disease or something done on purpose can also cause a baby to die suddenly and unexpectedly.

"Sleep-related causes of infant death" are those linked to how or where a baby sleeps or slept. These deaths are due to accidental causes, such as suffocation, entrapment, or strangulation. Entrapment is when the baby gets trapped between two objects, such as a mattress and a wall, and can't breathe. Strangulation is when something presses on or wraps around the baby's neck, blocking the baby's airway. These deaths are not SIDS.

Other things that SIDS is **not**:

- the same as suffocation and is not caused by suffocation

- caused by vaccines, immunizations, or shots

- contagious

- the result of neglect or child abuse

- caused by cribs

- caused by vomiting or choking

SIDS is not completely preventable, but there are ways to reduce the risk.

Ways to Reduce the Risk of SIDS and Other Sleep-Related Causes of Infant Death

We don't know exactly what causes SIDS at this time.

Scientists and healthcare providers are working very hard to find the cause or causes of SIDS. If we know the cause or causes, someday we might be able to prevent SIDS from happening at all.

More and more research evidence suggests that infants who die from SIDS are born with brain abnormalities or defects. These defects are typically found within a network of nerve cells that send signals to other nerve cells. The cells are located in the part of the brain that probably controls breathing, heart rate, blood pressure, temperature, and waking from sleep. At the present time, there is no way to identify babies who have these abnormalities, but researchers are working to develop specific screening tests.

But scientists believe that brain defects alone may not be enough to cause a SIDS death. Evidence suggests that other events must also occur for an infant to die from SIDS. Researchers use the Triple-Risk Model to explain this concept. In this model, all three factors have to occur at the same time for an infant to die from SIDS. Having only one of these factors may not be enough to cause death from SIDS, but when all three combine, the chances of SIDS are high.

Even though the exact cause of SIDS is unknown, there are ways to reduce the risk of SIDS and other sleep-related causes of infant death.

What Causes SIDS?

Research shows that there are several ways to reduce the risk of SIDS and other sleep-related causes of infant death:

Always Place Your Baby on His or Her Back to Sleep, for Naps and at Night, to Reduce the Risks of SIDS

Research shows that:

- Sleeping on the back carries the lowest risk for SIDS.

- Sleeping on the stomach or side carry the highest risk for SIDS.

- Babies who usually sleep on their backs but are then placed to sleep on their stomachs, such as for a nap, are at **very** high risk for SIDS.

The back sleep position is the safest position for all babies, including those born preterm or early. You should always place your baby on his or her back to sleep, for all sleep times—for naps and at night—to reduce the risk of SIDS.

Remember that **every sleep time counts**. Babies who usually sleep on their backs but who are then placed to sleep on their stomachs, for a sleep time like a nap, are at **very** high risk for SIDS.

That's why it is important for **everyone** who cares for your baby to place him or her on the back to sleep for all sleep times, including naps.

Can My Baby Choke If Placed on the Back to Sleep?

The short answer is no—babies are not more likely to choke when sleeping on their backs.

Use of Firm Sleep Surface, Such as a Mattress in a Safety-Approved Crib, Covered by a Fitted Sheet, to Reduce the Risk of SIDS and Other Sleep-Related Causes of Infant Death

Research shows that:

- Babies who sleep on soft surfaces, such as on an adult mattress, a couch, or an armchair, are at higher risk for SIDS and suffocation.

- Babies who sleep under a soft covering, such as a soft blanket or quilt, are at higher risk for SIDS and suffocation.

For these reasons, you should always place your baby to sleep on a firm sleep surface, such as a safety-approved* crib, bassinet, or portable play area. Use tight-fitting bedding, such as a fitted sheet, to help prevent your baby from getting tangled up in the bedding.

Do not use a car seat, carrier, swing, or similar product as your baby's everyday sleep area.

Never place your baby to sleep on soft surfaces, such as on a couch or sofa, or on pillows, comforters, quilts, or sheepskins. Do not place your baby to sleep on a waterbed, sofa, or soft mattress that allows the baby's head to sink into the surface.

Why Shouldn't I Use Crib Bumpers in My Baby's Sleep Area?

Bumper pads and similar products that attach to crib slats or sides are frequently used with the intent of protecting infants from injury. However, evidence does not support using crib bumpers to prevent injury. In fact, crib bumpers can cause serious injuries and even death. Keeping them out of your baby's sleep area is the best way to avoid these dangers

Room Sharing—Keeping Baby's Sleep Area Separate from Your Sleep Area in the Same Room Where You Sleep— Reduces the Risk of SIDS and Other Sleep Related-Related Cause of Infant Death

Room sharing—keeping baby's sleep area in the same room and next to where you sleep—is recommended by the AAP as a way to reduce the risk of SIDS and other sleep-related causes of infant death.

Your baby should also not sleep in an adult bed, on a couch, or on a chair alone, with you, or with anyone else.

Research also shows that:

- Babies who sleep in an adult bed with one or more adults are at higher risk for SIDS.

- Babies who sleep in an adult bed are at **significantly** higher risk for SIDS when they:

  - Are younger than 3 months of age

  - Share a bed with a current smoker (even if he or she does not smoke in bed) or if the mother smoked during pregnancy

  - Share a bed with someone who is very tired

  - Share a bed with someone who has used or is using medications or substances, such as alcohol or illicit drugs

  - Share a bed with someone who is not a parent, including other children

- Share a bed with more than one person

- Are placed on a waterbed, older mattress, sofa, couch, or armchair

- Are placed on a bed with soft bedding, including pillows, heavy blankets, quilts, and comforters

- Babies who are placed for sleep on adult bed, sofa, couch, or armchair are at serious risk for accidental suffocation, entrapment, injury, and death—regardless of whether they are alone or if they share the sleep area with someone.

For these reasons give your baby his or her own sleep area in the same room as you or others.

If you bring your baby into bed with you to feed, put him or her back in a separate sleep area, such as a safety-approved crib, bassinet, or portable play yard, in your room next to where you sleep when finished.

Keep Soft Objects, Toys, Crib Bumpers, and Loose Bedding out of Your Baby's Sleep, Area to Reduce the Risk of SIDS and Other Sleep-Related Causes of Infant Death

Research shows that:

- Loose bedding and other items placed under or over the baby or in the baby's sleep area could end up covering the baby's face, which could:

  - Put the baby at higher risk for suffocation or strangulation

  - Put the baby at higher risk for rebreathing air that is low in oxygen

  - Put the baby at higher risk of overheating

- Loose bedding and soft bedding, placed over or under the baby, such as quilts, comforters, and pillows increase the risk of SIDS regardless of sleep position.

It is reported that the majority of other sleep-related infant deaths are due to accidental suffocation involving pillows, quilts, and extra blankets. For these reasons, do not use pillows, blankets, quilts, sheepskins, stuffed animals, or crib bumpers anywhere in your baby's sleep area.

To Reduce the Risk of SIDS, Women Should:

Get regular healthcare during pregnancy

Research shows that:

- Babies of mothers who get regular healthcare during pregnancy are at lower risk for SIDS.

For this reason, start getting healthcare early in your pregnancy, and continue to get regular care throughout the entire pregnancy.

Not smoke, drink alcohol, or use illegal drugs during pregnancy or after the baby is born.

Research shows that:

- Babies of mothers who do **not** drink alcohol or use illegal drugs during or after pregnancy are at lower risk of SIDS.

- Babies who share a bed with a parent who uses alcohol or illegal drugs are at particularly high risk of SIDS.

For these reasons, you should not use alcohol and illegal drugs during pregnancy or after your baby is born.

To Reduce the Risk of SIDS, Do Not Smoke during Pregnancy, and Do Not Smoke or Allow Smoking around Your Baby

Research shows that:

- Babies of mothers who don't smoke have the lowest risk of SIDS.

- Babies of mothers who smoked during pregnancy are up to 3 to 4 times more likely to die of SIDS than babies whose mothers did not smoke during pregnancy.

- Babies whose caregivers smoke or who are exposed to secondhand smoke in their environment are at higher risk for SIDS than babies not exposed to secondhand smoke.

- Babies who share a bed with an adult smoker are at higher risk of SIDS.

- Babies who died of SIDS had higher nicotine concentrations in their lungs than did babies who died from other causes.

For these reasons, do not smoke during pregnancy or after the birth of your baby, and don't let others smoke around your baby.

Breastfeed Your Baby to Reduce the Risk of SIDS

Research shows that:

- Babies who are breastfed or fed with breast milk for the first 6 months of life are at lower risk of SIDS.

- Breastfeeding has many health benefits for mothers and babies.

For this reason, breastfeed your baby as much and for as long as you can.

If you bring your baby into your bed to breastfeed, make sure to put him or her back in a separate sleep area, such as a safety-approved crib, bassinet, or portable play area, in your room next to where you sleep when finished.

Give Your Baby a Dry Pacifier That Is Not Attached to a String for Naps and at Night to Reduce the Risk of SIDS

Research shows that babies who used pacifiers during their last sleep were at significantly lower risk for SIDS than were babies who did not.

For this reason, think about giving your baby a dry pacifier for sleep, but don't force the baby to use it.

Consider the following when using a pacifier:

- If you are breastfeeding, wait until your baby is used to breast-feeding before trying a pacifier.

- Because of the risk of strangulation, do not hang the pacifier around your baby's neck or attach it to his or her clothing with a string or cord.

- Do not coat the pacifier with anything sweet or sticky.

- Clean the pacifier often and replace the pacifier regularly.

- If the pacifier falls out of the baby's mouth during sleep, you don't have to put it back in the mouth during that sleep time.

Research shows that:

Babies who are breastfed or fed with breast milk for the first 6 months of life are at lower risk of SIDS.

- Breastfeeding has many health benefits for mothers and babies.

- For this reason, breastfeed your baby as much and for as long as you can.

If you bring your baby into your bed to breastfeed, make sure to put him or her back in a separate sleep area, such as a safety-approved crib, bassinet, or portable play area, in your room next to where you sleep when finished.

Do Not Let Your Baby Get Too Hot during Sleep

Research shows that:

- Some babies are more likely to die from SIDS if they are dressed in two or more layers of clothes for sleep.

- Babies who get too warm during sleep might sleep too deeply and be unable to wake themselves up, which could play a role in SIDS.

For these reasons, you should dress your baby in no more than one layer more of clothing than an adult would wear to be comfortable.

Babies who are too warm might sweat, have damp hair, have flushed or red cheeks, have a heat rash, or breathe rapidly (as if they are panting).

What if I want to use a blanket when putting my baby to bed?

Using a blanket is not recommended. In most cases, sleep clothing without a blanket is enough to keep baby warm during sleep. If you are concerned the room is not warm enough, consider an infant blanket sleeper.

If you choose to use a blanket, use it safely in the following way (sometimes called the "feet to foot" method):

- Place the baby with his or her feet at the end of the crib or sleep area.

- Tuck the ends of the blanket under the mattress.

- Keep the blanket away from the baby's face. The blanket should come no higher than the baby's chest or armpits to help ensure safety.

- Use only light sleep clothing—a diaper, onesie, T-shirt, or sleeper—under the blanket so the baby stays warm but doesn't get too warm during sleep.

Follow HealthCare Provide Guidance on Your Baby Vaccines and Regular Health Checkups

Following the recommended schedule for your baby's vaccines has a protective effect against SIDS. Research shows that immunizations reduce the risk of SIDS by 50%.

There is no evidence of a causal relationship between vaccines and SIDS.

For this reason, follow your healthcare provider's recommendations for vaccines and for regular health checkups for your baby.

Avoid Products That Claim to Reduce the Risk of SIDS and Other Sleep-Related Causes of Infant Death

Wedges, positioners, and other products that claim to reduce the risk of infant death have not been tested for safety or effectiveness. The U.S. Food and Drug Administration, the Consumer Product Safety Commission, and the American Academy of Pediatrics warn against using these products because of the dangers they pose to babies.

Parents and caregivers should also avoid using products made from foam rubber or Memory Foam™ because of the risk of suffocation.

Do Not Use Home Heart or Breathing Monitors to Reduce the Risk of SIDS

Research shows that home heart or breathing monitors that claim to be able to detect SIDS and other life-threatening events are not effective at detecting or reducing SIDS. For this reason, you should avoid using home monitor devices to detect and prevent SIDS.

Keep in mind that these heart and breathing monitors are different from "baby monitors," which allow caregivers to hear or see the baby from another room. Baby monitors are often useful for alerting caregivers that a baby is awake, but they do not detect or prevent SIDS.

In some cases, healthcare providers prescribe a home heart or breathing monitor for babies with certain medical conditions. These babies are under medical care for conditions not related to SIDS, and the monitors are **not** used to detect or reduce SIDS risk. If you have questions about using home heart or breathing monitors for medical conditions, talk to your baby's healthcare provider.

Give Your Baby Plenty Tummy Time When He or She Is Awake and When Someone Is Watching

Research shows that:

- Placing your baby on his or her tummy for short periods while the baby is awake and when someone is watching is an important part of healthy development.

- Supervised Tummy Time helps your baby's neck, shoulder, and arm muscles get stronger.

- When a baby is placed too often or for too long in the same position, pressure on the same part of the baby's head can cause flat spots. These flat spots are usually not dangerous, are not associated with long-term problems with head shape, and typically go away on their own once the baby starts sitting up. Tummy Time can help prevent those flat spots.

For these reasons, you should make sure your baby gets plenty of Tummy Time and use other ways to reduce the chance that flat spots will form on the back of your baby's head.

Chapter 49

Obstructive Sleep Apnea

What Is Obstructive Sleep Apnea?

Brief pauses in breathing during sleep are normal. But when breathing stops often or for longer periods, it's called sleep apnea.

When someone has sleep apnea, oxygen levels in the body may fall and sleep can be disrupted. You might think that only older people have sleep apnea, but kids and teens can develop it, too.

About Sleep Apnea

Sleep apnea happens when a person stops breathing during sleep ("apnea" comes from a Greek word meaning "without wind"). It is usually caused by something obstructing, or blocking, the upper airway. This is known as **obstructive sleep apnea (OSA)**.

OSA is a common, serious condition that can make kids miss out on healthy, restful sleep. If left untreated, obstructive sleep apnea can lead to learning, behavior, growth, and heart problems. In very rare cases, it can even be life threatening.

Less commonly, sleep apnea can happen when someone doesn't get enough oxygen during sleep because the brain doesn't send signals to the muscles that control breathing. This is called central sleep apnea. Head injuries and other conditions that affect the brain increase the risk of developing this type of apnea, which mostly affects older adults.

Causes

When we sleep, our muscles relax. This includes the muscles in the back of the throat that help keep the airway open. In obstructive sleep apnea, these muscles can relax too much and collapse the airway, making it hard to breathe.

This is especially true if someone has enlarged tonsils or adenoids (germ-fighting tissues at the back of the nasal cavity), which can block the airway during sleep. In fact, enlarged tonsils and adenoids are the most common cause of OSA in kids.

Risk factors for the development of OSA include:

- a family history of obstructive sleep apnea
- being overweight
- certain medical conditions, such as Down syndrome or cerebral palsy
- defects in the structures of the mouth, jaw, or throat that can narrow the airway
- a large neck (17 inches or more in circumference for men; 16 inches for women)
- a large tongue, which can fall back and block the airway during sleep

Symptoms

When breathing stops, oxygen levels in the body drop. This usually triggers the brain to briefly wake us up so that the airway reopens. Most of the time, this process happens quickly and we go right back to sleep without knowing we woke up. But with sleep apnea, this pattern repeats itself all night. So people who have it don't reach a deeper, more restful level of sleep.

Symptoms of OSA in kids include:

- snoring, often associated with pauses, snorts, or gasps
- heavy breathing while sleeping
- very restless sleep and sleeping in unusual positions
- bedwetting (especially if a child previously stayed dry at night)
- daytime sleepiness or behavioral problems

Because OSA makes it hard to get a good night's sleep, kids might have a hard time waking in the morning, be tired throughout the day, and have attention or other behavior problems. As a result, sleep apnea can hurt school performance. Teachers and others may think a child has attention deficit hyperactivity disorder (ADHD) or learning difficulties.

Diagnosis

If your child snores regularly, is a restless sleeper, is very sleepy during the day, or has other signs of sleep apnea, talk to your doctor. Your doctor might refer you to a sleep specialist or recommend a **sleep study**.

A sleep study (also called a polysomnogram) lets doctors check for OSA and record a variety of body functions while a child sleeps. Sleep studies also can help doctors diagnose central sleep apnea and other sleep disorders.

In the study, sensors are placed at a few spots on the child's body with a mild adhesive or tape. The sensors are wired to a computer to provide information while the child sleeps. Sleep studies are painless and risk-free, but patients usually need to spend the night in a hospital or sleep center.

During a sleep study, doctors monitor:

- eye movements
- heart rate
- breathing pattern
- brain waves
- blood oxygen level
- snoring and other noises
- body movements and sleep positions

Treatment

If enlarged tonsils or adenoids are thought to be causing the apnea, the doctor will refer your child to an ear, nose, and throat doctor (ENT). The ENT might decide that an operation called an adenotonsillectomy is needed to remove the tonsils and adenoids. This often is an effective treatment for OSA.

If tonsils and adenoids are not the cause of OSA or if symptoms of OSA remain after adenotonsillectomy, a doctor may recommend **continuous positive airway pressure (CPAP)** therapy. In CPAP therapy, a person wears a mask that covers the nose and mouth during sleep. The mask is connected to a machine that continuously pumps air into it to open the airways.

When excess weight is a factor in OSA, it's important to work with a doctor on diet changes, exercise, and other safe weight-loss methods. In mild cases of OSA, doctors may monitor a child for a period of time to see if symptoms improve before deciding on treatment.

Chapter 50

Bed Wetting (Enuresis)

What Is Enuresis?

The medical name for not being able to control your pee is enuresis. Sometimes enuresis is also called involuntary urination. Nocturnal enuresis is involuntary urination that happens at night while sleeping, after the age when a person should be able to control his or her bladder. (Involuntary urination that happens during the day is known as diurnal enuresis.)

There are two kinds of enuresis: primary and secondary. Someone with primary nocturnal enuresis has wet the bed since he or she was a baby (primary nocturnal enuresis is the most common form). Secondary enuresis is a condition that develops at least 6 months—or even several years—after a person has learned to control his or her bladder.

The bladder is a muscular receptacle, or holding container, for pee (urine). It expands (gets bigger) as urine enters and then contracts (gets smaller) to push the urine out.

In a person with normal bladder control, nerves in the bladder wall send a message to the brain when the bladder is full; the brain then sends a message back to the bladder to keep it from automatically

This chapter contains text excerpted from the following sources: Text under with the heading "What Is Enuresis?" is excerpted from "What Is Enuresis?" © 1995–2016. The Nemours Foundation/KidsHealth®. Reprinted with permission. June 2016; Text under the heading "Children and Bedwetting" is excerpted from "Urinary Incontinence in Children," National Institute of Diabetes and Digestive and Kidney Diseases (NIDDK), June 2012. Reviewed July 2016.

emptying until the person is ready to go to the bathroom. But people with nocturnal enuresis have a problem that causes them to pee involuntarily at night.

What Causes Enuresis?

Doctors don't always know the exact cause of nocturnal enuresis. They do have some theories, though, on what may contribute to someone developing the condition:

- **Hormonal problems**. A hormone called antidiuretic hormone, or ADH, causes the body to produce less urine at night. But some people's bodies don't make enough ADH, which means their bodies may produce too much urine while they're sleeping.

- **Bladder problems**. In some people with enuresis, too many muscle spasms can prevent the bladder from holding a normal amount of urine. Some teens and adults also have relatively small bladders that can't hold a large volume of urine.

- **Genetics**. Teens with enuresis often have a parent who had the same problem at about the same age. Scientists have identified specific genes that cause enuresis.

- **Sleep problems**. Some teens may sleep so deeply that they don't wake up when they need to pee.

- **Caffeine**. Using caffeine causes a person to urinate (pee) more.

- **Medical conditions**. Medical conditions that can trigger secondary enuresis include diabetes, urinary tract abnormalities (problems with the structure of a person's urinary tract), constipation, and urinary tract infections (UTIs). Spinal cord trauma, such as severe stretching of the spinal cord resulting from a fall, sports injury, auto accident, or other event may also play a role in enuresis, although this is rare.

- **Psychological problems**. Some experts believe that stress can be associated with enuresis. It's not uncommon to feel stressed out during the teenage years, and things such as divorce, the death of a friend or family member, a move to a new town and adapting to a new school and social environment, or family tension can feel overwhelming.

Doctors don't know exactly why, but more than twice as many guys as girls have enuresis. It is often seen in combination with ADHD.

How Is Enuresis Diagnosed?

If you're having trouble controlling your urine at night, talk to your doctor to learn more about nocturnal enuresis and to rule out the possibility of a medical problem.

In addition to doing a **physical examination**, the doctor will ask you about any concerns and symptoms you have, your past health, your family's health, any medications you're taking, any allergies you may have, and other issues. This is called the **medical history**. He or she may ask about sleep patterns, bowel habits, and urinary symptoms (such as an urge to pee a lot or pain or burning when you pee). Your doctor may also discuss any stressful situations that could be contributing to the problem.

The initial exam will probably include a **urinalysis** and urine culture. In these tests, urine is examined for signs of disease. Most of the time in people with nocturnal enuresis, these test results come back completely normal.

How Is It Treated?

Doctors can do several things to treat bedwetting, depending on what's causing it. If an illness is responsible, which is not very common, it will be treated. If the history and physical examination do not suggest a specific medical problem and the urine tests are negative, several behavioral approaches can be used for treatment:

- **Manage what you eat and drink before bed.** People with nocturnal enuresis can take some basic steps to prevent an overly full bladder by decreasing the amount of fluids they drink before going to bed. You can reduce the chances that you'll wet the bed by going to the toilet just before bedtime. It may help to avoid eating certain foods in the evening: Foods that can irritate the bladder include coffee, tea, chocolate, and sodas or other carbonated beverages containing caffeine.

- **Imagine yourself dry**. Using a technique called positive imagery, where you think about waking up dry before you go to sleep, can help some people stop bedwetting. Some people find that rewarding themselves for waking up dry also works.

- **Use bedwetting alarms**. Doctors and nurses sometimes prescribe bedwetting alarms to treat teens with enuresis. According to the National Kidney Foundation, 50% to 70% of cases of enuresis respond to treatment with these moisture alarms. With these alarms, a bell or buzzer goes off when a person begins to wet the bed. Then, you can quickly turn the alarm off, go to the toilet, and go back to sleep without wetting the bed too much. Don't get discouraged if the alarm doesn't help you stop wetting the bed immediately, though. It can take many weeks for the body to unlearn something it's been doing for years. Eventually, you can train yourself to get up before the alarm goes off or to hold your urine until morning. People who sleep very deeply may need to rely on a parent or other family member to wake them up if they don't hear the alarm. The key to bedwetting alarms is waking up quickly—the sooner a person wakes up, the more effective the behavior modification for telling the brain to wake up or send the bladder signals to hold the urine until the morning.

• Sometimes doctors treat enuresis with **medication**—although this is not usually the first course of action because no medicine has been proved to cure bedwetting permanently, and the problem usually returns when the medicine is stopped. Doctors sometimes prescribe a man made form of ADH to decrease urine buildup during the night. Other medications relax the bladder, allowing it to hold more pee.

If you're worried about enuresis, the best thing to do is talk to your doctor for ideas on how to cope with it. Your mom or dad can also give you tips on how to cope, especially if he or she had the problem during adolescence.

The good news is that it's likely that bedwetting will go away on its own. In fact, 15 out of 100 kids who wet the bed will stop every year without any treatment at all.

Children and Bedwetting

Why Does My Child Wet the Bed?

In most cases, the exact cause of bedwetting is not known. But many possible causes exist. Your child's bladder might be too small. Or the amount of urine produced overnight is too much for your child's bladder to hold. As a result, your child's bladder fills up before the night is over. Some children sleep so deeply that they don't wake up when they need to urinate. Others simply take longer to learn bladder control. Many children wet the bed until they are 5 years old or even older.

Bedwetting often runs in families. If both parents wet the bed as children, their child is likely to have the same problem. If only one parent has a history of bedwetting, the child has about a 30 percent chance of having the problem. Some children wet the bed even if neither parent ever did.

A child who has been dry for several months or even years may start wetting the bed. The cause might be emotional stress, such as the loss of a loved one, problems at school, a new sibling, or even toilet training too early.

Bedwetting is not your child's fault. Children rarely wet the bed on purpose. You can help your child by learning about the different causes and treatments for bedwetting.

How Can I Help My Child Stay Dry?

You can take several steps to help your child stay dry. Make sure your child drinks enough fluids throughout the day. A child who doesn't drink enough during the day may drink a lot before bedtime, causing wetness at night. Talk with your child's doctor about how much your child should drink each day. Have your child avoid drinks with caffeine, such as colas or tea. Drinks with caffeine speed up urine production. Give your child one drink with dinner and explain that it will be the last drink before going to bed. Make sure your child uses the bathroom just before bed. Many children will still wet the bed, but these steps may be helpful.

Children may feel bad about wetting the bed, so letting them know they are not to blame is important. Bedwetting is not a behavior problem. Scolding and punishment will not help your child stay dry. Be supportive. Praise your child for dry nights.

Most children grow out of bedwetting. Some children just take more time than others.

Should I Take My Child to See a Doctor?

Children younger than 5 do not need to see a doctor for bedwetting. Many children do not stay dry at night until age 7. A single episode of bedwetting should not cause alarm, even in an older child.

If your child is 7 years old or older and wets the bed more than two or three times in a week, a doctor may be able to help. If both day and night wetting occur after age 5, your child should see a doctor before age 7.

The doctor will ask questions about your child's health and the wetting problem, conduct a physical exam, and ask your child for a urine sample. The doctor will look for signs of health problems that can cause bedwetting, including the following:

- fever and bacteria in the urine—signs of infection

- weight loss—a sign of diabetes, a condition where blood glucose, also called blood sugar, is too high

- high blood pressure—a sign of a kidney problem

- poor reflexes in the legs or feet—a sign of a nerve problem

- a hard mass that can be felt in the stomach area—a sign of constipation, a condition in which a child has fewer than two bowel movements a week and stools can be hard, dry, small, and difficult to pass

- swollen tonsils, mouth breathing, or poor growth—a sign of sleep apnea, a condition in which breathing stops during sleep

The doctor may also ask your child about changes at home or school that may be causing emotional stress. In most cases, the doctor doesn't find any specific cause for bedwetting. If a health problem is found, the doctor will talk to you about treatment options. If your child is stressed, the doctor may be able to give your child strategies for dealing with the stress.

What Treatments Can Help My Child Stay Dry?

Treatments for bedwetting include bladder training, moisture alarms, and medicines. Talk with the doctor and your child about which ones to try.

Bladder Training

Bladder training can help your child hold urine longer. Write down what times your child urinates during the day. Then figure out the amount of time between trips to the bathroom. After a day or two, have your child try to wait an extra 15 minutes before using the bathroom. For example, if a trip to the bathroom usually occurs at 3:30 p.m., have your child wait until 3:45 p.m. Slowly make the wait time longer and longer. This method helps stretch your child's bladder to hold more urine. Be patient. Bladder training can take several weeks or even months.

Moisture Alarm

A small moisture alarm can be put in your child's bed or underwear. With the first drops of urine, the alarm triggers a bell or buzzer that wakes your child. Your child can then stop the flow of urine, get up, and use the bathroom. Waking also teaches your child how a full bladder feels.

Medicine

Medicine is available to treat bedwetting. The medicine used most often slows down how fast the body makes urine. Though medicine for bedwetting works well, wetting often returns when the child stops taking the medicine. If this occurs, keeping the child on medicine for a longer time may help.

Chapter 51

Pediatric Movement Disorders in Sleep

Babies between the ages of six and nine months sometimes begin to exhibit repetitive, rhythmic movements as part of the process of going to sleep. Some of the most common movements include body-rocking, head-rolling, and head-banging. Children who exhibit these behaviors may roll their heads forcefully from side to side, rise up on hands and knees and rock back and forth vigorously, or bang their heads repeatedly on a mattress, pillow, headboard, or side rail.

Although these violent movements can be alarming for parents and caregivers to witness, they are quite common, usually harmless, and tend to disappear gradually by the age of two or three. Parents often express concerns that head-banging or body-rocking will result in injury or brain damage, but this is rarely the case. In addition, many parents worry that these repetitive behaviors may indicate a developmental disability, yet they occur frequently among normal children. Parents should consult a pediatrician if the behaviors persist for more than a few months, or if the child nods or shakes their head frequently at other times, does not interact with other people, or shows evidence of developmental delays.

Researchers are not certain why children engage in body-rocking, head-rolling, and head-banging. They have determined that the behaviors occur three times more often in boys than in girls, and that most children outgrow the habit before they reach three years of age. Some experts believe that rocking offers babies comfort or pleasure because it simulates being carried in the womb or in a parent's arms. Others theorize that the behaviors are part of the natural process of mastering movement and gaining control of the body. Some claim that rhythmic motion helps babies to release stress, tension, or unspent energy and relax before going to sleep. For other children, head banging may provide a distraction from teething pain or an outlet for frustration or anger.

Coping with Repetitive Movements

Body-rocking, head-banging, and head-rolling can be distressing for parents and caregivers. In addition to feeling concern for the child's well-being, they may also feel frustrated or irritated by the noise or damage to furniture or walls. It is important to remember that babies who rock or bang their heads will usually fall asleep within a short time. Since most children simply outgrow the behavior over time, the easiest approach may be to do nothing and wait for it to go away. Reacting to the repetitive movements—even in a negative way—sometimes tends to reinforce the behavior. Other tips for dealing with body-rocking, head-rolling, and head-banging at bedtime include the following:

- engage in a relaxing bedtime routine that includes quiet time, cuddling, songs, nursery rhymes, or a story;
- place a mobile above the bed or an activity center on the side of the crib to provide interest and distraction;
- play soft, soothing music or white noise in the bedroom to promote relaxation;
- ensure that the child does not spend too much time in bed before it is time to sleep;
- check to make sure the child is not experiencing pain from teething, ear infection, allergies, or other sources;
- use a padded bumper on crib rails or headboards;
- pull the bed away from the wall and put a thick carpet or rubber pad under the legs—or put the mattress on the floor—to reduce movement and noise; or
- try changing the bedroom in which the child sleeps.

References

1. "Body-Rocking, Head-Rolling, and Head-Banging," Raising Children Network, August 25, 2014.

2. "Body-Rocking, Head-Rolling, and Head-Banging in Babies," World of Moms, October 10, 2014.

3. "Guide to Your Child's Symptoms: Rocking/Head Banging," American Academy of Pediatrics, 2001.

Chapter 52

Sleep Walking in Children

About Sleepwalking

Hours after bedtime, do you find your little one wandering the hall looking dazed and confused? If you have a sleepwalking child, you're not alone. It can be unnerving to see, but sleepwalking is very common in kids and most sleepwalkers only do so occasionally and outgrow it by the teen years. Still, some simple steps can keep your young sleep-walker safe while traipsing about.

Despite its name, sleepwalking (also called somnambulism) actually involves more than just walking. Sleepwalking behaviors can range from harmless (sitting up), to potentially dangerous (wandering outside), to just inappropriate (kids may even open a closet door and pee inside). No matter what kids do during sleepwalking episodes, though, it's unlikely that they'll remember ever having done it!

As we sleep, our brains pass through five stages of sleep—stages 1, 2, 3, 4, and REM (rapid eye movement) sleep. Together, these stages make up a sleep cycle. One complete sleep cycle lasts about 90 to 100 minutes. So a person experiences about four or five sleep cycles during an average night's sleep.

Sleepwalking most often occurs during the deeper sleep of stages 3 and 4. During these stages, it's more difficult to wake someone up, and when awakened, a person may feel groggy and disoriented for a few minutes.

Text in this chapter includes text excerpted from "Sleepwalking" © 1995–2016. The Nemours Foundation/KidsHealth®. Reprinted with permission.

Kids tend to sleepwalk within an hour or two of falling asleep and may walk around for anywhere from a few seconds to 30 minutes.

Causes of Sleepwalking

Sleepwalking is far more common in kids than in adults, as most sleepwalkers outgrow it by the early teen years. It may run in families, so if you or your partner are or were sleepwalkers, your child may be too.

Other factors that may bring on a sleepwalking episode include:

- lack of sleep or fatigue
- irregular sleep schedules
- illness or fever
- certain medications
- stress (sleepwalking is rarely caused by an underlying medical, emotional, or psychological problem)

Behaviors during Sleepwalking

Of course, getting out of bed and walking around while still sleeping is the most obvious sleepwalking symptom. But young sleepwalkers may also:

- sleeptalk
- be hard to wake up
- seem dazed
- be clumsy
- not respond when spoken to
- sit up in bed and go through repeated motions, such as rubbing their eyes or fussing with their pajamas

Also, sleepwalkers' eyes are open, but they don't see the same way they do when they're awake and they often think they're in different rooms of the house or different places altogether.

Sometimes, these other conditions may accompany sleepwalking:

- sleep apnea (brief pauses in breathing while sleeping)
- bedwetting (enuresis)
- night terrors

Is Sleepwalking Harmful?

Sleepwalking itself is not harmful. However, sleepwalking episodes can be hazardous since sleepwalking kids aren't awake and may not realize what they're doing, such as walking down stairs or opening windows.

Sleepwalking is not usually a sign that something is emotionally or psychologically wrong with a child. And it doesn't cause any emotional harm. Sleepwalkers probably won't even remember the nighttime stroll.

How to Keep a Sleepwalker Safe

Although sleepwalking isn't dangerous by itself, it's important to take precautions so that your sleepwalking child is less likely to fall down, run into something, walk out the front door, or drive (if your teen is a sleepwalker).

To help keep your sleepwalker out of harm's way:

- Try not to wake a sleepwalker because this might scare your child. Instead, gently guide him or her back to bed.

- Lock the windows and doors, not just in your child's bedroom but throughout your home, in case your young sleepwalker decides to wander. You may consider extra locks or child safety locks on doors. Keys should be kept out of reach for kids who are old enough to drive.

- To prevent falls, don't let your sleepwalker sleep in a bunk bed.

- Remove sharp or breakable things from around your child's bed.

- Keep dangerous objects out of reach.

- Remove obstacles from your child's room and throughout your home to prevent a stumble. Especially eliminate clutter on the floor (i.e., in your child's bedroom or playroom).

- Install safety gates outside your child's room and/or at the top of any stairs.

Other Ways to Help a Sleepwalker

Unless the episodes are very regular, cause your child to be sleepy during the day, or involve dangerous behaviors, there's usually no need to treat sleepwalking. But if the sleepwalking is frequent, causing problems, or your child hasn't outgrown it by the early teen years, talk to your doctor. Also talk to your doctor if you're concerned that something else could be going on, like reflux or trouble breathing.

For kids who sleepwalk often, doctors may recommend a treatment called scheduled awakening. This disrupts the sleep cycle enough to help stop sleepwalking. In rare cases, a doctor may prescribe medication to aid sleep.

Other ways to help minimize sleepwalking episodes:

- Have your child relax at bedtime by listening to soft music or relaxation tapes.

- Establish a regular sleep and nap schedule and stick to it—both nighttime and wake-up time.

- Make your child's bedtime earlier. This can improve excessive sleepiness.

- Don't let kids drink a lot in the evening and be sure they go to the bathroom before going to bed. (A full bladder can contribute to sleepwalking.)

- Avoid caffeine near bedtime.

- Make sure your child's bedroom is quiet, cozy, and conducive to sleeping. Keep noise to a minimum while kids are trying to sleep (at bedtime and naptime).

The next time you encounter your nighttime wanderer, don't panic. Simply steer your child back to the safety and comfort of his or her bed.

Chapter 53

Sleep Concerns among Teens

Why Do Teens Have Trouble Sleeping?

Research shows that teens need at least 8½ hours of sleep a night. You don't need to be a math whiz to figure out that if you wake up for school at 6:00 a.m., you'd have to go to bed at 9:00 p.m. to reach the 9-hour mark. Studies have found that many teens have trouble falling asleep that early, though. It's not because they don't want to sleep. It's because their brains naturally work on later schedules and aren't ready for bed.

During adolescence, the body's circadian rhythm (sort of like an internal biological clock) is reset, telling a teen to fall asleep later at night and wake up later in the morning. This change in the circadian rhythm seems to happen because a teen's brain makes the hormone melatonin later at night than the brains of kids and adults do. (Melatonin and another hormone, serotonin, help regulate a person's sleep–wake cycles.)

So, teens have a harder time falling asleep. Sometimes this delay in the sleep–wake cycle is so severe that it affects a person's daily activities. In those cases it's called **delayed sleep phase syndrome** or **"night owl" syndrome**.

Text in this chapter includes text excerpted from "Common Sleep Problems" © 1995–2016. The Nemours Foundation/KidsHealth®. Reprinted with permission.

This isn't the only reason teens lose sleep, though. Lots of people have **insomnia**—trouble falling or staying asleep. The most common cause of insomnia is stress. But all sorts of things can lead to insomnia, including physical discomfort (the stuffy nose of a cold or the pain of a headache, for example), emotional troubles (like family problems or relationship difficulties), and even an uncomfortable sleeping environment (a room that's too hot, cold, bright, or noisy). Exposing your eyes to excessive light at night—through mobile devices, for instance—also makes it harder to sleep.

It's common for everyone to have insomnia from time to time. But if insomnia lasts for a month or longer with no relief, then doctors call it **chronic**. Chronic insomnia can be caused by a number of different problems, including medical conditions, mental-health problems, medication side effects, or substance abuse. People with chronic insomnia usually can get help for it from a doctor, therapist, or other counselor.

Worrying about the insomnia can make it even worse for some people. A brief period of insomnia can build into something longer lasting when a person becomes anxious about not sleeping or worried about feeling tired the next day. Doctors call this **psychophysiologic insomnia.**

PLMD and RLS

People with periodic limb movement disorder (PLMD) or restless legs syndrome (RLS) find their sleep is disrupted by leg (or, less commonly, arm) movements, leaving them tired or irritable from lack of sleep.

In the case of PLMD, these movements are involuntary twitches or jerks: They're called involuntary because the person isn't consciously controlling them and is often unaware of the movement.

People with RLS actually feel physical sensations in their limbs, such as tingling, itching, cramping, or burning. The only way they can relieve these feelings is by moving their legs or arms to get rid of the discomfort.

Doctors can treat PLMD and RLS. For some people, treating an iron deficiency can make them go away; others might need to take other types of medication.

Obstructive Sleep Apnea

A person with obstructive sleep apnea temporarily stops breathing during sleep because the airway becomes narrowed or blocked.

One common cause of obstructive sleep apnea is enlarged tonsils or adenoids (tissues located in the passage that connects the nose and throat). Being overweight or obese also can put someone at risk for it.

People with this sleep disorder may snore, have difficulty breathing, and even sweat heavily during sleep. Because it disrupts sleep, a person may feel extremely sleepy or irritable during the day. People who show signs of obstructive sleep apnea, such as loud snoring or excessive daytime sleepiness, should talk to their doctor.

Reflux

In gastroesophageal reflux disease (GERD), stomach acid moves backward up into the esophagus, producing the uncomfortable, burning sensation known as heartburn. GERD symptoms can be worse when someone is lying down. Even if a person doesn't notice the feelings of heartburn during sleep, the discomfort it causes can still interfere with the sleep cycle.

Nightmares

Most teens have nightmares once in a while. But frequent nightmares can disrupt sleep patterns by waking someone during the night. The most common triggers for more frequent nightmares are emotional, such as stress or anxiety. Other things that can trigger them include certain medicines, and consuming drugs or alcohol. Sleep deprivation (getting too little sleep) also can lead to nightmares.

If nightmares are hurting your sleep, it's a good idea to talk to a parent, doctor, or counselor.

Narcolepsy

People with narcolepsy are often very sleepy during the day and have sleep "attacks" that may make them suddenly fall asleep, lose muscle control, or see vivid dreamlike images while dozing off or waking up. Someone's nighttime sleep may be disrupted, with frequent awakenings throughout the night.

Narcolepsy can be disturbing because people fall asleep without warning, making it hazardous to do things like drive. A person's school, work, or social life can be affected by the unusual sleep patterns.

Narcolepsy isn't common diagnosed in teens, but many cases go unrecognized. People usually first begin to have symptoms between the ages of 10 and 25, but may not be properly diagnosed until 10–15 years later. Doctors usually treat narcolepsy with medicines and life-style changes.

What Should I Do?

If you think you're getting enough rest at night and you're still feeling tired during the day, it's a good idea to visit your doctor. Excessive tiredness can be caused by all sorts of health problems, not just problems with sleep.

If a sleep problem is suspected, your doctor will look at your overall health and sleep habits. In addition to doing a physical examination, the doctor will take your medical history by asking you about any concerns and symptoms you have, your past health, your family's health, any medications you're taking, any allergies you may have, and other issues.

The doctor also might do tests to find out whether any conditions—such as obstructive sleep apnea—might be interfering with your sleep.

Chapter 54

Bruxism and Sleep

Bruxism is a type of movement disorder characterized by the grinding, gnashing, and clenching of the teeth. Many people may unconsciously grind or clench their teeth, but whether or not it qualifies as a case of bruxism depends largely on such factors as frequency, physical damage, and discomfort. The marked absence of clinical symptoms makes it difficult to estimate the prevalence of bruxism. Most cases go unreported, since the majority of "bruxers" remain unaware of their problem until a diagnosis can be made on the basis of visible signs of teeth wear. Bruxism is thought to affect an estimated 30 to 40 million people in the United States and tends to occur episodically during certain periods of a person's life. Bruxism can be either diurnal (daytime) or nocturnal (night). When people unconsciously clench their jaws during the day, it is called awake bruxism, and when they grind or clench their teeth while they are asleep, it is called sleep bruxism.

Prevalence of Sleep Bruxism

Since sleep bruxism (SB) is a type of parasomnia disorder that takes place during the night, it is consequently harder to control. While many people who grind their teeth during the night are not even aware of it, severe cases of sleep bruxism can have serious health consequences. According to reports, SB is more common in children than in adults. In most cases, the onset of SB is around one year of age, soon after the appearance of the primary incisors. The prevalence among adults is

---

"Bruxism and Sleep" @ 2016 Omnigraphics 2016. Reviewed July 2016.

nearly 12 percent, dropping to 3 percent in older individuals. Although, awake bruxism is more common among females, there does not appear to be any gender difference in SB prevalence.

Risk Factors

SB has been shown to have a wide range of causes. But long-term studies linking bruxism to its causal factors are still ongoing. Among the peripheral factors studied, the most important one is dental occlusion, which refers to the misalignment of the teeth in the upper and lower jaws. Certain pathophysiological factors have also been linked to SB, the most significant one being sleep arousal disorder. This condition is characterized by a sudden shift in the brain wave pattern during the transition from REM (rapid eye movement) sleep to non-REM sleep, or wakefulness, and is accompanied by an increase in respiratory rate and muscle activity. Bruxism has been shown to be a part of this arousal response.

Among all the factors that may contribute to sleep bruxism, the ones most extensively studied have been the psychosocial factors, which include stress and anxiety. Bruxing in children may often be traced to their emotional and psychological state. For instance, anxiety in children stemming from such causes as school exams, bullying, scolding from parents, or moving to a new neighborhood, may be a significant risk factor for SB. Some small children may grind their teeth as part of the teething process or due to frequent earaches. Among children, SB may tend to disappear on its own at puberty.

For adults, common sources of stress include workplace tensions, family problems, relationship issues, or anxiety about health conditions. Certain personality types tend to be more vulnerable to stress-related bruxism, including those who are highly aggressive, competitive, or hyperactive. The risk of developing bruxism can be increased by certain lifestyle factors, such as smoking, alcohol consumption, and drug use. Bruxism may also develop as a side effect of certain medications or as a symptom of neurological disorders like Huntington's disease and Parkinson disease. Studies have also shown that bruxism is often related to other sleep disorders, such as excessive snoring, pauses in breathing, or obstructive sleep apnea.

Symptoms and Diagnosis

The most common symptom of SB is rhythmic masticatory muscle activity (RMMA), or repetitive jaw muscle contractions. While mild to moderate muscle activity in bruxers may not cause any issues, severe cases could lead to dental problems, such as premature wearing of the teeth and dental implants, as well as temporomandibular dysfunction, which is pain and atrophy of the muscles and joints associated with chewing.

Bruxism is usually diagnosed through a visit to a dentist. During a regular checkup, the dentist will look for and inquire about the following symptoms:

- Damaged teeth

- Unusual teeth sensitivity

- Swelling and pain in the jaw or facial muscles around the mouth

- Tongue indentations

- Headaches or earaches

- Frequent awakening or poor quality of sleep

Treatment for SB

Treatments for bruxism should be selected to best fit the individual patient and the underlying cause of the disorder. When a dental problem is determined to be the cause of bruxism, a dental appliance, like a splint or mouth guard, might alleviate the condition. These devices help prevent the teeth from grinding together and also protect the tooth enamel from further damage. Various dental procedures can also be performed to correct misalignment of the teeth and jaw or address damage to the teeth from clenching and grinding. Cognitive behavioral therapy can also help patients deal with improper mouth and jaw alignment. Correcting the position and placement of the tongue, teeth, and lips can bring about a significant improvement in the condition. Biofeedback is another treatment method used to assess and alter the movement of the muscles around the mouth and jaw. The doctor may use monitoring equipment to help guide the patient toward overcoming the habit of clenching the jaw or grinding the teeth.

If the primary cause of bruxism is determined to be psychological in nature, a number of behavioral and related therapies may help alleviate the condition. Stress management is the foremost issue to be addressed in people with bruxism. Counseling sessions with experts can help patients develop coping strategies. Other common means of reducing stress include meditation, relaxation, exercise, and music. Hypnosis has also proven to be an effective treatment for people who grind their teeth at night. Most patients with bruxism tend to respond well with proper treatment prescribed by the appropriate professional.

References

1. "Causes of Bruxism," The Bruxism Association, n.d.

2. "Bruxism," The Nemours Foundation/KidsHealth, n.d.

3. Shilpa Shetty et al. "Bruxism: A Literature Review," *The Journal of Indian Prosthodontic Society* Volume 10 (3): 141-148, National Center for Biotechnology Information (NCBI), U.S. National Library of Medicine (NLM), January 22, 2011.

Part Seven

Clinical Trials on Sleep Disorders

Chapter 55

What Are Clinical Trials?

Clinical Trials

The National Heart, Lung, and Blood Institute (NHLBI) is strongly committed to supporting research aimed at preventing and treating heart, lung, and blood diseases and conditions and sleep disorders.

NHLBI-supported research has led to many advances in medical knowledge and care. For example, this research has uncovered some of the causes of various sleep disorders and ways to diagnose and treat these disorders.

The NHLBI continues to support research aimed at learning more about sleep and sleep disorders. The research will focus on sleep and the body's natural 24-hour cycle, the role of genes and the environment on sleep health, and ways to improve the prevention, diagnosis, and treatment of sleep disorders.

Much of this research depends on the willingness of volunteers to take part in clinical trials. Clinical trials test new ways to prevent, diagnose, or treat various diseases, conditions, and health problems.

For example, new treatments for a disease or condition (such as medicines, medical devices, surgeries, or procedures) are tested in volunteers who have the illness. Testing shows whether a treatment is safe and effective in humans before it is made available for widespread use.

This chapter includes text excerpted from "Clinical Trials," National Heart, Lung, and Blood Institute (NHLBI), March 29, 2012. Reviewed July 2016.

By taking part in a clinical trial, you may gain access to new treatments before they're widely available. You also will have the support of a team of healthcare providers, who will likely monitor your health closely. Even if you don't directly benefit from the results of a clinical trial, the information gathered can help others and add to scientific knowledge.

If you volunteer for a clinical trial, the research will be explained to you in detail. You'll learn about treatments and tests you may receive, and the benefits and risks they may pose. You'll also be given a chance to ask questions about the research. This process is called informed consent.

If you agree to take part in the trial, you'll be asked to sign an informed consent form. This form is not a contract. You have the right to withdraw from a study at any time, for any reason. Also, you have the right to learn about new risks or findings that emerge during the trial.

Chapter 56

A Method for Enhancing
Sleep in PTSD

Purpose

Sleep disturbance is nearly ubiquitous among individuals suffering from posttraumatic stress disorder (PTSD) and is a major problem among service members returning from combat deployments. The proposed study aims to test a novel, inexpensive, and easy to use approach to improving sleep among service members with PTSD.

Primary outcome measures will include not only PTSD symptom improvement but also include neuroimaging of brain structure, function, connectivity, and neurochemistry changes. The proposal is firmly grounded in the emerging scientific literature regarding sleep, light exposure, brain function, anxiety, and resilience. Prior evidence suggests that bright light therapy is effective for improving mood and fatigue, and our pilot data further suggest that this treatment may be effective for improving daytime sleepiness and brain functioning in brain injured individuals. Thus, this intervention, in our own research and in the work of others, has been shown to affect critical sleep regulatory systems. Improving sleep may be a vital component of recovery in these service members. Our approach would directly address this issue. Our preliminary data have shown that this approach is

This chapter includes text excerpted from "A Method for Enhancing Sleep in PTSD," ClinicalTrials.gov, January 29, 2016.

extremely well tolerated and is effective for improving sleep, mood, cognitive performance, and brain function among individuals with brain injuries.

Finally, the potential impact of this study is high because of the capability of transitioning the research to direct clinical application almost immediately. If the bright light treatment is demonstrated as effective, this approach would be readily available for nearly immediate large-scale implementation, as the devices have been widely used for years in other contexts, are already safety tested, and commercially available from several manufacturers for a very low cost. Thus, the impact of this research on treating PTSD would be high and immediate.

Study Type: Interventional

Study Design: Allocation: Randomized

Endpoint Classification: Efficacy Study

Intervention Model: Parallel Assignment

Masking: Double Blind (Subject, Outcomes Assessor)

Primary Purpose: Treatment

Official Title: A Non-Pharmacologic Method for Enhancing Sleep in PTSD

Estimated Enrollment: 90

Study Start Date: September 2014

Estimated Study Completion Date: January 2018

Estimated Primary Completion Date: January 2018 (Final data collection date for primary outcome measure)

Eligibility

Ages Eligible for Study: 18 Years to 45 Years (Adult)

Genders Eligible for Study: Both

Accepts Healthy Volunteers: No

Criteria

Inclusion Criteria:

- right handedness as assessed by the Edinburgh Handedness Inventory (EHS) (necessary to avoid mixed lateralization on brain imaging);

- For women: regular menstrual cycles (duration between 25 and 35 days with no more than 3 day variation between cycle (necessary to control brain metabolites on MR spectroscopy);

- SCID diagnoses and combat exposure consistent with PTSD

- ISI scale score of at least 8 or above

  Post first year evaluation w/low recruitment rates:

- recruit non-military participants who have also experienced traumatic incidents as part of their occupation (e.g., law enforcement, firefighters)

- include a broader range of post-traumatic cases, such as sexual trauma, domestic partner violence, assault, etc.

  Exclusion Criteria:

- History of head injury with loss of consciousness or post-traumatic amnesia, or major neurological illness;

- medical or neurologic condition that would confound interpretation of results, including alcohol (as verified via the Standard Drink handout for subjects) or drug abuse/dependence in the past 6 months, neurological disorders;

- mixed or left-handedness;

- abnormal visual acuity that cannot be corrected by contact lenses (necessary to see stimuli in scanner environment);

- IQ estimate less than 80;

- metal within the body, pregnancy, or other contraindication for MRI procedures;

- time since returning from deployment that exceeds 36 months;

- previous formal treatment with light therapy;

- history of light-induced migraine or epilepsy; medical complications that could elevate the risk of discomfort associated with light-therapy;

- use of medications that could affect functional neuroimaging results (e.g., fluoxetine, beta-blockers).

Patients currently taking other psychotropic medications (i.e., "treatment as usual") must be stabilized for at least 4-weeks prior to participation. Although participants will not be excluded from participation, detailed history and dosages will be documented and examined as appropriate in statistical analyses.

- ISI score of below 8.

- Participants will be excluded if they are currently taking or anticipate the need to take sleep-inducing medications (e.g., zolpidem) or supplements that have known effects on sleep (e.g., melatonin) during the course of the study.

Chapter 57

Cognitive Behavioral Therapy for Insomnia among Different Types of Shift Workers (CBT—Insomnia)

Purpose

The aim of the study is to compare the implementation and effectiveness of group and self-help based cognitive behavioral treatment for insomnia (CBT-I) delivered by occupational health services (OHS) in a randomized and controlled design (RCT) among different types of shift workers.

Study Type: Interventional

Study Design: Allocation: Randomized

Endpoint Classification: Efficacy Study

Intervention Model: Parallel Assignment

Masking: Open Label

Primary Purpose: Treatment

This chapter includes text excerpted from "Cognitive Behavioral Therapy for Insomnia among Different Types of Shift Workers (CBT-Insomnia)," ClinicalTrials. gov, August 13, 2015.

Official Title: Cognitive Behavioral Therapy for Insomnia Among Different Types of Shift Workers

Estimated Enrollment: 120

Study Start Date: January 2015

Estimated Primary Completion Date: December 2018 (Final data collection date for primary outcome measure)

Eligibility

Ages Eligible for Study: 20 Years to 60 Years (Adult)

Genders Eligible for Study: Both

Accepts Healthy Volunteers: No

Criteria

Inclusion Criteria:

- Chronic Insomnia (F51.0)

- Difficulty initiating and/or maintaining sleep for ≥ 30 minutes and/or the use of sleep promoting medicine on three or more nights per week for at least 3 months

- Motivation to treat insomnia with non-pharmacological methods

- Full-time shift work (at least 10 % of shifts are morning, evening and/or night shifts)

- Fluent Finnish (due to interventions)

Exclusion Criteria:

- Non-assessed or untreated somatic or mental illness which may explain insomnia

- Planned changes in the work (for example retirement)

Chapter 58

Improving Sleep in Veterans and Their CGs (SLEEP—E Dyads)

Purpose

This study addresses the neglected topic of sleep disturbance in older caregiving dyads-a topic that has important implications for the safety, health, functioning and quality of life of older Veterans living at home and being cared for by a family caregiver (CG). The purpose of the first phase of this study is determine the relationship between CG and care recipient (CR) sleep and describe the impact of dyadic sleep to daytime functioning and well-being for Veterans and their caregivers. The information from phase 1 will inform the next study phase in which the investigators develop and field test non-pharmacological, technology based, sleep hygiene, exercise and meditation interventions to improve sleep in Veteran caregiving dyads.

Study Type: Interventional

Study Design: Allocation: Randomized

Endpoint Classification: Efficacy Study

This chapter includes text excerpted from "Improving Sleep in Veterans and Their CGs (SLEEP—E Dyads)," ClinicalTrials.gov, April 13, 2016.

Intervention Model: Parallel Assignment

Masking: Open Label

Primary Purpose: Supportive Care

Official Title: Improving Sleep In Veterans and Their Family Caregivers

Estimated Enrollment: 260

Study Start Date: November 2010

Estimated Study Completion Date: July 2016

Estimated Primary Completion Date: June 2016 (Final data collection date for primary outcome measure)

Eligibility

Ages Eligible for Study: 18 Years and older (Adult, Senior)

Genders Eligible for Study: Both

Accepts Healthy Volunteers: Yes

Criteria

Inclusion Criteria:

- Care recipient must be age 60 and over and require assistance from the identified caregiver with more than one Activity of Daily Living or three or more Instrumental Activities of Daily Living,

- have a life expectancy of greater than or equal to six (6) months,

- have no plans for transitioning out of home in the next six months,

- and have approval from the primary care provider to participate in the research.

- Caregivers must live with care recipient

- Caregivers must obtain a negative mini-cog assessment or negative TICS-m assessment. Caregivers can be any relation (spouse, child, sibling, friend, etc.) to the care recipient so long as the two are cohabitating.

- Caregiver can be any age.

- For Phase 2 and Phase 3 of the study, either the care recipient or the caregiver must have difficulty sleeping as indicated by scores on the Insomnia Severity Index.

Exclusion Criteria:

- Parkinson's with tremor or other movement disorder that would invalidate actigraphy

- Untreated diagnosis of sleep apnea or restless leg syndrome

- Inability to tolerate actigraphy

- CG and CR sleep efficiency > 85% and/or both members of dyad report sleeping well

- Caregivers must have a negative screen with the Mini-Cog or the TICS-m to demonstrate cognitive capacity to provide informed consent

Chapter 59

Insomnia Self-Management in Heart Failure (HSS)

Purpose

Chronic insomnia may contribute to the development and exacerbation of heart failure (HF), incident mortality and contributes to common and disabling symptoms (fatigue, dyspnea, anxiety, depression, excessive daytime sleepiness, and pain) and decrements in objective and subjective functional performance.

The purposes of the study are to evaluate the sustained effects of CBT-I on insomnia severity, sleep characteristics, daytime symptoms, and functional performance over twelve months among patients who have stable chronic HF and chronic insomnia. The effects of the treatment on outcomes of HF (hospitalization, death) and costs of the treatment will also be examined.

A total of 200 participants will be randomized to 4 bi-weekly group sessions of cognitive behavioral therapy for CBT-I (behavioral was to improve insomnia and sleep) or HF self-management education.

Participants will complete wrist actigraph (wrist-watch like accelerometer) measures of sleep, diaries, reaction time, and 6 minute walk test distance. They will also complete self-report measures of insomnia, sleep, symptoms, and functional performance. In addition the effects on symptoms and function over a period of one year.

This chapter includes text excerpted from "Insomnia Self-Management in Heart Failure (HSS)," ClinicalTrials.gov, May 11, 2016.

Study Type: Interventional

Study Design: Allocation: Randomized

Endpoint Classification: Efficacy Study

Intervention Model: Parallel Assignment

Masking: Open Label

Primary Purpose: Treatment

Official Title: Cognitive Behavioral Therapy for Insomnia: A Self-Management Strategy for Chronic Illness in Heart Failure

Estimated Enrollment: 200

Study Start Date: October 2015

Estimated Study Completion Date: June 2020

Estimated Primary Completion Date: June 2019 (Final data collection date for primary outcome measure)

Eligibility

Ages Eligible for Study: 18 Years and older (Adult, Senior)

Genders Eligible for Study: Both

Accepts Healthy Volunteers: No

Criteria

Inclusion Criteria:

- stable chronic heart failure, chronic insomnia, English speaking/reading,

Exclusion Criteria:

- untreated sleep disordered breathing or restless legs syndrome, rotating/night shift work, active illicit drug use, bipolar disorder, neuromuscular conditions affecting the non-dominant arm end-stage renal failure, significant cognitive impairment, unstable medical or psychiatric disorders

Chapter 60

Music for Insomnia

Purpose

The aim of this study is to determine the effect of listening to music on sleep quality (subjective and objective), daytime dysfunction and neurophysiological arousal in patients with insomnia.

Study Type: Interventional

Study Design: Allocation: Randomized

Intervention Model: Parallel Assignment

Masking: Single Blind (Outcomes Assessor)

Primary Purpose: Treatment

Official Title: Better Night-Better Day: a Randomized Controlled Trial of Listening to Music for Improving Insomnia

Study Start Date: February 2015

Estimated Primary Completion Date: November 2015 (Final data collection date for primary outcome measure)

Eligibility

Ages Eligible for Study: 18 Years to 60 Years (Adult)

Genders Eligible for Study: Both

This chapter includes text excerpted from "Music for Insomnia," ClinicalTrials. gov, February 6, 2015.

Criteria

Inclusion Criteria:

- Insomnia diagnosis

Exclusion Criteria:

- Use of hypnotic medications
- Alcohol or substance abuse
- Pregnant or breastfeeding women
- Sleep apnea with an apnea hypopnea index (AHI) >5
- Clinically significant restless leg syndrome or periodic limp movement disorder

Chapter 61

Sleep Quality in Patients with Advanced Cancer

Purpose

The primary focus of this clinical study is the objective and subjective measurements of sleep quality in patients with advanced cancer using opioids. It also examines sleep disturbances and associations between sleep quality and symptoms in order to improve symptom management in patients with advanced cancer.

The overall aim of this study is to improve the clinical understanding of sleep quality in patients with advanced cancer using opioids and to improve the understanding of how sleep quality may best be measured in order to improve symptom management.

Study Type: Observational

Study Design: Observational Model: Cohort

Time Perspective: Cross-Sectional

Official Title: Sleep Quality in Patients With Advanced Cancer. A Comparison of Objective Assessments and Self-reports of Sleep Quality

Estimated Enrollment: 40

Study Start Date: October 2015

Estimated Study Completion Date: March 2017

This chapter includes text excerpted from "Sleep Quality in Patients with Advanced Cancer," ClinicalTrials.gov, May 4, 2016.

Estimated Primary Completion Date: March 2017 (Final data collection date for primary outcome measure)

Eligibility

Ages Eligible for Study: 18 Years and older (Adult, Senior)

Genders Eligible for Study: Both

Accepts Healthy Volunteers: No

Sampling Method: Non-Probability Sample

Study Population

Patients with advanced cancer using opioids (step III on the WHO pain ladder)

Criteria

Inclusion Criteria:

- A verified diagnosis of a malignant disease
- Presence of metastatic/disseminated disease
- Regularly scheduled oral, subcutaneous, transdermal or intravenous opioid treatment corresponding to step III at the WHO pain ladder with a duration of treatment not less than 3 days
- Able to comply with all study procedures
- Signed informed consent according to ICH Good Clinical Practice and national/local regulations

Exclusion Criteria:

- Not consenting to participation
- Not mastering the language used at the study centre
- Severe cognitive impairment as judged by the principal investigator
- Any reason why, in the opinion of the investigator, the patient should not participate
- Impaired use of the dominant arm
- Local anatomical illness or abnormalities precluding the use of polysomnography (e.g. facial tumour)
- having received chemotherapy for more than 4 weeks, having received the previous dose less than 5 days ago and receiving the next dose within the study period.

Chapter 62

Stroke-Sleep Disorders, Dysfunction of the Autonomic Nervous System and Depression

Purpose

The purpose of this study is to investigate sleep disordered breathing, autonomic dysfunction, and post stroke depression in acute and chronic stroke patients. Furthermore, to explore the interaction between these comorbidities, and their relation to stroke aetiology.

Study Type: Observational

Study Design: Observational Model: Cohort

Time Perspective: Prospective

Official Title: Stroke—Sleep Disorders, Dysfunction of the Autonomic Nervous System and Depression

Estimated Enrollment: 335

Study Start Date: March 2014

Estimated Study Completion Date: March 2020

This chapter includes text excerpted from "Stroke-Sleep Disorders, Dysfunction of the Autonomic Nervous System and Depression," ClinicalTrials.gov, February 11, 2016.

Estimated Primary Completion Date: March 2020 (Final data collection date for primary outcome measure)

Eligibility

Ages Eligible for Study: 18 Years and older (Adult, Senior)
Genders Eligible for Study: Both
Accepts Healthy Volunteers: No
Sampling Method: Non-Probability Sample

Study Population

The study population is recruited among patients admitted at the acute stroke unit at Glostrup university hospital.

Criteria

Inclusion Criteria:

- Clinical stroke either ischaemic or haemorrhagic

Exclusion Criteria:

- Transitory ischemic attac

- Congenital or acquired brain disease, other than stroke

- Dementia

- Mental retardation

- Fatal stroke or severe comorbidities with short expected life

- Pregnancy or breastfeeding

- Altered consciousness e.g. delirium or status epilepticus

- Other cause of the patient, according to the investigator believes, can not complete the study

Chapter 63

Treatment of Sleep Disturbances in Trauma-Affected Refugees (PTF5)

Purpose

The overall aim of this study is to examine the effects of sleep enhancing treatment in refugees with PTSD.

Study Type: Interventional

Study Design: Allocation: Randomized

Endpoint Classification: Efficacy Study

Intervention Model: Factorial Assignment

Masking: Open Label

Primary Purpose: Treatment

Official Title: Treatment of Sleep Disturbances in Trauma-affected Refugees: A Randomised Controlled Trial

Estimated Enrollment: 230

Study Start Date: March 2016

Estimated Study Completion Date: March 2019

Estimated Primary Completion Date: November 2018 (Final data collection date for primary outcome measure)

This chapter includes text excerpted from "Treatment of Sleep Disturbances in Trauma—Affected Refugees (PTF5)," ClinicalTrials.gov, May 2, 2016.

433

Eligibility

Ages Eligible for Study: 18 Years and older (Adult, Senior)
Genders Eligible for Study: Both
Accepts Healthy Volunteers: No

Criteria

Inclusion Criteria:

- Adults (18 years or older)

- Refugees or persons who have been family reunified with a refugee

- PTSD pursuant to the International Classification of Diseases ICD-10 research criteria

- Psychological trauma experienced outside Denmark in the anamnesis. Trauma is imprisonment or detention with torture (according to the United Nation definition of torture) or acts of cruel, inhuman and degrading treatment or punishment. Trauma can also be organised violence, long-term political persecution and harassment, or war and civil war experiences.

- Sleep disturbances/ PSQI >8

- Nightmares/ HTQ score on nightmare item ≥ "a little"

- Signed informed consent

Exclusion Criteria:

- Severe psychotic disorder (defined as patients with an ICD-10 diagnosis F2x and F30.1-F31.9). Patients are excluded only if the psychotic-like experiences are assessed to be part of an independent psychotic disorder and not part of a severe PTSD and/or depression

- Current abuse of drugs or alcohol (F1x.24-F1x.26)

- Known neurodegenerative disorder (Alzheimer's disease (AD), Parkinson's disease (PD), Levy-Body dementia (LBD))

- In need of admission to psychiatric hospital

- Pregnant and breastfeeding women and women of the reproductive age who wish to conceive during the project period.

- Allergy towards active ingredients or excipients in mianserin

- Lack of informed consent

Chapter 64

Bright Light Therapy for Treatment of Sleep Problems Following Mild Traumatic Brain Injury

Purpose

Mild traumatic brain injuries (mTBI) or "concussions" are an increasingly prevalent injury in the investigators society. Patients with post-concussion syndrome have been shown to have deficits on tests of short term memory, divided attention, multi-tasking, information processing speed, and reaction time, as well as alteration in mood and emotional functioning. Many patients have other vague complaints including fatigue, dizziness, irritability, sleep disturbances, and chronic headaches. Furthermore, sleep disruption of one of the most common complaints in patients suffering from traumatic brain injuries, with as many as 40 to 65% of patients with mTBI complaining of insomnia. Sleep problems in these patients are associated with poorer outcome, while resolution of the sleep disturbance is associated with improvement in cognitive functioning.

This chapter includes text excerpted from "Bright Light Therapy for Treatment of Sleep Problems Following Mild Traumatic Brain Injury," ClinicalTrials. gov, January 29, 2016.

435

Despite recent evidence of the correlation between sleep quality and recovery from traumatic brain injury, and the well-established role of sleep in neural plasticity and neurogenesis, there have been virtually no direct studies of the causal effects of sleep on recovery following mTBI. However, it is quite likely that sleep plays a critical role in recovery following brain injury.

A particularly promising non-pharmacologic approach that shows potential in improving/modifying abnormalities of the circadian rhythm and sleep-wake schedule is bright light therapy. For the proposed investigation, the investigators hypothesize that bright light therapy may be helpful in improving the sleep of patients with a recent history of mTBI and may also have other mood elevating effects, both of which should promote positive treatment outcome in these individuals. Bright light therapy may increase the likelihood that they will recover more quickly, benefit more extensively from other forms of therapy, and build emotional and cognitive resilience.

This study will also have a healthy control (HC)/effect localization arm that will assist in identifying and mapping the brain systems before and after light exposure so that researchers may develop further insights into the relationship between concussion, light exposure, sleep, and brain function. This healthy control arm will also provide brain targets for study in the analysis of the Main Study Arm.

Study Type: Interventional

Study Design: Allocation: Randomized

Endpoint Classification: Efficacy Study

Intervention Model: Parallel Assignment

Masking: Double Blind (Subject, Outcomes Assessor)

Primary Purpose: Treatment

Official Title: Bright Light Therapy for Treatment of Sleep Problems Following Mild Traumatic Brain Injury

Estimated Enrollment: 69

Study Start Date: April 2015

Estimated Primary Completion Date: December 2017 (Final data collection date for primary outcome measure)

Eligibility

Ages Eligible for Study: 18 Years to 50 Years (Adult)

Genders Eligible for Study: Both

Accepts Healthy Volunteers: Yes

Criteria

Inclusion criteria:

- Age range between 18 and 50.

- Subjects must be right handed.

- The primary language of the subjects must be English.

- Subjects have experienced a "concussion" or mTBI within the preceding 18 months, but no sooner that 4 weeks prior to their screening. The occurrence of a concussion or mTBI must be documented by a medical report or other professional witness documentation.

- If documented, Glasgow Coma Scale in the range of 13-15 following the injury.

- Subjects must have complaints of sleep difficulties that emerged or worsened following the most recent head injury.

- At least half of subjects must have evidence of sleep onset insomnia or delayed sleep phase disorder.

Exclusion criteria:

- Any other history of neurological illness, current Diagnostic Statistical Manual (DSM-IV) Axis I disorder, lifetime history of psychotic disorder, or head injury with loss of consciousness > 30 minutes.

- Complicating medical conditions that may influence the outcome of neuropsychological assessment or functional imaging (e.g., HIV, brain tumor, etc.)

- Mixed or left-handedness.

- Abnormal visual acuity that is not corrected by contact lenses..

- Metal within the body, claustrophobia, or other contraindications for neuroimaging.

- Less than 9th grade education.

- Excess current alcohol use (more than 2 instances of intake of 5+ drinks (men) when or 4+ drinks (women) when drinking in the past two months, and/or on average drinking > 2 drinks per day (men); > 1 drinks per day (women) during the past two months.

• History of alcoholism or substance use disorder.

• Significant use of illicit drugs.

• History of marijuana use within the past 6 weeks, use of marijuana before the age of 16, and/or use of > 20 marijuana cigarettes throughout the participant's lifetime.

Subjects who engage in shift-work, night work, or who have substantially desynchronized work-sleep schedules (i.e., sleeping later than 10:00 a.m. more than once a week) will be excluded.

Part Eight

Additional Help and Information

Chapter 65

Glossary of Terms Related to Sleep Disorders

acupuncture: A technique in which practitioners stimulate specific points on the body—most often by inserting thin needles through the skin. It is one of the practices used in traditional Chinese medicine.

anticonvulsant: A drug or other substance used to prevent or stop seizures or convulsions. Also called antiepileptic.

antidepressant: A name for a category of medications used to treat depression.

antihistamine: Drugs that are used to prevent or relieve the symptoms of hay fever and other allergies by preventing the action of a substance called histamine, which is produced by the body. Histamine can cause itching, sneezing, runny nose, watery eyes, and sometimes can make breathing difficult. Some of these drugs are also used to prevent motion sickness, nausea, vomiting, and dizziness. Since they may cause drowsiness as a side effect, some of them may be used to help people go to sleep.

apnea: Cessation of breathing.

benzodiazepine: A central nervous system depressant.

biological clock: It times and controls a person's sleep/wake cycle will attempt to function according to a normal day/night schedule even when that person tries to change it.

This glossary contains terms excerpted from documents produced by several sources deemed reliable.

biomarkers: A biological molecule found in blood, other body fluids, or tissues that is a sign of a normal or abnormal process, or of a condition or disease.

bone spurs: Small growths of bone that can occur on the edges of a joint affected by osteoarthritis. These growths are also known as osteophytes.

brain-wave rhythms: Patterns of electrical activity of the brain. They include: alpha rhythms (most consistent and predominant during relaxed wakefulness, particularly when your eyes are closed or you are in the dark, they cycle eighteen times per second); beta rhythms (usually associated with alert wakefulness, they are faster than alpha waves, cycling about thirteen to thirty-five times per second); delta rhythms (occurring chiefly in deep sleep stages 3 to 4, also known as slow sleep, they cycle less than four times per second); and theta rhythms (associated with the light sleep stages 1 and 2, these cycle four to eight times per second).

bright light therapy: It is used to treat seasonal affective disorder (SAD).

bruxism: A movement disorder characterized by grinding and clenching of teeth.

cartilage: A hard but slippery coating on the end of each bone. The breakdown of joint cartilage is the primary feature of osteoarthritis.

cataplexy: A sudden loss of motor tone and strength.

central nervous system (CNS): It includes the brain and the spinal cord.

central sleep apnea: It is caused by irregularities in the brain's normal signals to breathe.

chronic insomnia: A condition in which sleep problems occur at least 3 nights a week for more than a month.

circadian rhythms: Are physical, mental and behavioral changes that follow a roughly 24-hour cycle, responding primarily to light and darkness in an organism's environment.

cognitive-behavioral therapy: A blend of two therapies: cognitive therapy (CT) and behavioral therapy. It focuses on a person's thoughts and beliefs, and how they influence a person's mood and actions, and aims to change a person's thinking to be more adaptive and healthy.

collagen: A family of fibrous proteins that are components of cartilage. Collagens are the building blocks of skin, tendon, bone, and other connective tissues.

complementary and alternative medicine (CAM): It is the term for medical products and practices that are not part of standard medical care.

continuous positive airway pressure: A treatment that uses mild air pressure to keep the airways open.

corticosteroids: Powerful anti-inflammatory hormones made naturally in the body or man-made for use as medicine. Corticosteroids may be injected into the affected joints to temporarily reduce inflammation and relieve pain.

dopamine: A neurotransmitter present in regions of the brain that regulate movement, emotion, motivation, and feelings of pleasure.

enuresis: Involuntary urination during sleep.

estrogen: The major sex hormone in women. Estrogen is known to play a role in regulation of bone growth. Research suggests that estrogen may also have a protective effect on cartilage.

hypersomnia: A complaint of excessive daytime sleep or sleepiness.

hypnagogic hallucinations: Are visual and auditory perceptions that occur during sleep onset, while hypnopompic hallucinations occur on awakening.

hypnosis: A trance-like state in which a person becomes more aware and focused on particular thoughts, feelings, images, sensations, or behaviors.

hypothalamus: The area of the brain that controls body temperature, hunger, and thirst.

idiopathic: Seizure activity without a known cause that is controlled by medication or other means so that the person does not continue to have seizures.

insomnia: Not being able to sleep.

jet lag: A sleep disorder caused by traveling across different time zones.

Kleine-Levin syndrome: Is characterized by recurring but reversible periods of excessive sleep.

latency period: The time that passes between being exposed to something that can cause disease (such as radiation or a virus) and having symptoms.

L-Dopa: An amino acid precursor of dopamine with antiparkinsonian properties.

light therapy: It is used treat seasonal affective disorder.

magnetic resonance imaging (MRI): It provides high-resolution computerized images of internal body tissues. This procedure uses a strong magnet that passes a force through the body to create these images.

maintenance of wakefulness test (MWT): A daytime sleep study measures your ability to stay awake and alert. It's usually done the day after a PSG and takes most of the day.

melatonin: A natural hormone that plays a role in sleep.

multiple sleep latency test (MSLT): A daytime sleep study measures how sleepy you are. It typically is done the day after a PSG.

muscles: Bundles of specialized cells that contract and relax to produce movement when stimulated by nerves.

narcolepsy: A disorder that causes periods of extreme daytime sleepiness. The disorder also may cause muscle weakness.

neuron: A nerve cell that is the basic, working unit of the brain and nervous system, which processes and transmits information.

nightmare: A bad dream that brings out strong feelings of fear, terror, distress, or anxiety.

nocturia: Frequent urination of 2 or more times per night.

nocturnal myoclonus: Refers to night-time muscular spasm.

non-REM sleep: Stages of sleep ranging from light sleep to deep sleep.

nonsteroidal anti-inflammatory drugs (NSAIDs): A class of medications available over the counter or with a prescription that ease pain and inflammation. Commonly used NSAIDs include ibuprofen, naproxen sodium, and ketoprofen.

obstructive sleep apnea (syndrome): In this condition, the airway collapses or becomes blocked during sleep.

osteoarthritis: The most common form of arthritis. It is characterized by the breakdown of joint cartilage, leading to pain, stiffness, and disability.

osteotomy: A procedure that involves cutting and realigning bone, to shift the weight from a damaged and painful bone surface to a healthier one.

otolaryngology: A surgical specialty concerned with the study and treatment of disorders of the ear, nose, throat, respiratory and upper alimentary systems, and related structures of the head and neck.

parasomnia: It is defined as undesirable behavioral, physiological, or experiential events that accompany sleep.

periodic limb movement disorder: Causes repetitive jerking movements of the limbs, especially the legs. These movements occur every 20 to 40 seconds and cause repeated awakening and severely fragmented sleep.

polyp: Most colon cancers start as noncancerous growths called polyps.

polysomnogram: A sleep study that records brain activity, eye movements, heart rate, and blood pressure.

relaxation therapies: Also termed relaxation imagery; various methods or techniques for the alleviation of insomnia that help to relax the mind and the body and which can facilitate sleep onset.

REM sleep: It is the active or paradoxic phase of sleep in which the brain is active.

restless legs syndrome: A disorder that causes a powerful urge to move your legs. Your legs become uncomfortable when you are lying down or sitting. Some people describe it as a creeping, crawling, tingling or burning sensation. Moving makes your legs feel better, but not for long.

rheumatoid arthritis: A form of arthritis in which the immune system attacks the tissues of the joints, leading to pain, inflammation, and eventually joint damage and malformation. It typically begins at a younger age than osteoarthritis does, causes swelling and redness in joints, and may make people feel sick, tired, and feverish. Rheumatoid arthritis may also affect skin tissue, the lungs, the eyes, or the blood vessels.

seasonal affective disorder (SAD): A type of depression that occurs at a certain time of the year, usually in winter.

sedative: A drug that calms a person and allows her or him to sleep.

septum: The septum is the wall that separates the chambers on left and right sides of the heart. The wall prevents blood from mixing between the two sides of the heart.

serotonin: A neurotransmitter that regulates many functions, including mood, appetite, and sleep.

sleep apnea: A disorder involving brief interruptions of breathing during sleep.

sleep cycle: It is defined by a segment of non-rapid eye movement (NREM) sleep followed by a period of rapid eye movement (REM) sleep.

sleep debt: It develops when daily sleep time is less than an individual needs.

sleep deprivation: Sleep deprivation is a condition that occurs if you don't get enough sleep.

sleep hygiene: The promotion of regular sleep is known as sleep hygiene.

sleep medicine: The specialty concerned with conditions characterized by disturbances of usual sleep patterns or behaviors.

sleepwalking: Refers to doing other activities when you are asleep like: eating, talking, or driving a car.

snoring: Snoring is an example of sleep-disordered breathing – a condition that makes it more difficult to breathe during sleep.

somnambulism: Somnambulism is an arousal disorder that is usually benign, self-limited and only infrequently requires treatment.

stage 1 sleep: During stage 1, which is light sleep, we drift in and out of sleep and can be awakened easily. Our eyes move very slowly and muscle activity slows.

stage 2 sleep: When we enter stage 2 sleep, our eye movements stop and our brain waves (fluctuations of electrical activity that can be measured by electrodes) become slower, with occasional bursts of rapid waves called sleep spindles.

stage 3 sleep: In stage 3, extremely slow brain waves called delta waves begin to appear, interspersed with smaller and faster waves.

stage 4 sleep: The brain produces delta waves almost exclusively. It is very difficult to wake someone during stages 4, which are called deep sleep.

stimulant: Stimulants increase alertness, attention, and energy, as well as elevate blood pressure, heart rate, and respiration.

stimulus control: Stimulus control involves learning what social or environmental cues seem to encourage undesired eating, and then changing those cues.

teeth grinding: Teeth grinding is defined as an involuntary, non-functional, rhythmic or spasmodic gnashing, grinding, and clenching of teeth (not including chewing movements of the mandible), usually during sleep, sometimes leading to occlusal trauma. Causes may be related to repressed aggression, emotional tension, anger, fear, and frustration.

tendons: Tough, fibrous cords that connect muscles to bones.

tonsils: Glandular tissue located on both sides of the throat that helps the body to fight infection by trapping bacteria and viruses that enter through the mouth and nose.

X-ray: A procedure in which low-level radiation is passed through the body to produce a picture called a radiograph. X-rays of joints affected by osteoarthritis can show such things as cartilage loss, bone damage, and bone spurs.

Chapter 66

Directory of Resources Providing Information about Sleep Disorders

Circadian Rhythm Disorders

Circadian Sleep Disorders Network
4619 Woodfield Rd
Bethesda, MD 20814
Website: www.circadiansleepdisorders.org
E-mail: csd-n@csd-n.org

General

American Academy of Dental Sleep Medicine (AADSM)
2510 N. Frontage Rd.
Darien, IL 60561
Phone: 630-737-9705
Fax: 630-737-9790
Website: www.aadsm.org
E-mail: info@aadsm.org

Resources in this chapter were compiled from several sources deemed reliable; all contact information was verified and updated in July 2016.

American Academy of Sleep Medicine
2510 N. Frontage Rd.
Darien, IL 60561
Phone: 630-737-9700
Fax: 630-737-9790
Website: www.aasmnet.org
E-mail: AASMmembership@aasmnet.org

American Association of Sleep Technologists
2510 N. Frontage Rd.
Darien, IL 60561
Phone: 630-737-9704
Fax: 630-737-9788
Website: www.aastweb.org
E-mail: A2ZzzMagazine@AASTWeb.org

American Sleep Association (ASA)
1002 Lititz Pike
#229
Lititz, PA 17543
Website: www.sleepassociation.org

American Sleep Medicine Foundation (ASMF)
2510 North Frontage Rd.
Darien, IL 60561
Phone: 630-737-9700
Fax: 630-737-9790
Website: www.discoversleep.org
E-mail: asmfinfo@aasmnet.org

American Sleep Medicine, LLC
7900 Belfort Pkwy
Ste. 301
Jacksonville, FL 32256
Phone: 904-517-5500
Fax: 904-517-5501
Website: www.americansleepmedicine.com
E-mail: info@americansleepmedicine.com

American Thoracic Society
25 Broadway
New York, NY 10004
Phone: 212-315-8600
Fax: 212-315-6498
Website: www.thoracic.org
E-mail: ATSInfo@Thoracic.org

Better Sleep Council
501 Wythe St.
Alexandria, VA 22314-1917
Phone: 703-683-8371
Website: www.bettersleep.org
E-mail: mhuusimaki@sleepproducts.org

Center For Sleep and Wake Disorders
5454 Wisconsin Ave.
Ste. 1725
Chevy Chase, MD 20815
Phone: 301-654-1575
Fax: 301-654-5658
Website: ww.sleepdoc.com
E-mail: mail@sleepdoc.com

Cleveland Clinic
9500 Euclid Ave.
Cleveland, OH 44195
Toll-Free: 800-223-2273
Phone: 866-594-2091
TTY: 216-444-0261
Website: my.clevelandclinic.org
E-mail: sessled@ccf.org

Eastern Iowa Sleep Center
600 Seventh St. S.E.
Cedar Rapids, IA 52401
Phone: 319-362-4433
Fax: 319-362-4466
Website: www.iowasleepcenter.com

Eunice Kennedy Shriver *National Institute of Child Health and Human Development (NICHD)*
31 Center Dr.
Bldg. 31 Rm. 2A32
Bethesda, MD 20892-2425
Phone: 301-496-5133
Fax: 301-496-7101
Website: www.nichd.nih.gov
E-mail: prpl@mail.cc.nih.gov

KidsHealth
Website: www.KidsHealth.org
E-mail: PR@KidsHealth.org

Michigan Academy of Sleep Medicine (MASM)
3031 West Grand Blvd.
Ste. #645
Detroit, MI 48202
Phone: 313-874-1360
Fax: 313-874-1366
Website: www.masm.wildapricot.org
E-mail: kcarter@wcmssm.org

National Center on Sleep Disorders Research (NCSDR)
U.S. National Heart, Lung, and Blood Institute (NHLB)
Two Rockledge Centre Ste. 10038
6701 Rockledge Dr.
Bethesda, MD 20892-7920
Phone: 301-435-0199
Fax:301-480-3451
Website: www.nhlbi.nih.gov/about/ncsdr

National Fibromyalgia and Chronic Pain Association (NFMCPA)
31 Federal Ave.
Logan, UT 84321
Phone: 801-200-3627
Website: www.fmcpaware.org
E-mail: info@fmcpaware.org

National Heart, Lung, and Blood Institute Health Information Center (NHLBI)
NHLBI Health Information Center
P.O. Box 30105
Bethesda, MD 20824-0105
Toll-Free: 866-359-3226
Phone: 301-592-8573
TTY: 866-411-1010
Website: www.nhlbi.nih.gov
E-mail: NHLBIinfo@nhlbi.nih.gov

National Institute of Neurological Disorders and Stroke (NINDS)
NIH Neurological Institute
P.O. Box 5801
Bethesda, MD 20824
Toll-Free: 800-352-9424
Phone: 301-496-5751
TTY: 301-468-5981
Website: www.ninds.nih.gov
E-mail: NEXT@ninds.nih.gov

National Sleep Awareness Roundtable (NSART)
1010 N. Glebe Rd.
Ste. 420
Arlington, VA 22201
Phone: 703-243-1697
Fax: 202-347-3472
Website: www.nsart.org

National Sleep Foundation
1010 N. Glebe Rd.
Ste. 420
Arlington, VA 22201
Phone: 703-243-1697
Fax: 202-347-3472
Website: www.sleepfoundation.org
E-mail: nsf@sleepfoundation.org

Nocturna Sleep Care, Inc
Administration Office and Night Clinic
9077 S. Pecos Rd.
Ste. 3700
Henderson, NV 89074
Phone: 702-896-7378
Website: www.nocturnasleep.com
E-mail: referrals@nocturnasleep.net

Ohio Sleep Medicine Institute
4975 Bradenton Ave.
Dublin, OH 43017
Phone: 614-766-0773
Fax: 614-766-2599
Website: www.sleepohio.com
E-mail: info@sleepmedicine.com

Scottsdale Sleep Center
10277 N. 92nd St.
Ste. #103
Scottsdale, AZ 85258
Phone: 480-767-8811
Fax: 480-657-0737
Website: www.scottsdalesleepcenter.com
E-mail: info@thesleepcenteraz.com

Sleep Research Society
2510 N. Frontage Rd.
Darien, IL 60561
Phone: 630-737-9702
Website: www.sleepresearchsociety.org
E-mail: coordinator@srsnet.org

Sleep Services of America
890 Airport Park Rd.
Ste. 119
Glen Burnie, MD 21061
Phone: 800-340-9978
Fax: 410-790-6993
Website: www.sleepservices.net
E-mail: info@sleepservices.net

Spectrum Health Sleep Disorders Centers
100 Michigan St. N.E.
Grand Rapids, MI 49503
Toll-Free: 866-989-7999
Phone: 888-753-3752
Website: www.spectrumhealth.org
E-mail: patient.privacy@spectrumhealth.org

Talk About Sleep, Inc.
P.O. Box 146
Chaska, MN 55318
Phone: 866-657-5337
Website: www.talkaboutsleep.com
E-mail: info@talkaboutsleep.com

UT Sleep Center
1928 Alcoa Hwy
Ste. 119
Bldg. B
Knoxville, TN 37920
Phone: 865-305-8761
Website: www.utsleepdisorders.org
E-mail: utsleepcenter@mc.utmck.edu

Valley Sleep Center
P.O. Box 30388
Mesa, AZ 85275-0388
Phone: 480-830-3900
Fax: 480-830-3901
Website: www.valleysleepcenter.com

Washington University Sleep Medicine Center
Department of Neurology
1600 S. Brentwood Blvd.
#600 St.
St. Louis, MO 63108
Phone: 314-362-4342
Fax: 314-747-3813
Website: sleep.wustl.edu

Hypersomnia

Hypersomnia Foundation
5885, Cumming Hwy
Sugar Hill, GA 30518
Website: www.hypersomniafoundation.org
E-mail: info@hypersomniafoundation.org

Kleine-Levin Syndrome

Kleine-Levin Syndrome Foundation, Inc.
P.O. Box 5382
San Jose, CA 95150-5382
Phone: 408-265-1099
Website: klsfoundation.org
E-mail: dick@klsfoundation.org

Narcolepsy

Narcolepsy Network, Inc.
46 Union Dr.
#A212
N. Kingstown, RI 02852
Toll-Free: 888-292-6522
Phone: 401-667-2523
Fax: 401-633-6567
Website: www.narcolepsynetwork.org
E-mail: narnet@narcolepsynetwork.org

Wake Up Narcolepsy, Inc.
P.O. Box 60293
Worcester, MA 01606
Phone: 978-751-3693
Website: www.wakeupnarcolepsy.org
E-mail: info@wakeupnarcolepsy.org

Other Disorders Affecting Sleep

Alzheimer's Association
225 N. Michigan Ave.
Fl. 17
Chicago, IL 60601-7633
Toll-Free: 800-272-3900
Phone: 312-335-8700
TDD: 866-403-3073
Fax: 866-699-1246
Website: www.alz.org
E-mail: info@alz.org

American Gastroenterological Association (AGA)
4930 Del Ray Ave.
Bethesda, MD 20814
Toll-Free: 800-227-7888
Phone: 301-654-2055
Fax: 301-654-5920
Website: www.gastro.org
E-mail: member@gastro.org

American Parkinson Disease Association (APDA)
135 Parkinson Ave.
Staten Island, NY 10305
Toll-Free: 800-223-2732
Phone: 718-981-8001
Fax: 718-981-4399
Website: www.apdaparkinson.org
E-mail: apda@apdaparkinson.org

Anxiety Disorders Association of America (ADAA)
8730 Georgia Ave.
Ste. #412
Silver Spring, MD 20910
Phone: 240-485-1035
Fax: 240-485-1035
Website: www.adaa.org
E-mail: sgerfen@adaa.org

COPD Foundation
3300 Ponce de Leon Blvd.
Miami, Florida 33134
Toll-Free: 866-316-2673
Website: www.copdfoundation.org
E-mail: info@copdfoundation.org

National Center for Posttraumatic Stress Disorder
Website: www.ptsd.va.gov

National Institute of Mental Health (NIMH)
Science Writing, Press, and Dissemination Branch
6001 Executive Blvd.
Rm. 8184 MSC 9663
Bethesda, MD 20892-9663
Toll-Free: 866-615-6464
Phone: 301-443-4513
TTY: 866-415-8051
Fax: 301-443-4279
Website: www.nimh.nih.gov
E-mail: nimhinfo@nih.gov

National Multiple Sclerosis Society
733 Third Ave.
3rd Fl.
New York, NY 10017
Toll-Free: 800-344-4867
Website: www.nationalmssociety.org

Restless Legs Syndrome

Restless Legs Syndrome Foundation
3006 Bee Caves Rd.
Ste. D206
Austin, TX 78746
Phone: 512-366-9109
Fax: 512-366-9189
Website: www.rls.org
E-mail: info@rls.org

WE MOVE *(Worldwide Education and Awareness for Movement Disorders)*
204 W. 84th St.
New York, NY 10024
Phone: 844-734-2254
Fax: 212-875-8389
Website: www.wemove.org
E-mail: wemove@wemove.org

Sleep Apnea

American Sleep Apnea Association
1717 Pennsylvania Ave.
N.W. Ste. 1025
Washington, DC 20006
Phone: 202-280-2052
Fax: 888-293-3650
E-mail: egrandi@sleepapnea.org

Infant and Children Sleep Apnea Awareness Foundation, Inc.
P.O. Box 2328
New Smyrna Beach, FL 32170
Phone: 386-423-5430
Fax: 386-428-2001
Website: www.infantsleepapnea.org
E-mail: terrilynn@kidssleepdisorders.org

Nevada Sleep Diagnostics
8935 South Pecos Rd.
Ste. 22-D
Henderson, NV 89074
Phone: 702-990-7660
Fax: 702-990-7665
Website: www.nevadasleep.com

Sleep Apnea
1717 Pennsylvania Ave.
N.W. Ste. 1025
Washington, DC 20006
Phone: 202-280-2052
Fax: 888-293-3650
Website: www.sleepapnea.org
E-mail: asaa@sleepapnea.org

Index

Index

Page numbers followed by 'n' indicate a footnote. Page numbers in *italics* indicate a table or illustration.